WOMEN, HORMONES AND THE MENSTRUAL CYCLE

Women, hormones and the menstrual cycle

Herbal and medical solutions
from adolescence to menopause

Ruth Trickey

ALLEN & UNWIN

For Kirrian

First published in 1998
Reprinted twice in 1998, 1999, 2000

Allen & Unwin
9 Atchison Street, St Leonards NSW 2065 Australia
Phone: (61 2) 9901 4088
Fax: (61 2) 9906 2218
E-mail: frontdesk@allen-unwin.com.au
URL: http://www.allen-unwin.com.au

National Library of Australia
Cataloguing-in-Publication entry:

Trickey, Ruth, 1953– .
    Women, hormones and the menstrual cycle: herbal and medical
    solutions from adolescence to menopause.

    Includes index.
    ISBN 1 86448 525 6.

    1. Women—Health and hygiene. 2. Menstrual cycle. 3.
    Hormones. I. Title.

612.662

Set in 11/13 pt Sabon by DOCUPRO, Sydney
Printed and bound by Ligare Australia

Contents

Figures and tables

Figures

Tables

Boxes

Acknowledgments

I gratefully acknowledge the support provided by Deakin University during my period as Scholar in Residence in 1995 and 1996. In particular, I would like to thank Professor Robyn Rowland, former head of Deakin University's Department of Social Inquiry and the library staff, especially Elizabeth Broadfoot and Maria Shanahan, who collected the hundreds of research papers needed for this book.

Special thanks are also due to herbalist Ross Kalla for assistance with research and collating materials; consulting gynaecologist Dr Claire Pettersen for her valuable advice on the medical section; Jo Baevsksi for support and a space to work; and Kaz Cooke, who helped with editing and provided some much-needed humour.

Others who assisted in a myriad of different ways include Professor Andrew Sinclair from the Department of Applied Biochemistry, Royal Melbourne Institute of Technology; breast specialist, Dr Suzanne Neal; dermatologist, Dr Barbara Breadon; herbalists Dr Wojciech Kielczynski and Kerry Bone; naturopaths Michael Thomsen, Erin Collins, Colin Hammond, Susan Pitcher, Ondine Spitzer and Assunta Hunter; and Helga Kernke, who obtained and translated many of the German-language papers on herbal medicine. Thanks too, to Lauren Black for her extra research and study in the preparation of the plant illustrations for Chapter 19.

Thanks are also due to herbalist Isla Burgess and herbalist–GP Dr Nicki Baillie in New Zealand; chiropractors, Kay Hartley and Lee Hanton; Kate Herd; Jennifer Coate; Anne Trickey and the many other friends and family who gave time, support and assistance.

Ruth Trickey
Melbourne, September 1997

Introduction

An earlier menarche, better nutrition, less pregnancies and a longer life expectancy mean that today's woman will have many more periods in her lifetime than her ancestors did. The 'average' Australian woman can expect to menstruate from the age of twelve or thirteen until she is somewhere between 25 and 35 years old. She is then likely to become pregnant two or three times about every two years, breast-feeding for about three to nine months. Following her pregnancies, she can expect her cycle to remain fairly regular until she is about 50 years old when she will become menopausal.

All up, the average Australian woman will have about 30 years of regular menstruation, totalling between 360 and 400 periods.

Compared to this, women from earlier ages started to menstruate around fourteen or fifteen years old and were frequently married soon after. Child bearing began earlier and it was common for women to give birth many times if their fertility was not affected by sexually transmitted diseases, poor nutrition or indifferent health; or if they didn't die in childbirth. Contraception was not as reliable as it is today, and the spacing between pregnancies was influenced by breastfeeding—both because breast-feeding naturally reduced fertility, and because it was commonly held that a breast-feeding woman should abstain from sex. (Sex was believed to bring on a woman's period; and the return of the period was thought to deprive the baby of sustenance by diverting the breast milk—the 'white blood'—from the breasts to the womb.[1]) So, for most of their fertile years, these women were likely to be either pregnant or breast-feeding, and had an average of only 40 periods during their lifetime.

Both the menstrual cycle and menstruation itself are easily affected: diet, lifestyle and stress will all have an impact on the ease and regularity of the cycle. These associations have become less obvious with the modern-day tendency to take an aspirin or go on the Pill the moment the first problem arises. But there is an increasing understanding of the delicacy of the menstrual cycle, of its dependency on nutrition and harmony. Many women want to control or treat their menstrual difficulties with commonsense and common-place remedies which they can administer themselves, or use non-drug alternatives such as herbal medicines.

This doesn't mean that the Pill or aspirin are wrong—sometimes, and for some women, they are amongst the most convenient or appropriate choices. But it does mean that there are alternatives for those women who want to make it themselves, grow it in the garden, take something more natural, or adopt a lifestyle change.

The medical, surgical and herbal treatments for common menstrual disorders are covered in this book. No one treatment is more or less appropriate than another as an option—simply more or less appropriate for different women and in different situations.

The tenfold increase in the number of periods since the eighteenth century gives rise to more opportunities for problems to manifest, but a woman who is familiar with the events surrounding menstruation and who has access to appropriate information can often prevent a lot of sorrow by attending to deviations from her normal menstrual pattern quickly.

When problems have already arisen (which is, after all, when most of us seek written or professional advice), a range of possible treatments offered by natural therapists and doctors is discussed. This book is not a substitute for individual professional assessment and treatment, but is rather a guide to the options available.

Note

The information in this book is intended for *practical* application by herbalists and allied health-care practitioners, and may also be of value for those engaged in research or study. It can also be used as a guide to treatments for women suffering from menstrual complaints, but is not intended as a substitute for competent advice and guidance by a qualified practitioner.

Section A

Setting the scene

1

The history of natural medicine

Key words

abortifacient
Cold
Dry
elements
Hot
humoral theory
humour
Moist

phenomenology
pneuma
prana
qi
qualities
temperament
vital force

THE EARLY TRADITIONS

Three cultures, the Chinese, the Indian and the Greco-Roman, developed and described remarkably similar systems for explaining human physiology and recognising health and disease. These systems had a central 'elemental' basis (Air, Earth, Fire, Water, Metal) and a vital force.

Clearly, to oversimplify the comparisons between these traditions does not give credit to the effect of the distinct geographical, cultural and religious convictions that were integral to the evolution of these concepts. However, so remarkably similar were their beliefs that they can be broadly summarised as follows:

- The belief in a vital force as the living and generative energy in the body. The vital force generates heat, circulates throughout the body, and is necessary for life and procreation.
- Deficiencies of the vital force are associated with poor health, slow recovery from illness and early death.
- Incorporated within this understanding, is a wider concept that the macrocosm (the world) reflects the microcosm (the individual).

Table 1.1 The three major medical systems from antiquity

System	Vital energy	Element	Season or quality	Organ system or constitutional type
Greco-Roman	Pneuma	Air	Hot & Moist/Spring	Sanguine
		Fire	Hot & Dry/Summer	Choleric
		Water	Cold & Moist/Autumn	Phlegmatic
		Earth	Cold & Dry/Winter	Melancholic
Chinese	Qi	Wood	Wind/Spring	Liver
		Fire	Heat/Summer	Heart
		Earth	Damp/Late Summer	Spleen
		Metal	Dry/Autumn	Lung
		Water	Cold/Winter	Kidney
Ayurvedic	Prana	Air	Dry/Autumn	Vata
		Fire/Water	Hot/Moist Spring/Summer	Pitta
		Water/Earth	Moist/Heavy Winter/Spring	Kapha

- The elements Earth, Air, Fire, Water and (in the Chinese system) Metal and Wood are described as being the constituents of all life forms.
- Ill-health is influenced by the relative preponderance of one or more of the elements.
- All life forms are made of identical 'elements' and are subject to the same universal laws, celestial influences and patterns of change.
- Each of these life forms, as part of the greater whole, is in no way superior to any other life form.
- Extremes in environmental factors are evident in many diseases.

The medicine of early cultures was based on observation. Groups of symptoms were seen to form repetitive patterns, and these were related to observed phenomena in the universe. These patterns were associated with environmental factors, and as the philosophies evolved, greater complexity was introduced which described the workings of a vital force, *qi* or *prana*. The humoral theory was the name given to the Greco-Roman system. Much of this system has survived as the traditional medicine of India and Pakistan, called Unani, or Tibb in Middle Eastern countries.

Astrology was intimately connected with the humoral laws: an individual's physiology and outer anatomy was believed to be continually influenced by the constellations of the zodiac. The humoral fluids, like the ocean tides, were under the dominion of the planets and the moon. Disease, regarded primarily in terms of disturbance of the humoral balance, was caused by a change in the body fluids and could either be related to the positions of the planets or moon, the quality of the diet, or to a loss of body fluids, such as sweat, menstrual blood or urine.The humoral theory is phenomenological. In other words, it is based on the careful observation and classification of phenomena

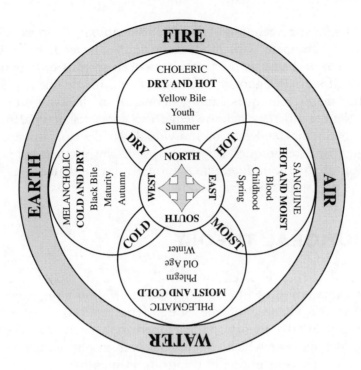

Figure 1.1 The humoral theory

according to their Qualities and the Elements which govern them. To the modern observer they can be seen as a valid attempt to classify the patient and their condition in order to match an appropriate treatment, or to correct an imbalance.

A diagnosis using the phenomenological approach is based on those things that are apparent during a consultation and unaided physical examination—and *only* those things (blood tests, X-rays and swabs to identify bacteria have no role in this type of diagnosis). The 'phenomena' form part of an overall symptom picture which reveal the person's physical, emotional and constitutional tendencies. Disease and the symptoms of disease are considered to be part of the whole picture, not something set apart.

The complaint and the individual are treated simultaneously by counterbalancing the qualities of a disease and the qualities of the individual with the opposite qualities in the herbs to be prescribed. Using the qualities, a herbalist can choose between similar herbs and match them more appropriately to the individual and their condition, limiting side effects and enhancing the therapeutic outcome.

There is a renewed interest in medical systems based on phenomenology. Chinese medicine, in particular, is seen to be somehow special and better because it follows this approach. Western herbal medicine has also started to rediscover the herbal qualities and their application to contemporary herbal medicine.

As a diagnostic technique, the phenomenological approach could never hope to compete with modern medicine. Instead, both are used by the modern herbalist as the two interwoven strands of diagnosis and treatment. Modern diagnostic techniques are invaluable to diagnose *disease*, but these techniques cannot define all of the symptoms seen in practice. Neither do they acknowledge the concepts of vitalism which in part explain the tendency of individuals to develop disease. Traditional diagnostic techniques fill the gaps in the picture by providing information about the *individual*. A modern-day herbalist uses both to treat the patient and their complaint.

THE HUMORAL THEORY

The humoral theory evolved over millennia and finally became the dominant explanation of human physiology at almost the same time in history that the Chinese of the Song dynasty (960–1279 AD) were refining the Yin/Yang theory. It developed as a complete system with many interlocking laws which sought to represent physiology as a group of four interactive and mutually opposing elements.

'Humoral' refers to the semi-gaseous fluids or 'humours' and is sometimes translated to mean 'body fluids', however, humours cannot be equated to any scientifically identified body constituent. In health, the humours were present in a state of relative balance while in ill-health one of the humours became relatively more dominant. The four humours were Blood, Phlegm, Yellow Bile, and Black Bile and they gave each individual an unique constitutional type or temperament, for example, Choleric people were fiery and quick-witted; Phlegmatic were slow and even-tempered.

The four elements of Earth, Air, Fire and Water together with the four qualities of Hot, Cold, Moist and Dry represented an overall picture of the humoral balance of the individual. The nature or temperament was believed to be directly influenced by the dominant element. A predominance of air was related to Blood and the Sanguine (cheerful) temperament; Fire to Yellow Bile and the Choleric (irritable) temperament; Water to Phlegm and the Phlegmatic (even or unexcitable) temperament; and Earth to Black Bile and the Melancholic temperament.

The elements were also present in food and drink which were made of varying combinations of Air, Earth, Fire and Water. Everything taken into the body would contribute to the humoral balance because digestion transformed the elements into the appropriate humours. A diet lacking in balance would contribute to disease by affecting the humoral balance. When other factors had initiated the humoral imbalance, the diet could be manipulated to regain health.

Galen (c. 129–c. 200 AD) was responsible for elaborating the Greek concept of the *pneuma*, or vital energy. He described a 'vital *pneuma*' as being carried by the arteries to all organs and as the active force involved in respiration and the production of heat and energy. The 'psychic *pneuma*' activated the mind and was produced by the vital *pneuma* in the blood vessels in the base of the brain. The transformation of the vital *pneuma* into psychic *pneuma* involved purification through a network of capillaries.

When it came to recognising and treating illness, a diagnosis was made by closely observing the individual for combinations of signs and symptoms. A correlation was made between observed phenomena in the universe and the patterns of disharmony in the person. For example, the observation that fats and oils became thick or hardened with increasing cold was taken as an indication that Cold would cause the body fluids to become thick and movement to be difficult. To treat this condition, Hot remedies were used to counterbalance the Cold. Other observations associated heat with redness, and cold with a purplish discolouration. This led to the association of bright red blood with Heat, and purplish, dark or maroon blood with Cold.

Choosing and categorising herbs occurred in much the same way. Plants which had a pungent and spicy taste were believed to be Heating as well as Drying because heat was seen in nature to dry more efficiently than cold. If a plant grew close to water like the willow, it was believed to be Cooling and Moistening. On the basis of this observation, willow was used for colds, fevers, and inflammatory joint problems to alleviate fever and reduce inflammation in the joints. Today we know that willow is indeed anti-inflammatory, and can reduce temperatures because of its ability to yield salicylate after ingestion.

According to the humoral theory Hot and Cold are the active, primary qualities, and Dry and Moist are the passive, secondary qualities. All of the factors which influence life and health, including the four humours, the elements and temperaments, the organs, and the seasons, contain at most, two of the qualities. For example the qualities Hot and Dry are inherent in the Choleric temperament, the Yellow Bile humour, the Fire element, and the season of summer.

Schematically, the humoral theory was represented with the qualities and the elements organised around two circles. Each element is composed of two qualities: Fire is Hot and Dry, Earth is Dry and Cold, Water is Cold and Moist and Air is Moist and Hot.

Affinities between the qualities—Hot, Moist, Cold and Dry—are read clockwise around the circle; while oppositions between these qualities are represented as being diagonally opposite: Hot is the opposite of Cold, and Moist is the opposite of Dry.

Affinities between the elements of Fire, Air, Water and Earth are also read clockwise around the circle. The elements in opposition to each other are represented as being opposite in the diagram: Fire is the opposite of Water, and Air is the opposite of Earth.

The four elements were believed to form the structure of all earthly objects. Change occurred when the qualities combined in different ways,

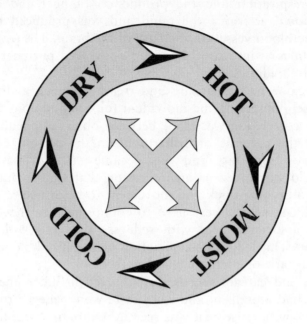

Figure 1.2 The qualities

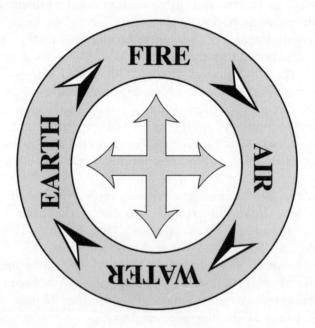

Figure 1.3 The elements

or the changing proportions of the elements transformed into another humour. This change was governed by the principles of attraction and repulsion which were respectively believed to be the forces of creation and unity; and destruction and diversity. (These laws are similar in many aspects to the laws of Yin and Yang.) See Appendix 1 for further details of the qualities, the elements, the temperaments and physiology according to the humoral theory.

HERBS: THE EARLIEST MEDICINE

Herbal medicine is as old as humanity itself. Evidence that plants may have been used as medicines as early as sixty thousand years ago came from the recent discovery of the pollens of common plant medicines at the burial site of a Neanderthal man in a cave in Iraq. Marshmallow, grape hyacinth, yarrow, ephedra, all in use today, were placed beside him, perhaps as decorative offerings, or perhaps for his journey to the afterlife.[1]

According to available knowledge, virtually all peoples throughout the world have used some form of plant medicine. Of those who still use herbal remedies as their source of medicine, many seem to share common traits. Almost all have an individual to whom the knowledge of specific plants is entrusted and who will pass on the information only to selected initiates. Many make a distinction between men's and women's knowledge and use of medicines.

Over centuries, careful observation revealed that there were optimum times to pick plants and administer medicines according to the phases of the moon, seasons or times of day; and that some parts of the plant were more effective than others. It soon became clear that different plants were more effective when administered in certain ways. Gradually the doctoring and supply of herbs developed into recognised professions: the physician became the early doctor and the apothecary became the pharmacist.

The first recorded herbal text was written in Ancient Greece, in the fourth century BC by Diocles of Carystius, a pupil of Aristotle. Herbals were initially probably written for the apothecaries. In the first century AD, Dioscorides wrote his famous *De Materia Medica*. The selection of plants, many of them previously unknown, and the precise way he wrote his text made the work so popular that it is still copied and quoted today.

Sufficient numbers of the valuable texts from the Arabs, Greeks, Romans and Egyptians have survived to give a good indication of the practice of herbal medicine by the scholarly and educated. But much of the early practice of women's medicine was continued as an oral tradition. It was either passed on from one initiate to another by the priestesses and wise women to be used in strict accordance with the current law; or in the case of the common and everyday remedies, passed on from mother to daughter. This seems to have been especially true of contraceptive practices.

Birth control, or the absence of, has always had important consequences for women so it is highly likely they have sought to control their fertility throughout all of history. Certainly there is evidence that rates of reproduction have been limited by one means or another since as early as 200 BC[2]. Restrictions in sexual activity and barrier contraceptives were used, and there is also evidence for the use of herbal remedies as contraceptives and abortifacients from as early as the first Egyptian medical documents.

One of the most compelling written pieces of evidence comes from the writings of Soranus, a Greek writer on gynaecology around 100 AD. He distinguishes between a contraceptive which: 'does not let conception take place' and an abortive which: 'destroys what has been conceived' and comments that 'it is safer to prevent conception from taking place than to destroy the foetus'. A number of common plants including pomegranate (*Punica granatum*), the giant fennel (*Ferula opopanax*), rue (*Ruta graveolens*), juniper (*Juniperus communis*) and asafoetida (*Ferula asafoetida*) were all mentioned as being in common use in Europe.

But while some writers mention the use of these agents, there is little clear advice on the correct dosage, times of administration or even the way to take the remedies. Were they, for instance, to be used as pessaries, or taken orally? John Riddle, Professor of History at North Carolina State University, who has studied these issues extensively, has a possible explanation:

> . . . ancient physicians, all those cited thus far being male, did not fully understand the procedures for taking the anti-fertility agents. In no account, medical or non-medical, is there sufficient detail to permit efficient administration . . . Thus knowledge of anti-fertility plants, and how and when to take them, appears from the evidence—scant though it is—to belong to a female culture. Some of the medicinal plants were also salad plants. The implication . . . is that women were eating plants, such as rue and dill, from the same bowl as men who may not even have been aware of what was going on. One must suppose women knew what to eat, when and how often, and they would appear not to have learned this through books.[3]

Science and medicine have remained sceptical of the effectiveness of plants for contraceptive purposes. In recent times, scientists have found that the seeds of Queen Anne's lace (*Daucas carota*) have contraceptive qualities and stop implantation of the embryo as well as inhibit the production of progesterone. The regular consumption of the common pea, *Pisum sativum*, is reportedly responsible for the low birth rate in Tibet.[4]

What was once common knowledge about herbal contraception, passed on through word of mouth, is lost to today's herbalist. Early writing and current use both support the view that herbs taken as contraceptives seem efficient, and may even be relatively safe. Further investigation into their mode of action, the correct dosage and timing of administration may yet provide enough information to enable their confident prescription.

In sharp contrast to contraception, fever management was an important aspect of treatment for the early physicians and a vast body of instruction can be found in the literature. Infectious diseases were a cause of high mortality for all, but particularly for the young and the infirm, and prior to the use of antibiotics, even minor conditions had the potential to cause death. Elaborate systems for the differentiation of febrile conditions were developed which were based on removing the offending environmental agent, and stimulating the individual's vitality.

Traditional practices for the management of colds, viruses and flus are still recommended by herbalists: acute illness with high temperatures where the person feels cold are treated with Hot herbs and fluids to encourage a subjective sense of heat and to allow the 'fever to break'. This is in direct opposition to the recommended 'take an aspirin and go to bed' advice commonly given today. Herbalists believe that the body attempts to generate heat to overcome viral or bacterial invasion and that assisting this process may shorten the course of the illness.

All traditional medicine has developed a specific language and philosophy on which to base its diagnostic and treatment rationales. Lack of vitality, catarrhal complaints, lymphatic congestion, toxicity or liverishness are all characteristic of herbal medicine, but are often understood by the public: for example, most of us know about being liverish and have an idea of what it means to lack vitality. In many cultures these concepts become so entwined with the language and a common understanding of health and disease, that only a thin line exists between 'common sense' and the knowledge of the practitioner. As a result, these concepts become difficult to articulate; they are just 'known' and as a result may not be taught or even conceptualised as concise and recurring syndromes.

> Constitutional [Holistic] Herb Therapy is widely practiced in China, Tibet, India, Japan, and Southeast Asia; its theories and methods have been written about in various Asian languages. The concept is so ingrained in everyday Asian life that herbalists there have not concerned themselves with comparing Constitutional Therapy with other kinds of therapy. As a result, it is not easy to find a book devoted to this subject even in the cultures where it is practiced.[5]

Over the past 50 years, herbal medicine in the West has changed its focus from the individual to be more interested in specific constituents and their impact on diseases. Detailed information is now available on the outcomes of a herbal medicine and it is possible to prescribe precisely for a number of complaints. Partly, this has been related to the increasing use of herbal remedies by medical practitioners in Europe and Japan, but it has also been associated with a lapse in the traditional language and philosophy of herbal medicine on which it originally based its rationale for diagnosing and treating disease.

One of the most basic tenets of the natural practitioner is the focus on the individual; on why there is disease, rather than what disease; on the vitality and constitutional type rather than the strain of bacteria, the type of cancer, the exact level of some blood component. To do anything less is to betray those people who have turned to herbal medicine for a more holistic solution to their health care. It is vital that herbalists retain their traditional understanding of patho-physiology. A herbalist without this understanding might just as well be a doctor using herbs.

ADMINISTERED FROM HOME . . .

During the seventeenth century in Europe and America, women who managed large houses, were titled or married to churchmen, saw it amongst their duties to provide basic health care. For these women, it was their religious and social responsibility to attend to not only their family and the members of their household, but also to their neighbours and the local villagers. The apothecaries were often quite a distance away, and the services of a physician were expensive and not always available. 'A good reliable herbal—like a sound basic cookery book— was the first essential of the young housewife . . .'[6] these herbals were used to identify the plants and their uses and to assist with the preparation of the herbal creams, extracts, syrups and poultices.

Some of these women took to their role with vigour and enthusiasm. This was, after all, one of the few pursuits other than housewife open to the women of the time and many of these women were obviously talented and became well respected. Some had extensive 'still-rooms'; the rooms where they extracted herbal vinegars and wines, made oint-ments, dried their herbs, distilled oils and made their perfumes, pomades and household goods.

Eventually, books were compiled from the collected recipes and advice of some of the more famous of these women; some became best-sellers. Usually, no distinction was made between books for culinary and medical advice and the manuals written for housewives included mixtures of medical and cookery recipes. *The English House-wife*[7] was one of these books which included advice on common ailments such as toothache, anaemia or 'green sickness', jaundice, epilepsy, diarrhoea, skin diseases and hernias alongside recipes for custards, jams and potted meat loaf.

This tradition was continued in Australia, initially with books pub-lished overseas, such as *The Family Doctor*,[8] but eventually by Australian publishing houses. John Broadbent, 'practical medical herb-alist' of Melbourne wrote two for the general market: *The Australian*

Botanic Guide (1887)[9] and *Botanic Multim in Parvo* (1899). Although not general household books, both reflected the trend for home treatment which had been employed in the English households.

Many of the books, both those published here and overseas, gave a wide variety of advice on cookery, hygiene and herbal or other remedies for a surprising range of conditions.[10] Mrs Lance Rawson's book, *Australian Enquiry Book of Household and General Information* (1910),[11] in the tradition of *The English House-wife*, encompassed cookery, preserving, embroidery, swimming lessons, farming tips, building and decorating as well as health and hygiene. Even as late as 1939, the *Ladies·Handbook of Home Treatment*[12] gave advice on diet, convalescence, douches and instruction for personal hygiene, although by this time, the use of herbal and other natural remedies had disappeared to be replaced by a more chemical approach (the use of mercury, lead, arsenic and copper had been increasingly popular since the late 1500s).

These books are excellent chronicles of the fading tradition of tending to family and friends in the home. Australian women, probably because of their isolation, seem to have been keen advocates of this tradition; utilising common household remedies to make, amongst other things, their own cough medicines, cold and flu remedies or chest poultices. Today, the possibility of treating complaints with common and natural ingredients contributes to the popularity of natural medicine. These remedies, rather than being passed over as 'old wives tales', are proving to be effective and safe and enable people to once again be involved in their own health-care at a fundamental level.

THE HOLISTIC PHILOSOPHY AND HEALTH

The workings of the human body are much more involved than can be discovered by breaking it down into its constituent parts and placing it under a microscope to see how it works. There are a myriad of influences on each individual that will contribute to their overall condition. Recently, the holistic philosophy with its emphasis on the body-mind continuum and a belief in the body to heal itself, has had far-reaching influences throughout medicine. Table 1.2 outlines the major differences between the 'old and new paradigms'.

> 'Holistic', when that adjective is properly applied to health care, refers to a qualitatively different approach, one that respects the interaction of mind, body, and environment. Beyond the allopathic approach of treating the disease and the symptoms of disease, it seeks to correct the underlying disharmony causing the problem.[13]

Table 1.2 The major differences between the old and new paradigms of medicine and health

Assumptions of the old paradigm of medicine	Assumptions of the new paradigm of health
Treatment of symptoms	Search for patterns and causes, plus treatment of symptoms
Specialised	Integrated, concerned with the whole patient
Emphasis on efficiency	Emphasis on human values
Profession should be emotionally neutral	Profession's caring is a component of healing
Pain and disease are wholly negative	Pain and disease are information about conflict, disharmony
Primary intervention with drugs, surgery	Minimal intervention with 'appropriate technology', complemented with full armamentarium of non-invasive techniques (psychotherapies, diet, exercise)
Body seen as a machine in good or bad repair	Body seen as a dynamic system, context, field of energy within other fields
Disease or disability seen as a thing, entity	Disease seen as process
Emphasis on eliminating symptoms, disease	Emphasis on achieving maximum wellness, 'meta-health'
Patient is dependent	Patient is (or should be) autonomous
Profession is authority	Profession is therapeutic partner
Body and mind are separate; psychosomatic illness is mental, may be referred to psychiatrist	Body/mind perspective; psychosomatic illness is a province of all health-care professionals
Mind is a secondary factor in organic illness	Mind is primary or coequal factor in *all* illness
Placebo effect shows the power of suggestion	Placebo effect shows the mind's role in disease and healing
Primary reliance on quantitative information (charts, tests, dates)	Primary reliance on qualitative information, including patient's subjective reports and professional's intuition; quantitative data an adjunct
'Prevention' largely environmental: vitamins, rest, exercise, immunisation, not smoking	'Prevention' synonymous with wholeness: work, relationships, goals, body-mind-spirit

Source: The Aquarian Conspiracy[14]

Treating holistically is about treating individuals with conditions and not just about treating diseases. But it is more than that. It is also about validating an individual's perception of their health. Take for example, the case of a woman with lower pelvic pain. Every reasonable investigation has been performed and nothing is found. Her doctor tells her that there is nothing wrong with her, but from her perspective, she is still in pain. Is it true to say there is nothing wrong? From a holistic perspective there may be no disease, but something *is* wrong because she is experiencing pain and pain indicates some form of disharmony.

This demonstrates another of the important differences between the two paradigms. Medicine usually sees health as an absence of a disease, and defines illness in terms of discernible and diagnosed disease states. Holism sees health as the sense of positive wellness in conjunction with the absence of disease and makes a further distinction between being ill and having a disease. See box 'Signs of health'.

SIGNS OF HEALTH

What is health? Although we often think of ourselves as being healthy if we're not sick, healthy individuals, along with having no overt signs of disease, no pain, complete digestion and clear skin, show other signs of balance, harmony, happiness and wellness.

This description of health would be recognised by any practitioner or student of traditional medicine, and describes those features of health that we often know, but don't articulate:

- The stature is erect and held with ease.
- The skin is clear, smooth and lustrous. To the touch it is warm, firm and slightly moist.
- The individual is within the normal weight range for their age, build and height.
- The normal body processes such as digestion, evacuation of the bowels, urination and menstruation proceed normally and occur without excessive discomfort.
- The bodily excretions such as sweat, urine, faeces, menstrual blood and saliva are of normal consistency, colour and do not have unusually strong or unpleasant odours.
- The appetite is normal and there is hunger in the mornings.
- The desire for fluids is balanced: it increases in hot weather and with exercise, and the preference is for fluids which are neither too hot nor too cold.
- The emotions are balanced and even. There is neither too much anger, joy, fear, boldness, impulsiveness nor procrastination, and the emotions are maintained in a state of equilibrium.
- Sleep is balanced with wakefulness, and is not interrupted by excessive or disturbing dreaming. Dreams that occur are pleasant, uplifting and filled with optimism.
- The mind is quick, alert and imaginative; the memory is good.
- The limbs move easily, with strength and precision.
- The blood vessels can be seen in the flesh and are neither too deep, nor do they bulge out.
- The hair is lustrous and is neither too thin nor too coarse. It grows in the correct places and does not grey or fall prematurely.

A disease is a condition which can be defined by the presence of a number of reproducible signs, such as abnormal blood tests or X-rays, but illness is a subjective sense of feeling sick or being unwell which may or may not be related to a disease. Functional disorders fall into this category. The organs may not be functioning correctly, but as yet, there are no appreciable signs of changes at a cellular level and routine tests remain within the normal range.

A muscle cramp is an example of this type of problem. The muscle is not diseased, even though the excruciating pain indicates otherwise. Instead, the problem has arisen because the muscle is behaving abnormally. There may be a number of stimuli that have initiated this response, they may be transient and never recur. But the cramp is real and the body is indicating the presence of some sort of disharmony.

Many gynaecological conditions are classed as functional disorders, including most types of period pain and many of the conditions associated with hormone imbalance such as premenstrual syndrome (PMS). Many of the syndromes described by natural therapists are also functional disorders, for example, functional hypoglycaemia and adrenal exhaustion. It is not possible to diagnose these conditions with blood tests, but their response to traditional treatments is reproducible and predictable.

Complementary medicine

'Never before in history have so much effort and so much money been expended on medical care; nevertheless, there appears to be a constant number of patients whose suffering medical science has been virtually powerless to alleviate . . . In a study of the patients treated by group medical practices in Hamburg, half were classified as chronically ill; 30–40% were said to be suffering from 'neurotic ailments,' and a mere 10–20% of patients responded 'correctly' to the standard medical procedure . . .'[15]

Complementary medicine can be defined as the use of any or all of the possible disciplines of health-care, including orthodox medicine, for a particular complaint. The term came into being because the term 'alternative medicine' was so problematic, implying that natural medicine was the alternative to the dominant, orthodox medicine. But the problem still remained. It was natural medicine that was ultimately referred to as 'complementary', and the question has to be asked: 'complementary to what?'.

The problem is, of course, that many orthodox practitioners think that complementary means that natural therapists complement them, instead of believing that all disciplines complement each other.

There are many problems for the conventionally trained practitioner if they consider adopting a complementary approach, not the least of which is the concept of 'co-equal partners in health and disease' outlined in Table 1.2. Medicine has taken an authoritative role in the therapeutic process for so long that it is now difficult for most doctors (and many natural therapists) to be more interactive in their consultation styles.

The best complementary medicine must be interactive. There is no one system of intervention that will work for every person; neither is it reasonable to expect that a condition will always respond favourably to a treatment, even if this has been the case for other individuals many times in the past. It is even possible that someone will respond successfully to a treatment once and then never again, or that they will only respond intermittently.

In an interactive consultation the decision-making can be shared as to which of the complex array of possible disciplines might be useful. Most individuals are familiar with associated causes of their complaint: for example, they know that stress will aggravate their irritable bowel syndrome, but they might also need advice on how to change their diet to improve their condition. Becoming involved in the treatment strategies improves compliance to the treatment, assists positive outcomes and helps people to understand how to intervene on their own behalf when or if the condition arises again.

Most clients have an opinion on the factors contributing to their illness and are usually relieved to be treated with the 'professional as the therapeutic partner' approach described by Marilyn Ferguson (see Table 1.2). Even though the condition may be more complex than can be dealt with using self-care strategies, many are willing to contribute to their eventual recovery. Some explanation and a range of options are usually all that most people ask for. Unfortunately, many practitioners do not seek an opinion from their clients or ask them how they can best be helped, thus missing a valuable opportunity to allow their clients to become involved in their health-care.

> Western science can be criticised for insensitivity, for arrogance, for storming Heaven—but the fact remains that it is humble, and humility is integral to the best scientific thought. For all its misuses, the idea of progress implies that not everything has been achieved, that more is yet to come. In order to remain science, science must believe that what it discovers tomorrow may undermine and revolutionise everything it believes today. Western science . . . is necessarily receptive to the new.[16]

Referrals

Three aspects of examination are not normally performed by natural therapists and referral to a doctor is needed. While this does not constitute complementary medicine, it is desirable that it occur harmoniously:

- Routine screening procedures such as breast examination and Pap smears.
- Gynaecological examinations which are performed vaginally and involve internal palpation of the pelvic organs.
Pathology tests such as blood tests, swabs or urine tests; and radiological examinations such as ultrasounds and X-rays.

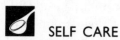 SELF CARE

Although this book has a self-care focus it is intended that it be used in combination with consulting a trained practitioner.

Each of the conditions has a section which deals with what can be done at home. For some conditions there may be very little, but for others, like endometriosis, the deciding factor between a successful and prolonged reduction in symptoms will often depend upon the self-care aspect of the treatment.

The 'self help' movement started in earnest in the 1970s and was a move to encourage women to take responsibility for their health and to encourage them to become more involved in the decision-making about treatments proposed by their doctors.

Self care is about an individual learning about their own body and learning to recognise early signs that something is changing that may need attention.

- Breast and cervical screening programs are offered as free services for Australian women. These are an integral part of self care. Breast self-examination (BSE) pamphlets are available from most GP's surgeries and should also be available at natural therapist's clinics. BSE should be performed after every period: most breast lumps are found by women noticing breast changes.
- Cervical screening for dysplasia or cervical cancer will also detect sexually transmitted diseases (except chlamydia) as well as vaginal infections. The Pap smear is performed by doctors and nurse clinics which specialise in women's health issues. An internal pelvic exam-ination should also be performed to detect changes in the pelvic structures, particularly the ovaries. 'The Well Woman's Check List', which describes these procedures, is included in Chapter 3.

NATURAL MEDICINE IN AUSTRALIA AND THE WESTERN WORLD

Natural therapies have enjoyed a renaissance in Australia and around the world. Not only do many people seek the advice of a natural therapist of one kind or another—25 per cent of Australians in 1984 when the last extensive survey was taken—but they are increasingly likely to choose a natural therapist as their first choice rather than as a last resort. Although many of the treatments have been around for millennia, the new terms and (sometimes) extraordinary list of disciplines that are described under the term 'natural therapies' leave some with an understandable level of bewilderment.

Natural medicine is a generic term that denotes the use of any of the therapeutic disciplines that do not use drugs or invasive techniques. In Australia, the common disciplines are: naturopathy, herbal medicine, homoeopathy, acupuncture and Traditional Chinese Medicine (TCM), aromatherapy, all of the massage therapies, osteopathy and chiropractic.

Practitioners who use natural therapies may specialise in one area, for example, they may be a homoeopath or herbalist; or they may train in a variety of disciplines. A practitioner who uses the multi-disciplinary approach has usually trained as a naturopath. Naturopathy is not made up of a specified group of disciplines and each of the colleges may train their students differently. As such, it is necessary to ask practitioners who call themselves natural therapists or naturopaths which disciplines they use before making an appointment.

The quality of training is extremely varied and there are no regulations in Australia governing the practice of natural therapies. (A butcher could prescribe herbs and be within the law!) Many practitioners are not happy with this state of affairs and most belong to professional associations as a way of giving an indication of their educational standing and to demonstrate their commitment to improving the status of their profession. A list of these associations and their educational requirements is provided on page 20.

Table 1.3 gives a brief description of the most common disciplines practised in Australia.

The contemporary natural therapist evaluates a broad range of information before making a diagnosis. Traditional theories emphasise the maintenance of *health*; the diagnosis of patterns of disharmony; the understanding of the 'constitutional type'; correct living and a healthy internal environment. Science and modern medicine emphasise an understanding of *disease* and its processes; how to diagnose diseases and then to prescribe specific remedies for its eradication.

National Herbalists Association of Australia (NHAA)
Contact: President, David McLeod
ph: (02) 4973 4107/4857
Require 700 hrs in an approved course of study.

Victorian Herbalists Association (VHA)
Contact: Secretary
P.O. Box 205
Clifton Hill 3068
or ph: 014 868 461
Require 1500 hours in an approved course of study.

Australian Natural Therapists Association (ANTA)
Contact: National Administration Officer
ph: 1800 817 577
Require 700 hours in an approved course of study. Individual practitioners can apply.

Australian Traditional Medicine Society (ATMS)
Contact: (02) 9809 6800
Assesses individual college curricula. Consumers should ring for more information.

Table 1.3 The most common natural medicine disciplines practised in Australia & New Zealand

Discipline	Definition
Naturopathy	The use of any or all of the techniques listed below, usually within a holistic framework
Herbal medicine	The prescription of herbs for the treatment of complaints Prescriptions are usually based on the philosophical doctrine of medical herbalism rather than being used as a substitute for drugs
Homoeopathy	Based on the law of the minimum dose and 'like cures like', homoeopathy is the treatment of disease by minute doses of remedies that in healthy persons would produce symptoms like those of the disease
Acupuncture	The insertion of specialised acupuncture needles to regulate and stimulate the body's energy flow or qi
Traditional Chinese Medicine (TCM)	The use of acupuncture and herbs, and the manipulation of the flow of qi with massage and specific exercises
Aromatherapy	The use of 'essential oils' as therapeutic agents either orally, in an oil burner or applied to the skin
Massage	Massages may be relaxing or 'therapeutic' A therapeutic massage involves deep tissue massage for the relief of injury, muscular spasm and tension A relaxation massage is usually more gentle and is designed to relieve stress
Chiropractic and osteopathy	The mobilisation and manipulation of the skeletal structures along with the strengthening and stretching of the muscular components of the body

The fundamental principle guiding the philosophy of the natural therapist is the belief in the body's innate capacity to heal and repair itself, given the correct environment (nutritionally, physically and emotionally). The type of treatments suggested will depend on the discipline used by the practitioner as well as their philosophy. Not every practitioner will adopt a holistic approach, nor will they always involve their clients in the decisions about treatments. However, while the actual delivery of the treatment will vary, the belief that restoring the patient to normal health is more important than the treatment of any particular disease, will (or should) remain constant.

Section B

The way things are

2

Anatomy

Key words

corpus albicans
corpus luteum
endometriosis
endometrium
fimbria
follicle
follicular atresia
follicular phase

fornix
genitalia
luteal phase
myometrium
perineum
peritoneum
primary follicle
secretory phase

THE EXTERNAL ORGANS

The vulva and Bartholin's glands

The vulva is the term for a woman's external genitalia. It is a collective
term for the labia minora and majora, the vaginal and urethral openings,
the clitoris and the Bartholin's glands. The boundaries of the vulva are
the mons pubis (the pubic mound) at the front of the body, and the
perineum at the back.

The labia majora are the large fleshy skin folds that encompass the
inner structures of the vulva. Pubic hair grows on the external surfaces,
and the inner surfaces are lined with mucus membranes which also cover
the smaller, inner labia called the labia minora. The mucus membranes
are well supplied with small mucus-producing glands which lubricate
the area during sexual activity.

The labia minora are joined together at the front to form the
covering for the clitoris. This covering is sometimes called the clitoral
hood or the prepuce. Within the folds of the labia minora are the

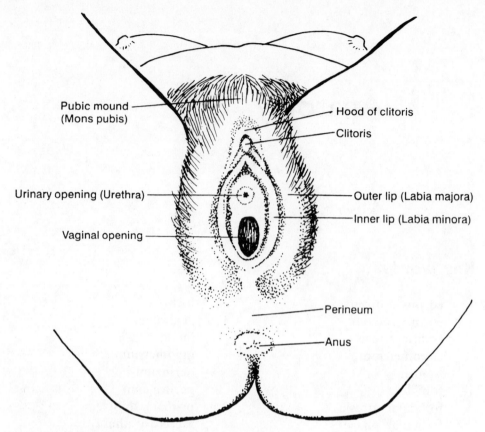

Labels on figure:
- Pubic mound (Mons pubis)
- Hood of clitoris
- Clitoris
- Urinary opening (Urethra)
- Outer lip (Labia majora)
- Inner lip (Labia minora)
- Vaginal opening
- Perineum
- Anus

Figure 2.1 The anatomy of the female genitalia

urethral and vaginal opening. Also within the labia minora and quite near to the vaginal opening are the Bartholin's glands. These glands also secrete mucus to lubricate the vagina during sexual arousal.

THE INTERNAL ORGANS

The uterus

The uterus is a muscular organ and uterine muscle—myometrium—is one of the strongest muscles in the body. This organ can stretch to accommodate a developing foetus and to rhythmically contract during childbirth. The strength of the muscular contraction also affects the volume of the menstrual and post-delivery blood loss and has an impact on the severity of period pain.

Normally the uterus is about the size and shape of a slightly flattened pear. Fibroids, polyps, a current pregnancy or repeated pregnancies can all cause an increase in uterine size or shape. These changes might be discovered during a pelvic examination and will usually require follow-up investigations if this is the first time the change has been discovered. A uterus which is larger than usual is sometimes referred to as a 'bulky' uterus.

The lining of the uterus, the endometrium, is shed as menstrual fluid. It develops due to the influence of the ovarian hormones oestrogen and progesterone. During the first part of the cycle, just after menstruation, the endometrium is at its thinnest and oestrogen causes the lining to change and develop. If ovulation occurs, progesterone is produced in increasing amounts and the endometrium not only thickens, it changes in structure and becomes 'glandular'. Regular shedding of the endometrium is an indication of hormonal change, but not necessarily of ovulation. (Menstruation can occur without prior ovulation.)

Fallopian tubes

The Fallopian tubes, otherwise known as the oviducts or *egg ducts,* are muscular and are lined with microscopic hairs called cilia. Rhythmic contractions along the Fallopian tubes convey the ovum into the uterus. These contractions also partially prevent the 'backflow' of menstrual blood, however, some blood normally flows back along the tubes and into the pelvic cavity during each period. This is called 'retrograde menstruation', and was once believed to be abnormal and the cause of endometriosis. The contractions of the Fallopian tubes are also thought to have a role to play in keeping any infected matter from reaching the pelvic cavity where it could cause peritonitis.

The cilia in the Fallopian tubes are microscopic structures that are hair-like and line the entire length of the tube. Like the cilia in the lung, their continual wave-like motion propels any matter in one direction; in this case toward the uterus. Their main function is to assist the ovum to move along the length of the tube and their activity is enhanced by the presence of oestrogen which stimulates increased activity of the tiny hair-like projections. They, like the muscular activity of the tubes, may also be involved in protection against pelvic infection.

On average, the tubes are about 10 cm long and end in small finger-like projections called fimbria. Fimbriae are like tiny fingers. They are delicate structures, usually in motion, sweeping the ovum into the end of the Fallopian tube. Because they can create tiny waves and currents in the fluid around the ovary, the egg is drawn into the end of the tube where the muscular action and the cilia take over. Damage to the fimbriae from infection, surgery, endometriosis, or adhesions can dramatically affect the normal functioning of these structures and can cause infertility. Amazingly, it has been shown that the activity of the fimbriae is so pronounced that they can cause the ovum from one ovary to be drawn toward the opposite tube where fertilisation and normal tubal transport can occur.

The tubes are funnel-shaped structures which widen at the ovarian end where they partially encircle the ovary, and narrow at the uterine end where they are only about the width of a fine needle. Fortunately, infection and adhesions are more likely to effect the wider end of the tube, but even so, any alteration of the internal diameter of the tube is likely to affect fertility or increase the chances of an ectopic pregnancy.

The ovaries

There are two ovaries, each an oval shape and about the size of a small, slightly flattened hen's egg. Enlarged ovaries can develop due to conditions such as endometriosis, where the endometrium can implant in the ovarian tissue and form endometrial or 'chocolate' cysts; polycystic ovaries where there are too many cystic follicles growing in the ovaries; other types of ovarian cysts or ovarian cancer. An internal pelvic examination and an ultrasound are used to determine whether any increase in ovarian size needs further examination or surgery.

The ovary is not attached to the end of the Fallopian tube, but to the uterus by the ovarian ligament. This is a fibromuscular cord which attaches the ovary to the uterus just below the entrance of the Fallopian tube. The suspensory ligament of the ovary also attaches the ovary to the side wall of the pelvis and contains the ovarian blood vessels, lymphatic vessels and nerves.

The ovaries and the entire pelvic cavity are covered by a membrane called the peritoneum which can be imagined as two layers of plastic (like cling wrap) lying over the posterior and anterior surfaces of the pelvic cavity with the organs, blood vessels and ligaments in between. In states of ill-health such as infection and bleeding into the pelvic cavity, the peritoneum will become inflamed and/or irritated and will cause the pain characteristic of these conditions.

The cervix

The lower third of the uterus is the tubular cervix, about half of which protrudes down into the vagina—the other half of the cervix is above the vaginal attachment. The cervix is sometimes called 'the neck of the womb' and is important because it is prone to cancerous change. The cervix can also become infected or inflamed and can sometimes bleed. All of these problems can be detected with a speculum examination, a swab to detect bacteria or a Pap smear. This procedure is explained on pages 49–50 in the 'Well Woman's Check List'.

The cervical opening is normally tightly closed except during childbirth, and allows for the outward passage of the menstrual fluid and the entry of sperm. Women who have not yet given birth have a cervical opening that is round, but after a vaginal delivery, the cervix has a flattened opening.

The vagina

The vagina is situated between the rectum (the opening from the bowel) and the urethra (the opening from the bladder). It is the structure via which the uterine secretions shed during menstruation are conveyed to the outside. Vaginal tissue, being primarily muscular, can also stretch to many times its normal size during the birth of a baby and then return to normal.

The upper portion of the vagina surrounds the cervix, somewhat like an umbrella, and the recesses that are created between the vaginal wall and the cervix are called the fornices. A fornix (plural fornices) is an arch-like space or recess formed between two structures. The fornices are important because they are relatively thin-walled and allow the internal abdominal organs to be felt during a physical examination (sometimes called internal palpation). The posterior fornix, which is formed by the back wall of the vagina and the cervix, is longer than the other fornices and is called the pouch of Douglas. See Figures 2.2 and 2.3.

The pouch of Douglas is lined with peritoneum. This is a common place for endometrial tissue to grow when a woman has endometriosis. Infected fluid or pus can also collect in the pouch of Douglas if a woman has a pelvic infection.

THE MICROSCOPIC STRUCTURE OF THE OVARY AND ENDOMETRIUM

Ovary

Structure

The microscopic structures of the ovary are constantly changing. At any time during the menstrual cycle, ovum in different stages of development, maturation or disintegration are present. (See Figure 2.4.)

The actual time when a given follicle starts to mature is not known. Some believe that a follicle starts to develop several cycles before the cycle in which it ovulates; others, that maturation starts when obvious

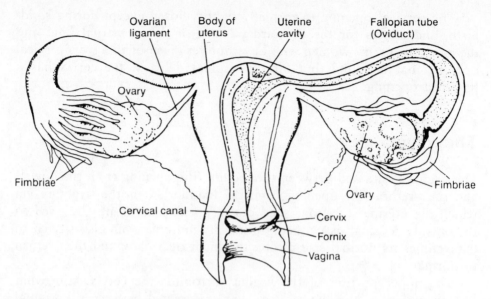

Figure 2.2 Internal reproductive organs

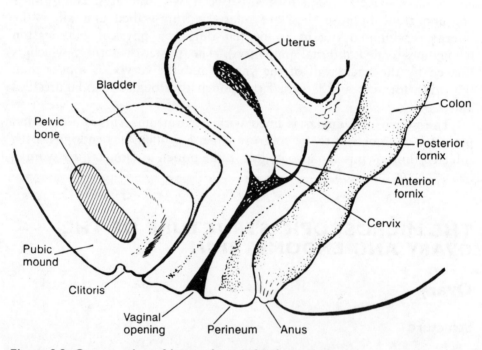

Figure 2.3 Cross-section of internal reproductive organs

changes occur in the late luteal phase of the preceding cycle. A number of the primordial follicles (eggs-in-waiting) start to develop together, but between day eight and twelve in the follicular phase, one has become the primary follicle. The others degenerate and are reabsorbed before reaching maturity (follicular atresia). The primary follicle produces the

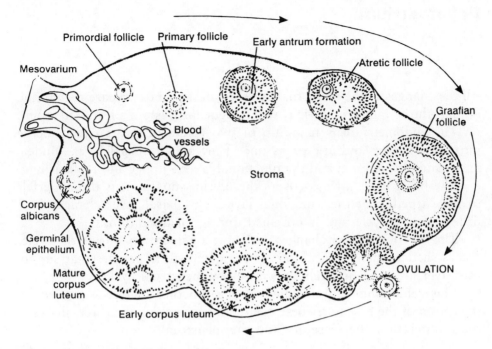

Figure 2.4 Ovarian follicle maturation

ovum, which is expelled into the pelvic cavity at ovulation on about day thirteen or fourteen.

The primary follicle containing the ovum grows rapidly and, at ultrasound, can be seen as a blister-like protrusion on the surface of the ovary. This maturing follicle is also known as a Graafian follicle. The ovum is released gently along with the follicular fluid and does not burst from the enlarged follicle, as was once believed. It is now thought that enzymes 'digest' the follicle wall and assist with the rupture of the membrane around the ovum.

The structure left behind, the corpus luteum, is the 'yellow body' which secretes the hormones oestrogen and progesterone into the blood-stream. It is by far the largest structure within the ovarian tissue and can be seen on an ultrasound scan. After about fourteen days, the corpus luteum dies and about one day later the period starts. The old corpus luteum becomes scar tissue known as the corpus albicans. Healthy ovaries contain many of these 'scars' indicating the ovulation has occurred normally.

Provided ovulation takes place, this same sequence of events recurs every month. As a woman ages and menopause approaches, the follicles are less responsive to the hormonal stimulation. The ovary has fewer primordial follicles left, and eventually no more of them will ripen and produce ovum.

Endometrium

Structure

All the changes in the menstrual cycle are designed to prepare the uterine lining—the endometrium—in case it's needed to sustain a fertilised ovum.

The endometrium is made up of two layers of tissue which merge into one another and appear as one. They are the basal layer—underneath and unchanging; and the functional layer—upper and replenishing.

The basal layer always covers the uterine muscle; it is the underfelt to the carpeting of the functional layer. This basal layer changes very little during a cycle and is not shed during menstruation.

The functional layer changes with hormonal activity during the cycle, and is shed as menstrual blood. Microscopic spiral arteries that supply this layer are shed and rebuilt with every menstrual cycle.

This rebuilding and shedding of the functional layer is caused by the action of the hormones oestrogen and progesterone in three phases—the proliferative, the secretory and the menstrual.

The proliferative phase

The proliferative phase in the endometrial cycle corresponds exactly to the follicular phase of the ovarian cycle and the production of oestrogen—so when the ovum is maturing, so is the uterine lining. The length of this phase is variable. It starts immediately menstruation has stopped, between about days three and six of the cycle, and is completed when ovulation occurs.

Proliferation of cells is one of the major effects of oestrogen, and this is nowhere more evident than on the endometrial cells which line the uterus. Most of the functional layer of the endometrium is shed during menstruation. The basal layer is then resurfaced by the rapidly growing endometrial cells. Within two days of the end of menstruation, or by about day eight of a cycle, the endometrium has completely resurfaced the uterine wall. During the remaining four days or so before ovulation, the endometrium thickens from about 1 mm at the end of the period to about 6 mm by ovulation.

Endometrial thickening occurs because of a combination of events. Supportive tissue (stroma) in the functional layer becomes thickened and spongy. Glands develop within the stroma, ready to secrete mucus and glycogen which would assist with the growth of any fertilised ovum. (See Figure 2.5.) Blood vessels start to develop within the endometrium to provide nutrients to the developing tissues—towards the end of the proliferative phase, these small arteries start to show early signs of spiral formation.

The secretory phase

The secretory phase of the endometrium and the luteal (post-ovulatory) phase of the ovary occur simultaneously. Once ovulation has occurred, the corpus luteum starts to produce large amounts of progesterone. Oestrogen continues to be produced. See Figure 2.5.

Progesterone and oestrogen act together on the already oestrogen-primed endometrium causing it to become a 'secretory' tissue. The glandular structures enlarge and become more convoluted. They also start to produce and secrete larger amounts of glycogen.

The arteries also develop rapidly during this phase. They become much more tortuous than they were in the proliferative phase and take on the typical spiral shape indicative of progesterone activity. Veins also increase in size and tend to form large venous 'lakes' amongst the endometrial tissue.

The supportive stromal tissue becomes even more spongy and the endometrium thickens further. If fertilisation occurs, the fertilised ovum arrives in the uterus to find the cavity filled with thick glycogen-rich tissue where it can embed and develop. If fertilisation does not occur, the endometrium, which has by now reached a thickness of about 8 mm, will be shed during menstruation.

The menstrual phase

After about fourteen days of producing oestrogen and progesterone the corpus luteum degenerates and the production of these hormones falls. The endometrium becomes fragile and starts to break down.

A number of factors occur together to initiate the shedding of the endometrium. One of the first is thought to be the loss of the sponginess within the stromal tissue which causes the endometrium to collapse on itself and cut off its own blood supply. Prostaglandins also play a role in the initiation of menstruation. Levels increase during the secretory phase and this stimulates the uterine contractions to become stronger and more frequent. (Very weak uterine contractions occur throughout the whole cycle.) The spiral arterioles are also effected by prostaglandins and tend to constrict and further deprive the endometrium of its blood supply.

The combination of these factors causes the tissue to degenerate and the functional layer comes away from the basal layer of the endometrium. Uterine contractions assist with the expulsion of the spent endometrial lining through the cervical opening and menstruation begins.

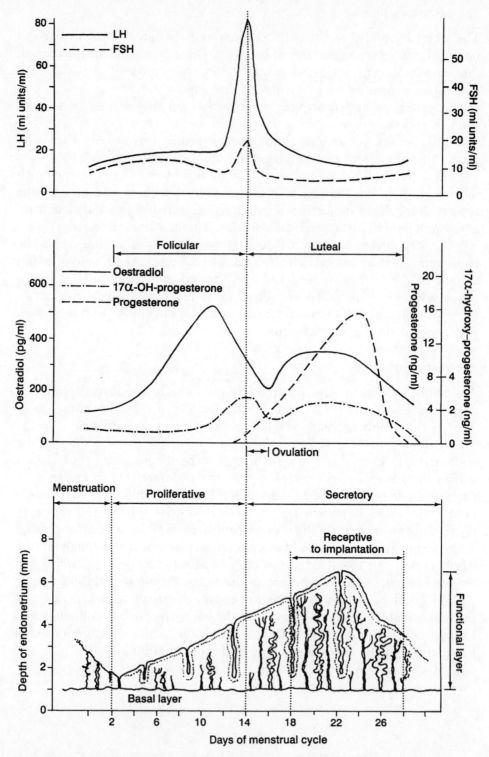

Figure 2.5 The endometrial cycle in relation to plasma levels of ovarian steroid hormones

3

Menstruation and the menstrual cycle

Key words

adhesions
amenorrhoea
corpus luteum
embryo
emmenagogue
endometrium
fertilised ovum
foetus
FSH (follicle-
   stimulating hormone)

GnRH
   (gonadotrophin-
   releasing hormone)
LH (luteinising
   hormone)
nervine
prostaglandins
ovum
spasmolytic

ATTITUDES TO MENSTRUATION

There are many myths, taboos, mistakes, and just plain silly nonsense about periods to be found written, thought or passed on from woman to woman. In the past, ideas about menstruating women and the power of menstrual blood were so extreme that they now seem amusing and quaint. These attitudes have changed for the better, we believe. But have they changed enough?

Around the second century AD, Pliny made his enduring contribution to the understanding of menstruation and its effects. Amongst other powers, he believed a menstruating woman could sour wine, make vines wither, cause fruit to drop from trees, kill bees, blunt knives, discolour mirrors and make dogs rabid. He was by no means the first. Around the fourth century BC, Democritus wrote that 'a girl in her first menstruation should be led three times around the garden beds so that any caterpillars there would instantly fall and die . . . .'.[2]

The prevailing belief was that menstrual blood was extremely poisonous and toxic, not only to the menstruating woman, but to anyone else in the vicinity. It was even thought to be the origin of period pain, because its toxicity caused pain by harming the tissues it touched. Having sex with a menstruating women was also forbidden on pain of death, either by contact with the blood itself, or by Church decree. At any rate, a child born from such an act would be deformed, leprous, have red hair, or be a girl!

For centuries, the scholarly wrote of the inherent weakness and toxicity of women, especially menstruating women. Irrefutable evidence of woman's weakness could be found simply by comparing the male and female anatomy: the male was the standard of normalcy, the female his inferior 'other half'. This could be seen in the anatomy of the male and female genitals—the male perfect and complete with genitals turned outward; the female imperfect, incomplete and with genitals turned inward.

The origin of menstrual blood was comfortably accommodated within the philosophies of the humoral theory which described bodily excretions as the means by which an individual retained a state of homoeostasis. Hippocrates (first century BC) and all of the physicians after him, thought of women as Colder and Moister than men. Women, therefore, did not sweat or grow hair on their face or body (both signs of greater body heat—animals grew horns instead) and had to menstruate to rid their bodies of 'unprofitable blood'. This was supposedly substantiated by the observation that women labourers (who sweated), and 'coarse' women (who grew hair and probably had polycystic ovarian disease) had lighter periods or did not menstruate at all.

Later, another somewhat contradictory theory was put forward by Galen in the second century. He suggested that women, being weaker than men, could not use all of the blood that they concocted from food, and menstruated regularly to rid themselves of the 'plethora' (excess of blood). He observed that women who ate rich and moist food bled more than women who ate coarse and difficult-to-digest foods. Hunger, he noticed, also affected menstruation, and women who were starving didn't menstruate at all.

Believing as they did that menstruation was necessary to purify the blood, *not* menstruating was viewed with grave concern—a condition requiring prompt action. The popular medical texts of the Middle Ages were crammed with remedies for 'stopped menstruation'. There were believed to be a variety of causes: the blood might be too thick to flow easily, or the uterine muscle too 'tough' to let the blood pass. The unknown author of the *Medieval Woman's Guide to Health* listed diet, stress and overwork amongst the causes of failing to menstruate '. . . being awake too much, thinking too much, being too angry or too sad, or eating too little'.[3]

Stoppage of the menses was believed to have frightening consequences: the humoral imbalance created noxious vapours which rose to
the head and caused melancholia, suicidal thoughts and insanity, or
'mother fits', a type of epilepsy (the mother was the word for the uterus).
The cure was blood-letting, which must have been worse than useless
when the cause was anaemia as it often was. Still, menstruating or at
least some form of purgation of the blood was considered necessary for
a woman's health, and so blood-letting or leeches were used as treatments until the start of this century.

With all of the beliefs about amenorrhoea, imagine the difficulty
when a woman became menopausal. Deprived of the necessary monthly
loss, she was believed to become so poisonous that just by looking into
the cradle, she could damage the eyes of a baby. Menopausal women
were often called witches and were thought to be capable of extraordinary feats.

Unusual theories about menstruation prevailed into the nineteenth
century. An American medical professor at Harvard wrote in 1873 that
although he believed women had the right to do anything they were
physically capable of, they should not study. The reproductive system
of the female, he said, was incapable of normal development while a
woman was engaged in academic pursuits, because the female body was
incapable of doing two things well at the same time. This argument was
used to deny higher education to women who wanted it.[4]

Myths persist today. Some religions still isolate or ban women from
churches during menstruation, and chefs have been known to prevent
women from entering their kitchen in case they were menstruating and
curdled their sauce or soufflé by their very presence. In the 1970s and
1980s, a number of books on natural therapies advocated the long-term
use of the 'pure' fruit and vegetable only diet. One of the benefits of
this diet, the authors claimed, was that women who stayed on it long
enough stopped menstruating—and menstruation, they would have us
believe, was only necessary when a woman's body needed purification.
As late as 1993, an American scientist put forward the (new) theory
that menstruation was necessary to cleanse the body and remove sperm-
borne pathogens.[5]

We modern women menstruate for about three years in a lifetime,
about ten times more often than our forebears. Even so, we study and
continue to menstruate, and on average our growth isn't stunted and
we are quite sane.

It is important that our understanding of menstruation is not tangled
up with some outdated notion of the inherent weakness and uncleanli-
ness of women. Most of us are quite happy to have a period once a
month, despite the slight nuisance value, knowing that our monthly
period is a normal biological event.

THE 'NORMAL' PERIOD

What is a period?

A period is the regular shedding of the endometrium—the lining of the uterus—which occurs every month for most women. Menstrual loss looks like blood, but is composed of other tissues and secretions from the inside of the uterus. These consist of small amounts of blood from the capillaries that feed the muscular wall of the uterus; mucus from the glandular cells found in the endometrium; small amounts of tissue from inside the uterus; and the remnants from the structures within the endometrium. These elements are all shed during menstruation.

Most textbooks and doctors talk about periods in relation to pregnancy: 'If pregnancy does not occur, menstruation will commence', with the implication that pregnancy is the normal and expected event and that menstruation is the abnormal event. This may be the case physiologically, but many women in our society don't think of menstruation as a missed opportunity to conceive, but rather as a relief because they know they're *not* pregnant.

> As menstruation only occurs if a woman is not pregnant, some male authors refer to it as the 'weeping womb', suggesting the womb is shedding tears at the disappointment of a failed conception. Whilst there are numerous women who are trying to conceive, many a woman has shed a tear when her period has failed to arrive. Women are most often relieved when their periods arrive and maybe this is why another universal term is the 'woman's friend'.[6]

Some common names for the period include 'Fred'; 'on the rags' (women used rags before pads and tampons were available, and some still do); the 'curse'; 'that time of the month'; 'women's trouble'; or the 'monthlies'. Younger women seem less inclined to use these terms to describe their periods, perhaps because they have had a more liberal education and feel less embarrassed about menstruating.

THE MENSTRUAL CYCLE

For all of her menstruating years, a woman produces variable levels of the sex hormones which establish the regular nature of the menstrual cycle. Under normal circumstances, these hormone levels do not fall below a certain level, known as the 'baseline', and it is the hormonal variations *above* that level which create the cyclic variability. The endocrine glands responsible for hormone production and cycle regulation are the hypothalamus, the pituitary and the ovaries. (Sometimes known as the 'hypothalamic-pituitary-ovarian unit' or the 'hormonal axis'.) See Figure 3.1.

The endocrine glands work together as an integrated unit, sending messages via hormones and utilising a mechanism called the 'feed-back loop'. The hypothalamus produces gonadotrophin-releasing hormone (GnRH) which is recognised by the pituitary; the pituitary produces luteinising hormone (LH) and follicle-stimulating hormone (FSH) to signal the ovaries; and the ovaries secrete oestrogen and progesterone which are recognised by the hypothalamus. Fluctuations in the production of the hormones from each of the endocrine glands signals the next gland in the chain to vary its hormone production. This is the feed-back loop in action.

The hypothalamus responds to both high and low levels of the ovarian hormones oestrogen and progesterone. When oestrogen drops during the period, the hypothalamus secretes GnRH. This signals the pituitary to release FSH which is responsible for the initiation of follicular growth in the ovary.

This stage of the menstrual cycle is often called the follicular phase in recognition of the growth of the follicles. Between ten and twenty may begin to develop, but only one of these will become dominant and mature completely to become an ovum, or egg. The others degenerate (this process is called atresia) and by the time of ovulation the mature follicle is the only one to remain.

While the follicles are developing, they produce more and more oestrogen which stimulates the endometrium to develop or proliferate. This is the origin of another term for the first half of the menstrual cycle: the 'proliferative' phase.

The vaginal secretions are also changing during this phase of the cycle. From being alkaline and very scant, the rising oestrogen levels induce the vaginal secretions to produce more glycogen (sugar). This is acted on by normal vaginal bacteria to produce lactic acid. Vaginal acidity reduces the incidence of infection. The high levels of oestrogen prior to ovulation also convert the mucus around the cervix to copious 'egg-white' secretions referred to as 'fertile mucus'.

Oestrogen levels continue to increase while the ovum develops in the most mature follicle. Eventually, the increasing levels trigger the secretion of GnRH from the hypothalamus which in turn signals a simultaneous surge of both LH and FSH, thought to trigger the release of the ovum. Ovulation occurs, FSH levels drop sharply and LH starts to decline slowly.

Ovulation is followed by the luteal phase. This stage of the cycle takes its name from the corpus luteum which is the remnant of the follicle where the ovum developed. Under the influence of LH, the corpus luteum now starts to secrete increasing quantities of progesterone and, after an initial drop, fairly constant levels of oestrogen.

Progesterone further influences the endometrium which started to develop under the influence of oestrogen, causing it to develop glandular structures and blood vessels which are capable of nourishing a developing embryo. An alternative name for this stage of the cycle is the 'secretory phase' in reference to the secretory structures which develop in the endometrium.

LH is in part responsible for maintaining the normal function of the corpus luteum, but increasing progesterone levels lead to a steadily declining production of LH. If fertilisation does not occur the corpus luteum regresses after about fourteen days, probably due to the activity of prostaglandins. This leads to a decline in the levels of the hormones secreted by the corpus luteum and the eventual shedding of the endometrium which is at all times dependant on the levels of hormones for its development, health and maintenance. When the level of oestrogen reaches a low enough point, the hypothalamus releases GnRH and the cycle starts again.

Counting the days

The first day of the menstrual cycle is always the first day of the properly established period. (Premenstrual spotting is not counted and is considered to be part of the previous cycle.) The days between the first day of the period and ovulation are called the follicular phase. This phase is usually described as being fourteen days long (but varies from woman to woman). When ovulation occurs, the luteal phase begins.

The luteal phase is usually also about fourteen days long and is all of the days between ovulation and the proper beginning of the next period. It seems likely that a healthy corpus luteum is responsible for the accepted normal length of the luteal phase. Corpus luteum is Latin for the 'yellow body' which is the hormone-producing structure left on the surface of the ovary after the ovum has been expelled. Figure 3.1 shows these phases.

THE RANGE OF 'NORMAL'

'Normal' is a strange term to use for the menstrual cycle and periods, because the range is so wide and there are so many exceptions that fit the description of a 'normal' period. The 'textbook period', so described because it appears in every textbook as the description of a menstrual cycle, is 28 days long with a period lasting three to five days. The inherent assumption is that the luteal phase (the time between ovulation and menstruation) will be fourteen days long, and that the follicular

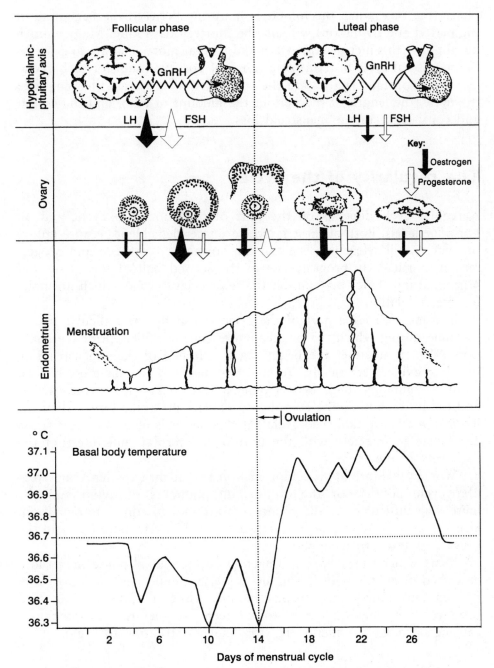

Follicular phase

Luteal phase

Hypothalmic-pituitary axis

GnRH

GnRH

LH   FSH

LH   FSH

Key:

Oestrogen

Progesterone

Ovary

Endometrium

Menstruation

Ovulation

°C

37.1 —

37.0 —

36.9 —

36.8 —

36.7 —

36.6 —

36.5 —

36.4 —

36.3 —

Basal body temperature

| | 2 | 6 | 10 | 14 | 18 | 22 | 26 |

Days of menstrual cycle

Note: Pulsatile release of GnRH stimulates an increase in LH and FSH by the pituitary in late follicular phase and is followed by a pre-ovulatory surge. Both LH and FSH are low in luteal phase, as shown by arrows in diagram.
Oestrogen starts to rise in follicular phase, progesterone in the early luteal phase and both continue to affect the endometrium until menstruation. The temperature reflects the activity of progesterone.

Figure 3.1 The menstrual cycle

phase (the time when the follicle is maturing between the beginning of the period and ovulation) will also be fourteen days long. Many women do not have this menstrual pattern and it is far more accurate to describe the menstrual cycle in terms of a range of possible times for each event.

The important factors are the regularity of the cycle, the length of the cycle, the length of the period, the amount of pain, and the colour and consistency of the menstrual loss.

The regularity of the cycle

A regular cycle depends on the time of ovulation in a cycle, and on hormone levels. Both of these factors are inter-dependent because failure to ovulate will affect the levels of the hormones oestrogen and progesterone (particularly progesterone in the second half of the cycle) and hormonal imbalance may inhibit the sequence of events which normally initiates ovulation.

The most variable part of the cycle is usually the follicular phase, the time during which the ovum matures in the follicle prior to ovulation. Women at either the beginning or the end of their menstruating life may ovulate erratically. Younger women may not have established regular 'communication' between the hormonal systems in the ovaries and the brain, and so the stimulus to ovulate may take longer than for women with an established cycle. At this age it is also easier for stress or change to interfere with the hormonal interplay and interrupt the regularity of the cycle.

Women who are approaching menopause might experience an irregular cycle because of the diminishing numbers of ovum and the increasing difficulty for the pituitary hormones to stimulate ovulation. Stress is also likely to alter the regularity of the cycle more easily in the years leading up to menopause.

Some women may have a longer or shorter luteal phase than those described in the textbooks. The luteal phase is dependent on a normally formed and functioning corpus luteum which usually survives and produces hormones for twelve to fourteen days before it disintegrates, causing hormone production to stop and menstruation to begin.

Missing a period

Pregnancy is the most usual cause of a missed period if a woman has had unprotected sex. Pregnancy tests are available from chemists, supermarkets or doctors, and will give an accurate result within days of conception. Blood tests can be accurate as early as ten days after fertilisation of the ovum has occurred, but waiting until fourteen days is usually recommended to be absolutely sure of not getting a false negative test.

Many women who miss a period (and who are not pregnant) fear that they may have some sort of illness, but a missed period is often a hormonal or ovulatory 'hiccough' caused by stress. The hormonal axis is very delicate and can be easily interfered with by either pleasant or unpleasant experiences. The same physiological response occurs in times of increased exercise, physical hardship or extremes of emotion, and so trips overseas, weddings, relationship break-ups, shock, grief, falling in love, hard work and illness are all commonly associated with missed periods.

A missed period due to stress is rarely a serious problem and the cycle will usually re-establish a normal pattern once the episode is over (unless the woman becomes so worried about the changes in her cycle that she aggravates the hormone balance by being even more stressed!).

Many women will completely stop menstruating when travelling and for some time after their return home. This can be because of a 'pleasurable' stress, but the rapid weight loss due to illness, poor diet or irregular patterns of sleep and activity common amongst travellers may be the real culprits. Women who intend to travel for many months or years may need to be cautious about their lifestyle and dietary patterns so that they maintain a regular pattern and avoid the problems associated with lack of periods, including loss of bone density.

Some women who have irregular periods wrongly assume that they can't get pregnant, but missing a period or even a series of periods does not necessarily imply infertility. Ovulation can spontaneously occur at any time and a woman can become pregnant if she has not used contraception. The difficulty here, of course, is that the woman who has not had a period for months will not be expecting one, and if she becomes pregnant may not realise for some time. She may discover that she is pregnant when it is too late to safely have an abortion; or she may have behaved in ways that are harmful to a developing embryo. Women who intend to have sexual intercourse, but don't want to get pregnant need to consult a Family Planning Clinic or local doctor about options for contraception.

Missing a period for more than six months is called amenorrhoea and the reasons are dealt with in Chapter 13.

The length of the cycle

The usual range for a menstrual cycle is between 21 and 35 days. This *usual* range is only a guide; some women will have cycles that are regularly longer or shorter than this pattern.

Doctors will often be uninterested in cycle lengths that fall outside the 21–35 day range when women have no evidence of serious disease.

Herbalists, however, may view this as a sign that the body is not functioning as well as it might and will look for more subtle signs of ill health. These might include evidence of stress, poor nutrition, abnormal body weight to height ratio, or poor 'Liver' function (see page 256). If none are evident and the woman is full of vigour with no clinical signs of ill health, but with a regularly long or short cycle, she is demonstrating her own normal pattern.

There may be health implications from abnormally short or long cycles. Very short cycles can be associated with erratic ovulation and may be an indication of mid-cycle bleeding which is not really a period at all. Very long cycles can be a problem when women are trying to conceive. Some women will have regularly irregular cycles. This is usually a sign of erratic ovulatory patterns, which, although not 'normal', really doesn't constitute a serious medical problem.

Very short or very long cycles which are accompanied by signs of ill health indicate a need to consult a health care practitioner; and so do any deviations from the expected pattern of the woman's own cycle.

The duration of a period

Between three and five days is the accepted duration of a normal period. Periods that last for fewer days may be related to a number of systemic conditions including thyroid disorders, anaemia and low body weight. These and other reasons for light periods will be discussed in later chapters.

Longer periods may be an indication of hormonal imbalance, and in particular a failure to ovulate because progesterone normally helps to stop excess bleeding because of its effect on the uterine lining. Very long periods can also be a sign of systemic disorders and some gynaecological conditions and will also be discussed under 'Erratic bleeding' (Chapter 12). The length of a period does not include those days when pre- or post-menstrual spotting occurs. Spotting near the time of a period can be an indication of gynaecological problems and may need to be investigated; and any spotting between periods should always be reported.

The volume of the flow

A normal menstrual loss is said to be 50 mL and a heavy period is anything over 80 mL, but because no one measures their menstrual loss and neither do their practitioners, these are mostly meaningless figures. It is far easier to talk in terms of a *need* to change sanitary protection. The word 'need' is important here: the need and not the desire to change is most indicative of the amount of menstrual loss.

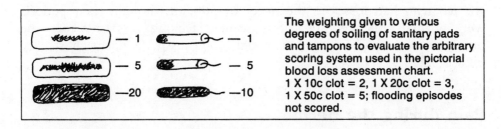

The weighting given to various degrees of soiling of sanitary pads and tampons to evaluate the arbitrary scoring system used in the pictorial blood loss assessment chart.
1 X 10c clot = 2, 1 X 20c clot = 3, 1 X 50c clot = 5; flooding episodes not scored.

Name: Jane   **Day Start:** 1 / 6 / 97

PADS	1	2	3	4	5	6	7	8
(light pad)	||	|		|	|	||		
(medium pad)	||	̶H̶H̶T̶	|||	||	|			
(heavy pad)	|||	||						
Clots/flooding		(10)x2 (50)x4	(10) 4x					

TAMPONS	1	2	3	4	5	6	7	8
(light tampon)	|		|		|		|	
(medium tampon)	|	||	|||	||	||	|		
(heavy tampon)		||||	||					
Clots/flooding								
Daily total	88	135	59	21	17	7	1	

Total Score: 328

A pictorial blood loss assessment chart (PBAC) completed by a patient who had menorrhagia and objective measured menstrual blood loss of 287 mL. Her calculated score was 328 mL.

Figure 3.2 Pictorial blood loss assessment chart (PBAC)

Many practitioners are sceptical about the accuracy of a woman's self-assessed menstrual loss. A number of large studies show that women who reported excess menstrual loss actually had a huge difference in blood volume when this was measured. Some women who were losing around 10 mL thought that they were bleeding heavily, while other women who had losses in the order of 300 mL thought their periods were normal! An accurate self-assessment technique is to record the number of used pads using a 'pictorial blood loss assessment chart'. See Figure 3.2.

Pain during the period

It may be usual for women to experience pain during their periods, but it is certainly not desirable and often not normal. Beware of the comment 'it's normal and you'll just have to put up with it', or 'it's part of being a woman'. No amount of pain is truly normal as the pain response is a survival mechanism indicating that something has gone wrong.

Period pain usually only occurs in a cycle when ovulation has occurred, and period pain often only starts in earnest about two years after the period has begun, that is after ovulation has become regular. This is why an occasional period can be uncharacteristically pain-free— ovulation failed to occur in that cycle.

Symptoms of pelvic discomfort, heaviness or mild pain during a period are often greatly improved by eating well, exercising regularly and stress reduction. Stronger, crampy pain can also be helped by lifestyle changes, and although it seems more serious, this type of pain is not necessarily associated with a gynaecological disease, but may be related to abnormal cramping of the uterine muscle caused by a prostaglandins imbalance. This is called primary dysmenorrhoea and is discussed in Chapter 14.

An investigation should be made of any strong pain prior to bleeding, pain which is situated on one side of the body and pain not directly associated with the period. But *any* pain which is worrying or interfering with day-to-day activity warrants investigation and treatment. It's not a case of 'grin and bear it'.

Heavy loss without pain

The most usual reason for a painless period (when pain has been a normal feature of a period), is failure to ovulate. This type of bleeding can happen at any time, but is common around menopause. Natural therapists view the associated heavy loss as an indication of a lack of uterine tone and give herbs to strengthen the uterine muscle and the mucus membranes.

Heavy loss with pain

In the past, the menstrual loss was considered to be so toxic that it could cause pain simply by coming in contact with the body parts! The suggested treatments were often diets to cleanse the system, reduce the toxicity of the blood, and thereby control the pain. In many cases these recommendations would have been successful because altering the diet can change the prostaglandins levels which are responsible for pain.

We know today that both heavy loss and pain can be caused by prostaglandins imbalance and/or over-stimulation of the uterine lining from oestrogens. Herbalists treat these symptoms by regulating the hormones, treating the 'Liver' to improve excretion of oestrogen and modifying the diet to alter the prostaglandins ratio.

Very slight loss with strong crampy pain

These symptoms are associated with uterine muscle spasm and prostaglandins imbalance. To a natural therapist, these symptoms indicate the need for medicines to relax and calm the uterine muscle in particular, but may also indicate an overall need for calming and soothing remedies around the time of the period. Spasmolytics and nervines are prescribed for these symptoms.

Colour and consistency of menstrual loss

For natural therapists, the type of menstrual loss is important and is often used diagnostically and as an indication of the type of remedy, or even which remedy, to give.

Medical practitioners are less interested in the exact nature of menstrual loss because medicine does not have a tradition of using this type of information to make a diagnosis or decide between treatments. This does not make one or the other system better or more thorough; they are just based on entirely different systems and require different sorts of information to assist with prescriptions.

The following is a list of *associations* and does not represent a diagnostic system in and of itself. These signs would need to be accompanied by at least two other signs or symptoms of disease before they could be even assumed to relate to a pathology.

Bright red blood

Generally bright blood is seen to be an indication that the period is normal, although very bright and fiery-looking blood was historically seen to occur more often when there was too much Heat. This might either be a localised problem, for example an infection in the pelvic organs, or a tendency to be constitutionally Hot or Choleric.[7] Bright red blood might indicate the need for Cooling herbs or for astringents.

Dark, brown or thick blood

Dark blood which is thick, looks too old or is brown is thought to be caused by sluggishness of the menstrual flow. Some women have a very dark red loss and this is quite normal and indicates that their blood quality is good.

Very sluggish, dark blood indicates a need for uterine tonics which regulate uterine muscular activity; emmenagogues which increase the expulsive ability of the uterus; or spasmolytics which help the uterine muscle relax.

Watery, thin or pale blood

Very thin (pale pink) blood can mean poor blood quality and indicates a need for blood enriching herbs, or hormone regulation.

Pale menstrual loss can also be associated with deregulation of the hormone balance—especially when the woman is weak, tired, exercising excessively or eating poorly. Watery menstrual loss is common after surgical procedures which involve the uterus, such as terminations and curettes.

Clots

Clots generally indicate excessive flow and are formed when the anti-clotting factors normally present in menstrual blood are unable to keep the blood in a fluid state because of the volume of the loss. Clots may indicate the need for an improvement in uterine tone with either emmenagogues or astringents.

A period 'out of the ordinary'

Most women will have at least one 'strange' period in their menstruating lives; some will have many. The cycle may be unusual, the flow different from what is normally expected; pain may be a new or different feature; or the colour and consistency of the flow might change.

The important questions include:

- Is pregnancy a possibility?
- Are there other signs of ill health?
- Has there been a stressful episode (either pleasurable or difficult)?

If the answer to either of the first two questions is yes, then it is wise to seek medical advice. If the third option is a possibility, relax, wait for another cycle and see what happens. Worrying about an unusual period might delay the onset of the next one.

(A menstrual diary is included on page 116.)

THE WELL WOMAN'S CHECK LIST

Pelvic examinations

These are performed every year. They involve two procedures, a vaginal speculum examination and an examination of the size and shape of the pelvic organs by hand. Although some doctors will use stirrups, many will ask the woman to lie on her back with her knees bent. Remaining as relaxed as possible will definitely lessen any discomfort and make the examination much easier to perform for the doctor. Although no-one's idea of good fun, a pelvic examination should not be overly painful unless the woman has a vaginal or pelvic infection, adhesions or an acute complaint. If it is, and the doctor has found nothing wrong, another doctor should be sought to perform the examination in the future.

Vaginal speculum examination is performed by inserting a speculum in the vagina so that the lower portion of the cervix can be viewed. A Pap smear may be taken at the same time.

A bi-manual pelvic examination, so called because two hands are used, is performed to feel the size and shape of the pelvic organs. Two fingers of a gloved hand are inserted into the vagina and the other hand is placed over the lower abdomen. The uterus can be felt between both hands and, if the woman is relaxed, it is fairly easy to tell whether it is normally situated, can move easily, and is the right size. Pain on movement indicating endometriosis, infection or adhesions; unusual swellings, enlargement of the ovaries, uterine fibroids, pregnancy and tumours can be detected using this method.

Pap smear

A Papanicolaou smear (named after the physician who invented it) is used to screen for cervical cancer. Cells are gently scraped from the surface of the cervix with a specially designed wooden spatula, smeared onto a glass slide, 'fixed' with a special chemical (usually sprayed on), and sent to a pathology laboratory for examination. The procedure should be painless, but can be a little uncomfortable, especially if the woman is not relaxed or the doctor is hurried.

The cervical cells are examined under a microscope and graded according to the type of cells and whether they have undergone any changes. Table 3.1 gives the standard classification for cell changes. Pap smears can be inaccurate. The most frequent problem is that the cells are classed incorrectly. A Pap smear result may indicate dysplasia (changed cells) when the correct diagnosis is carcinoma in situ (cancer of the cervix), or carcinoma may really be benign changes. Sometimes altered cells are not detected at all, but this happens much less often. When changes are found in a Pap smear, a colposcopy is suggested.

A Pap smear should be taken every two years unless directed otherwise by the woman's doctor.

Table 3.1 Standard classification for cervical cell changes

Class	Common names given to the cell changes
I	Normal, benign cells, negative smear
II	Benign, inflamed, atypical cells, atypical metaplasia
III	Mild or moderate cervical intraepithelial neoplasia (CIN), mild or moderate dysplasia, CIN type I or II
IV	Severe cervical intraepithelial neoplasia (CIN), severe dysplasia, CIN type III, carcinoma in situ
V	Malignant, invasive cancer

Breast checks

Breast checks should involve regular, monthly self-examination after each period (called breast self-examination and often abbreviated to BSE), and an annual check by the woman's doctor. If a doctor does not routinely check a woman's breasts, another should be found.

The examination is performed to detect the presence of lumps or any changes in breast tissue. Most women detect breast changes themselves. They know the 'normal' feel of their own breasts and are in a unique position to detect change and detect it early. About 80 per cent of breast lumps are not cancerous, but even when a breast lump is caused by cancer, the earlier it is found, the better the outlook.

Breast examination involves two phases: visual examination and palpation (physical examination) of the breast tissue. It should be practised after every period, from the beginning of menstruation, and regularly every month after menopause. Figure 3.3 shows the accepted technique for breast self-examination.

1. The map

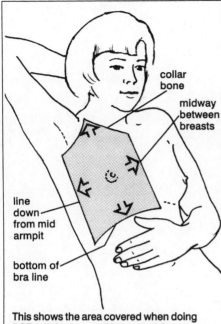

collar bone

midway between breasts

line down from mid armpit

bottom of bra line

This shows the area covered when doing BSE: all the breast tissue must be covered and not just the breast mound. The area examined extends from the collar bone to the bottom of the bra line and from midway between the breasts to an imaginary line down the middle of the armpit.

2. The vertical strip

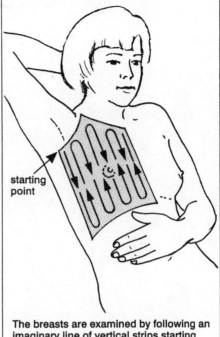

starting point

The breasts are examined by following an imaginary line of vertical strips starting from the armpit and working down and up across the breast.

3. Feeling the breast

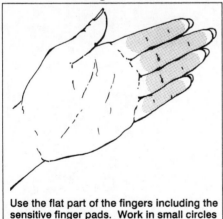

Use the flat part of the fingers including the sensitive finger pads. Work in small circles about five centimetres across.

4. The pressure

Use two pressures to feel the breast at each spot.

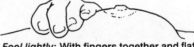

Feel lightly: With fingers together and flat, make the first circle with light pressure to feel for anything near the surface of the skin.

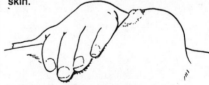

Feel firmly: At the same spot, make a second circle pressing quite firmly to feel any lump deep in the breast.
Firm pressure should not cause discomfort, but the ribs can usually be felt.

Source: Adapted from *The New Breast Self-Examination Technique*, Anti Cancer Council of Victoria

Figure 3.3 Breast self-examination (BSE)

Section C

Maintaining order and balance

Hormones and prostaglandins are both found throughout the body, but are different in that hormones are transported via the bloodstream to act at distant sites (oestrogen to bone, for example), while prostaglandins are produced and act in the same tissue (uterine muscle, for example). Hormones orchestrate the big picture via a continual ebb and flow which ensures that ovulation and menstruation occur rhythmically and regularly.

Prostaglandins are very much more local—the small picture substances. Almost within the time it takes to take one breath, prostaglandins are formed, act and then are broken down again. Their role is to regulate the activity of certain tissues, like muscles, by stepping up or calming down muscular activity.

It is possible to follow and understand the complex interplay between the different hormones and the various types of prostaglandins, but it's not essential. For those who are not interested in the nuts and bolts of how the body works, the parts of the book that explain problems and how to deal with them give enough information without needing to learn about the intricate inner workings of the body. But if you're the sort of person who would like a guide through the complexities of hormones and prostaglandins, read on. One thing's for certain, comments like 'it's just your hormones' or 'that's caused by a prostaglandins imbalance' will never be an adequate explanation again!

4

Hormones

Key words

anabolic
androstenedione
aromatisation
beta-glucuronidase
competitive inhibition
cortisol
deconjugated oestrogen
dehydroepiandrosterone
dihydroxytestosterone
dopamine
endogenous oestrogen
feed-back loop
glucocorticoids
2-hydroxyoestrone
16-hydroxyoestrone

hypothalamus
neurotransmitter
oestradiol
oestriol
oestrone
peripheral conversion
phyto-oestrogen
pituitary gland
pregnenolone
prolactin
receptor site
steroid hormone
transcortin
xeno-oestrogen

MAINTAINING AN ORDERLY MENSTRUAL CYCLE

Maintaining hormonal regulation is something like putting on a complicated stage play with each of the different hormones having different roles to play. Hormones—the microscopic substances carried in the blood and detected by blood tests—are the actors, directors and managers in the monthly play called the menstrual cycle. The managers, directors and actors in this play must perform in perfect synchrony for each act to proceed successfully. The hormonal 'actors' are all 'steroid hormones'. The steroids—androgens, oestrogens and progesterones—

have a central component made from cholesterol and are structurally similar. Each hormone has minor changes in configuration which give it characteristic effects within the body.

The body metabolises steroid hormones step by step from cholesterol according to need. This may mean that a hormone starts out as pregnenolone (a precursor of progesterone), changes into progesterone, then to testosterone and finally into oestradiol (see Figure 4.1). As the steroids change, they play out the role suitable for that hormone. This cycle might continue with the hormone (seemingly) at the end of the line changing into a different form, into another type of hormone, or being broken down and excreted from the body.

Hormone production is regulated by the 'feed-back loop'. The feed-back loop describes the hormonal communication between the hypothalamus, the pituitary gland and the ovaries which controls the level of hormones produced. The level of each hormone constantly see-saws with its hormonal partner. When the level of one hormone rises, information is relayed to turn off the production of its hormonal partner. When the level drops, the feed-back control is activated and production of the partner hormone is switched on again. All steroid hormones are regulated by this type of feed-back loop.

Two examples include the two major hormones involved in the menstrual cycle, progesterone and oestrogen (actors). Both have 'trigger' hormones in the feed-back loop (directors).

- Progesterone production is triggered by luteinising hormone (LH) which stimulates the corpus luteum in the ovary to produce progesterone.

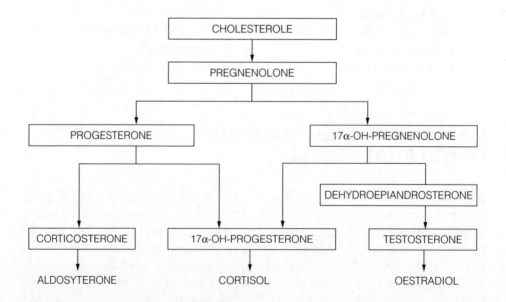

Figure 4.1 Steroid hormone pathways

- Oestrogen is produced when follicle-stimulating hormone (FSH) stimulates the follicle to produce oestrogen. A rise in oestrogen shuts off the production in FSH; a fall turns it back on again.

Hormones also have a mechanism for interacting with their target cells. To do this, they 'dock' onto a specialised part of cells with hormonal sensitivity called receptor sites.

For the 'menstrual' play to proceed smoothly, the hormones must remain in some sort of balance with each other, making their entrance at the right time and responding to cues. Oestrogen must remain at suitable levels in relation to progesterone and androgen; and all of the different types of oestrogen should be in balance with each other. For the period to occur at the right time, the balance of oestrogen must drop, then after ovulation, rise again.

The managers

The hypothalamus is situated in the base of the brain and produces a number of 'releasing' and 'inhibiting' hormones. The manager hormones of most interest in menstrual cycle regulation are gonadotrophin-releasing hormone (GnRH) and prolactin-inhibiting hormone (PIH, also known as dopamine).

Gonadotrophin-releasing hormone (GnRH)

The hypothalamus receives various messages from hormones and chemicals in the blood, and from the nervous system. The hypothalamus processes all of these pieces of information and sends messages to the nearby pituitary gland in the form of intermittent pulses of GnRH every 60 to 90 minutes. The pulsatile release of GnRH increases mid-cycle and around menstruation, indicating to the pituitary that it's time to increase the production of FSH and LH.

Dopamine—prolactin-inhibiting hormone (PIH)

In non-lactating women, the hypothalamus also secretes dopamine to prevent the production of prolactin (the hormone responsible for breast milk production). Dopamine, a neurotransmitter secreted by the hypothalamus, powerfully inhibits prolactin secretion. A long list of substances including many drugs, inhibit either dopamine production or uptake, block dopamine receptors, or cause dopamine depletion and can lead to a rise in prolactin.

The directors

The pituitary gland is also sensitive to messages in the form of hormones and nerve impulses. The pituitary produces the gonadotrophins (FSH and LH) and prolactin—our directors. 'Gonadotrophin' is an easier term to understand if it is broken down into meaningful parts. A gonad is the ovary (or the testis in the male) and '-trophin' is a derivative of trophic which means to stimulate or make grow. A gonadotrophin then, is a hormone that stimulates or 'directs' the ovarian cells.

Luteinising hormone (LH)

The levels of LH increase slowly in response to the low levels of oestrogen during the follicular phase of the cycle. These low oestrogen levels are sensed by the hypothalamus which sends GnRH messages of increasing amplitude to the pituitary. Just before mid-cycle, a dramatic surge in both oestrogen and LH, and a corresponding increase in FSH, initiate the beginning of ovulation. The exact mechanism by which ovulation is induced by LH and FSH is unknown, but somewhere between 18 and 36 hours after the gonadotrophin surge, ovulation occurs. (See Figure 3.1.)

LH stimulates both oestrogen and progesterone production by the ovary. In the luteal phase, the increasing amounts of progesterone inhibit the release of LH from the pituitary gland, and the levels remain low until progesterone levels drop when the corpus luteum degenerates and menstruation begins.

Follicle-stimulating hormone (FSH)

Follicle-stimulating hormone does exactly what its name suggests it should; it stimulates the growth and development of the ovarian follicle—the structure which contains the developing ovum. Levels of FSH increase in the follicular phase of the cycle and stimulate an increase in the number of oestrogen-producing cells in the developing follicle.

Oestrogen and FSH are connected by the feed-back loop—the initial rise in oestrogen triggers the release of GnRH and a surge in FSH. A few hours later, when oestrogen levels are even higher, FSH production is turned off. Just before menstruation, when oestrogen levels fall, the hypothalamus senses the change, sends out GnRH messages to the pituitary and FSH begins to rise again.

Prolactin

Prolactin is the hormone responsible for lactation and affects the breast, stimulating growth during pregnancy and then milk production in response to suckling. Non-pregnant women have low levels of prolactin (inhibited by dopamine from the hypothalamus) which normally increase slightly at night, with stress, and during the luteal phase of the menstrual cycle.

The actors

The ovary and the adrenal gland produce the steroid hormones oestrogen, androgen and progesterone. These 'actor' hormones initiate tissue changes within the ovary, the bodily changes associated with physical development and the changes in the endometrium which result in menstruation.

Oestrogen

There are three main oestrogens—oestradiol, oestrone and oestriol. When people talk about oestrogen or oestrogen levels, they usually mean the cumulative effect of these three in the body, even though each one has a different role to play. Oestrogens have hormonal and growth-enhancing effects which are most obvious during puberty when they first stimulate the development of the reproductive system. They are responsible for the deposition of body fat around the abdomen, hips and breasts; and stimulate the growth of the uterine muscle and the lining of the uterus (the endometrium). The maintenance of the structure of skin and blood vessels, and the strength of bones is influenced by oestrogen throughout life.

One of the most important functions of oestrogen is to stimulate an increase in the number of cells (proliferation) where there are oestrogen receptors. Oestrogen also initiates an increase in the number of receptors on each cell. So not only are there more cells produced in an oestrogen-rich environment, but they also contain more oestrogen receptors. This leads to an escalating ability for oestrogen to stimulate cell growth, and an increased number of places for oestrogens to interact with the cells.

The lifespan of the oestrogens

Every month after the period, the ovaries start to secrete oestrogen in the active form (oestradiol). Some oestradiol is converted into a weaker oestrogen called oestrone, and then both oestradiol and oestrone are secreted into the bloodstream and travel to oestrogen-sensitive cells to stimulate cell growth. Ovarian oestrogen production reaches a peak just prior to ovulation, then remains elevated during the second phase of the menstrual cycle, and falls just before menstruation.

A second source of oestrogen is derived from the conversion of androgens into oestrone by the aromatase enzyme. This process is referred to as 'peripheral conversion' or 'aromatisation'. Aromatisation occurs in the hair follicles, the skin, the brain, the bone and bone marrow, muscle and fatty tissue. Muscle and adipose (fatty) tissue are the major conversion sites—about 25 per cent occurs in the muscle and 10–15 per cent in the fat. Post-menopausal women derive almost all of their oestrogen (oestrone) from the aromatisation of androgens in fatty tissue and muscle.

Before menopause most of the oestrogen is manufactured by the ovaries, but a percentage of oestrogen is always contributed by the aromatisation of androgens into oestrone. Thin women who are pre-menopausal may be deprived of this important secondary source of oestrogen and can sometimes develop menopausal symptoms, such as hot flushes and vaginal dryness. They may stop ovulating and menstru-ating.

Oestradiol is further converted into two types (metabolites) by enzymatic conversion. These are 2-hydroxyoestrone—the 'good' or pro-tective oestrogen; and 16-hydroxyoestrone which is thought to have stronger growth-promoting potential and may even damage cellular genetic make-up—the 'bad' oestrogen. Researchers have found that 16-hydroxyoestrone is in higher concentrations in the breast tissue of women with breast cancer.[1]

These two metabolites cannot be produced at the same time. As yet all of the factors which favour the production of 2-hydroxyoestrone are unknown, however, the levels of 16-hydroxyoestrone have been shown to increase in the presence of chemical contaminants (xeno-oestrogens) which have an oestrogenic effect.[2] They are discussed below.

All of the different sources of oestrogen have the potential to interact with target cells but, eventually, all will pass through the liver. In the liver, oestrogens are changed (conjugated) into different forms which are less active and which are excreted (in the bile) into the intestine. Once there, a number of things might happen. Some of the conjugated oestrogens will be excreted in the faeces in this form, but some will be acted on by enzymes called beta-glucuronidase which are produced by intestinal bacteria. These enzymes have the capacity to change the oestrogen back into an active form (known as deconjugated oestrogen) which might either be excreted in the faeces as well, or might be reabsorbed back into the bloodstream. This is called the entero-hepatic (entero—intestine, hepatic—liver) circulation of oestrogen and is shown in Figure 4.2.

All of the oestrogen circulating in the blood will eventually pass

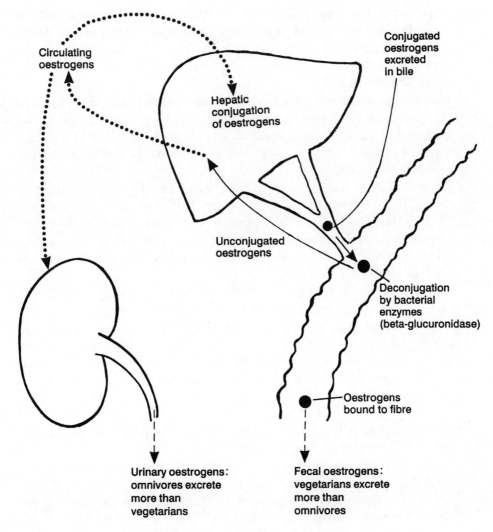

Figure 4.2 The entero-hepatic circulation of oestrogens

Labels in figure:

Circulating oestrogens

Conjugated oestrogens excreted in bile

Hepatic conjugation of oestrogens

Unconjugated oestrogens

Deconjugation by bacterial enzymes (beta-glucuronidase)

Oestrogens bound to fibre

Urinary oestrogens: omnivores excrete more than vegetarians

Fecal oestrogens: vegetarians excrete more than omnivores

through the kidney where it is changed into the very weak oestrogen found in the urine called oestriol. It forms the basis of some pregnancy tests and can be used to determine the health of the placenta during pregnancy. Oestriol is a very weak oestrogen, being about 80 times less potent than oestradiol, so while it contributes to the oestrogen pool, in comparison to oestradiol and oestrone, its effects are closer to that of some of the plant hormones.

The 'oestrogen pool'

Any discussion about oestrogen should not only include those oestrogens produced in the body, but also a diverse group of other substances which have oestrogenic effects. These include the phyto-oestrogens produced in plants, which have many desirable and therapeutic attributes; and the less desirable 'environmental oestrogens', which are consumed as foods or as contaminants of foods, such as pesticides. The oestrogenic effect of all of these different types of 'oestrogens' must be considered in the overall oestrogen equation.

An oestrogenic effect is caused by any substance which has the ability to connect to an oestrogen receptor site. Oestrogen receptors can 'recognise' and accept any substance, even a chemical, which has a molecular structure similar to endogenous oestrogen (the oestrogen produced in the body).

The potential to cause a strong oestrogen-like effect is dependent on the chemical 'fit' between the oestrogenic substance and the receptor site. If the substance is chemically similar to oestrogen and is recognised by the receptor, the oestrogenic effect is strong—if its chemical structure is slightly dissimilar to oestrogen and the fit is less than ideal, the oestrogenic effect is weakened.

The phyto-oestrogens cause different effects depending on whether a woman is pre- or post-menopausal. In pre-menopausal women, many of the plant oestrogens are weaker than the oestrogens produced in the body. This means that they have an *anti*-oestrogenic effect because they occupy receptor sites and prevent the stronger oestrogens from being able to exert their usual effects. Once a women is post-menopausal, however, and has very little oestrogen, plant oestrogens are thought to exert an *oestrogenic* effect by virtue of the fact that they are the most dominant oestrogens in an oestrogen-poor environment and are able to occupy all of the empty receptor sites.

During menopause, women can reduce their menopausal symptoms by increasing their dietary intake of phyto-oestrogens, or taking medicinal herbs. Pre-menopausal women with endometriosis or fibroids can reduce an excessive oestrogenic effect by selectively introducing foods that compete with their own over-stimulatory ovarian oestrogen. See Table 18.2, page 317.

As well, a number of common conditions are associated with a low consumption of phyto-oestrogens. In particular, breast cancer and endometrial cancers in women have been linked to the persistent over-stimulation of cells which can occur when plant oestrogens are not available to occupy some of the receptor sites instead of the more stimulatory endogenous oestrogens. This is termed 'competitive inhibition'.

The picture with the 'environmental oestrogens' (xeno-oestrogens) is less clear. This large group of chemical compounds includes the pesticides such as endosulphan, toxaphene, dieldrin and chlordecone;[3] the polychlorinated biphenols (PCBs)[4] found in a range of products such as hydraulic fluid, neon tubes and the pesticides DDT and DDE;[5] plastics such as nonylphenol released from 'soft' plastics and modified polystyrene;[6] and bisphenol-A, a plastic found in the 'lacquer' used to coat metal cans for preserved food.[7]

These chemicals are found throughout the food chain and tend to accumulate in fatty tissue. Ingestion of pesticides increases when diets are high in foods from animals at the top of the food chain; for example flesh from animals that eat smaller animals, or animals that continually consume contaminated feed or water. Vegetables containing residues of pesticides are likely to contain lower levels, and organically-grown produce less again.

Food wrapped or stored in plastic, particularly when the plastic is soft (like food wrap) or has been heated, can easily become contaminated with these xeno-oestrogens. This is a particular problem with high fat-containing foods because xeno-oestrogens are soluble in fats. Xeno-oestrogens can also be taken in by breathing air contaminated by chemicals from industry or the burning of rubbish, or by drinking contaminated water.

The health implications of these chemicals is unknown. Levels of DDT are higher in fibroid tissue than normal tissue[8] and pre-natal exposure may alter sexual maturation of the foetus (particularly males) and influence fertility in later life.[9] Xeno-oestrogens can increase the levels of 16-hydroxyoestrone, a metabolite of oestrogen which has been associated with breast cancer.

Research into the effects of xeno-oestrogens on the risk of developing oestrogen-dependent cancers in women, however, has produced conflicting results. While some researchers found no link between exposure to xeno-oestrogenic insecticides,[10] others have proposed that combinations of these chemicals may have profound biological implications. They found that while xeno-oestrogens singly had little biological effect, combinations of these compounds exerted effects 1000 times more potent than any one chemical alone.[11]

Endogenous oestrogens are only biologically active during the years of sexual maturity, have a life expectancy measured in days, and fluctuate from month to month with the menstrual cycle. Xeno-oestrogens, however, are ubiquitous contaminants in the food chain. Exposure to them starts with foetal development, they persist in the body for decades, and their levels continue to accumulate with advancing years. It is very likely that all of the effects of environmental oestrogens have yet to be identified.

Progesterone

Progesterone is the hormonal precursor of many of the other steroid hormones including the glucocorticoids, oestrogen and testosterone and so plays an important biological role not only in menstruation and reproduction, but also in a number of other metabolic processes.

In the reproductive organs, progesterone is 'secretory'. It stimulates cellular and structural changes in organs containing progesterone-sensitive tissue like the breast and the uterus so that these tissues become capable of secretory functions. In the uterus, progesterone stimulates the production of glandular structures in the endometrium which can produce sugars and also generates the production of blood vessels so that the endometrium can support a developing embryo. When fertilisation does not occur and the corpus luteum degenerates, the level of progesterone falls, the endometrial tissue disintegrates and is shed as menstruation.

In the breast, progesterone initiates glandular changes in the tissue so that the breast is capable of secreting milk. Progesterone also keeps the levels of androgens (circulating in women at low levels) in check—when progesterone levels are high, androgens are low, but once progesterone production slows or stops, as occurs in the post-menopausal years, androgen levels increase. The change in the progesterone and androgen ratio may account for the loss of scalp hair and the growth of facial hairs seen in some elderly women.

Progesterone has other actions that include improved fat metabolism, an increase in bone density, a mood-elevating effect and a natural diuretic action. It also helps to prevent both cancerous and benign breast changes by counter-balancing the effects of oestrogen in the breast, and has the same protective and counter-balancing effect on the endometrium.

Progesterone is also the precursor hormone to the production of corticosteroids which have many important biological roles throughout the body including the maintenance of stable blood sugar, the reduction of inflammation and the capacity to withstand stress.

The lifespan of a progesterone

The primary source of progesterone is from the corpus luteum—the remnant egg sac—in the ovary. Small amounts are also secreted by the adrenal gland. Cholesterol is the starting molecule for progesterone production in both the ovary and the adrenal gland. In a step-by-step process cholesterol is converted into pregnenolone and then to progesterone. The progesterone might then be converted into any one of the other steroid hormones including oestradiol, oestrone, testosterone or cortisone.

Progesterone circulates in the blood and interacts with cell receptors, but eventually it will pass through the liver where it is inactivated and excreted into the bile and urine.

Androgens

Androgens are hormones, secreted in both males and females, and are the hormones responsible for masculinisation. When the secretion of androgens is inappropriately high, such as polycystic ovarian disease (see Chapter 16), abnormalities of the menstrual cycle and the reproductive function can occur, along with male pattern hair growth, deepening of the voice and loss of the female body contours, including a decrease in breast size.

Testosterone is the most abundant androgen found in the blood of normal women. It is also the most potent. Of the total volume, 25 per cent originates from the ovary, 25 per cent from the adrenal gland and 50 per cent is derived from the conversion of other adrenal or ovarian hormones. In muscle, testosterone acts directly on the androgen receptors to produce growth-promoting (anabolic) effects.

Androstenedione is the principal pre-hormone, transformed at several sites including the liver, fat, and skin, to re-enter the circulation as testosterone. Conversion is believed to occur in the tissues so that cells which are receptive to androgens have a local supply, ruling out a need for high blood levels of androgens which may have undesirable effects. Androstenedione is produced in both the ovary and the adrenal gland, the amount from each source seeming to vary with time of day and phase of ovarian cycle.

Dihydrotestosterone (DHT) is produced from testosterone and androstenedione and an excess is believed to cause masculinising effects in women such as male-pattern hair growth, acne and hypertrophy (enlargement) of the clitoris.

Dehydroepiandrosterone (DHEA) and DHEA sulphate are secreted by the adrenal gland, with very small amounts also from the ovary. They are less biologically active than the other androgens and their role is not clear, however, levels of DHEA decline with age. Some DHEA is converted into testosterone in the tissues. DHEA sulphate is easily measured and provides a reliable means for evaluating abnormal adrenal androgen levels.

Androstenediol is moderately androgenic and is the intermediate hormone between the formation of testosterone from DHEA. In hirsute women the levels of androstenediol is twice that of normal women.

The carrier proteins

Most of the steroid hormones circulate in the plasma bound by proteins (albumins and globulins). Each hormone appears to have a specific binding globulin or carrier protein which is responsible for its transport. When the hormones are bound to the globulins, they are less able to interact with target tissues than when they are floating 'free' in the plasma. They are also protected from inactivation and break down.

Sex hormone-binding globulin (SHBG)

SHBG is synthesised in the liver and its production is increased by oestrogen, and by an excess of thyroid hormone. It can bind to oestrogens and androgens. A number of factors lower SHBG production. These include obesity, excessive levels of testosterone, the administration of progestogens, glucocorticoid hormone excess as seen in Cushing's syndrome, growth hormone excess (acromegaly), and thyroid hormone deficiency. The level of SHBG controls oestrogenic activity by reducing the amount of 'free' oestrogen that can interact with target cells.

Cortisol-binding globulin (CBG)

CBG, also known as transcortin, is the carrier protein for both cortisol and progesterone. More than 90 per cent of progesterone is bound to CBG which regulates the amounts of available progesterone in the same way that SHBG does for oestrogen and androgen.

5

Maintaining hormonal balance

Key words

basal body temperature
3 beta-dehydrogenase
betacarotene
betaglucuronidase
competitive inhibition
coumestrol
lignan
luteal phase defect

methionine
relative hormone
  imbalance
saponin
steroidal saponin
triterpenoid saponin
xeno-oestrogens

In health, hormones (and prostaglandins) act together to initiate the responses which culminate in a normal menstrual cycle. Many gynaecological complaints can become apparent when hormone levels change.

These changes can be related to an absolute deficiency of a hormone (when a woman becomes menopausal for example); or a 'relative' deficiency (a hormone may be relatively lower than it ought to be, or relatively lower in relation to other hormones). This is believed to occur, for example, if a woman has premenstrual syndrome (PMS), when relatively low levels of progesterone in relation to oestrogen are thought to give rise to a range of premenstrual symptoms.

On the other hand, hormone levels can be too high, exposure to them can be excessively prolonged, or they can occur at levels that are too high in relation to other hormones. Women with endometriosis and fibroids, for example, are thought to be exposed to relatively high levels of oestrogen for too long.

TOO MUCH OESTROGEN

Women today, compared with women of earlier eras, are relatively over-exposed to the stimulatory effects of oestrogen because the modern lifestyle seems to impair oestrogen excretion via the liver and bowel, and favour higher circulating levels of available (biologically active) oestrogens in the blood. Environmental oestrogens can also be introduced into the body and are emerging as significant risks for disease development. Modern women are also affected more by oestrogen simply because they have more periods per lifetime.

Oestrogen excess does not occur because the ovaries make too much oestrogen—on the contrary there is usually a problem with availability and clearance of oestrogen. Symptoms may include heavier than usual menstruation, longer than usual menstrual periods, and premenstrual tension. An increased incidence of menorrhagia, endometriosis, fibroids, fibrocystic breast disease and breast and endometrial cancer have all been associated with relative oestrogen excess.

Excessively high levels of oestrogen are *comparative* and cannot be detected on a single blood test. Researchers speculate that an imbalance may be the mechanism of disease initiation and test their hypothesis by comparing blood levels and/or the length of oestrogen exposure (time when periods started, number of pregnancies, breast-feeding, menopause etc.) of large numbers of well women with those who have the oestrogen-dependent complaint.

Diet and obesity increase the availability of oestrogen

Diet

Epidemiological studies have identified diets containing excessive amounts of refined carbohydrate, low levels of dietary fibre and high levels of saturated fats with an increased risk of oestrogen-dependent conditions including cancers.

Fat intake

Saturated animal fats encourage the growth of intestinal bacteria which produce an enzyme called beta-glucuronidase.[1] This enzyme converts oestrogen into a form that can be re-absorbed from the bowel and women who eat more fat have significantly higher blood levels of oestrogen than those on low fat diets.[2] Conversely, reducing fat intake leads to lower oestrogen levels.[3] A high-fat intake has been linked with benign breast disease, breast cancer, heavy menstruation, endometriosis and fibroids. See page 281 for sources of saturated fats and optimum dietary intakes.

Obesity

Obesity is not just being overweight or carrying a few extra kilos. Women at increased risk are substantially overweight and are in the highest percentile of the body mass index.[4] Obesity can disrupt the menstrual cycle by interfering with normal ovulatory function and is also associated with elevated oestrogen levels. More fatty tissue means a greater ability to convert androgens into oestrogens in fatty tissue and can lead to an increased risk of breast cancer,[5] fibroids,[6] and endometriosis.[7]

There is also a suggestion that the type of obesity may play a role. Women with a high distribution of upper body fat (high waist measurement), tend to have lower levels of SHBG, and therefore more free oestrogen.[8]

Xeno-oestrogens

Xeno-oestrogens are chemical substances with oestrogen-like effects. Exposure to these chemicals is life-long and continual and they have been implicated in an increase in the incidence of oestrogen-dependent cancers, and possibly also fibroids. They are discussed on pages 62–3.

Dietary and lifestyle changes to reduce oestrogen levels

Diet

Fibre

Dietary fibre reduces oestrogen levels in the blood and urine,[9] possibly by influencing the enzymes produced by intestinal bacteria (beta-glucuronidase). A diet which is high in fibre and low in fat reduces both the activity of this enzyme and the amount of (deconjugated) oestrogen able to re-enter the bloodstream. Vegetarians have significantly lower bacterial enzyme activity than meat eaters because they tend to have a higher fibre diet and a lower intake of fats generally.

The fibre which occurs as a component of whole food is preferable to fibre-only breakfast cereals which provide no other advantageous nutrients.

Cultured milk products and yoghurt

The bacteria in yoghurt, *lactobacillus acidophilus*, also reduces the activity of beta-glucuronidase[10] which suggests a positive effect on oestrogen excretion from eating yoghurt and fermented milk products.[11] Researchers found that eating these foods is associated with a lower incidence of breast cancer which they attributed either to the reduced re-absorption of oestrogen or to other immune-enhancing effects of the *lactobacillus* bacteria.[12]

Phyto-oestrogens

Phyto-oestrogens or plant oestrogens have diverse effects on oestrogens. They can prevent oestrogens produced in the body from binding to their receptor sites via a mechanism called 'competitive inhibition'. They are also capable of slowing down the conversion of androgens to oestrogen that normally occurs in fatty tissue;[13] and they can make oestrogen relatively unavailable by increasing levels of oestrogen's carrier protein, SHBG.[14] Oestrogen bound to SHBG is relatively unavailable to bind to the oestrogen receptors.

The steroidal saponins are a specialised group of phyto-oestrogens found in many of the medicinal plants used for gynaecological complaints. They have a similar structure to the steroid hormones. Their precise action is unknown, but they seem to interact with receptors in the hypothalamus and pituitary glands and increase fertility and ovulation (and, therefore progesterone production). They are primarily indicated for complaints associated with oestrogen excess and progesterone deficiency.

The cabbage family

Constituents found in the cabbage family vegetables and herbs (the indoles) can increase the rate at which the liver changes oestrogen into the water soluble form which can be excreted in the faeces.[15] Indoles also competitively inhibit oestrogen[16] and seem to inhibit the growth of breast cancer cells.[17]

The cabbage family vegetables can be consumed regularly by women who have oestrogen-dependent conditions. They include all cabbages, broccoli, brussels sprouts and radicchio. *Capsella bursa-pastoris* is a medicinal herb from this family which is used for abnormal uterine bleeding.

Protein intake

Higher intakes of protein improve metabolism of oestrogen in the liver.[18] Since many conditions are associated with excess protein intake, it is recommended that protein be taken in the form of grains, legumes and low-fat meat and that it constitute no more than 60 g daily.

Vitamin B$_6$

Vitamin B$_6$ apparently has indirect effects on oestrogen. In vitamin B$_6$ deficiency, tissues in the uterus and breast have been shown to have increased susceptibility to the stimulating effects of oestrogen, and B$_6$-deficient women with breast cancer have a poorer survival rate.[19]

The positive effects of B$_6$ may occur because the vitamin behaves like a pharmacological agent and alters the bodily changes induced by oestrogen excess.[20]

Alcohol

The effects of alcohol on oestrogen metabolism and oestrogen-related disorders are complex. Moderate alcohol consumption (one glass of beer, one glass of wine or one shot of spirits daily) has been associated with reduced levels of oestrogen, and a lower incidence of uterine cancer (particularly in overweight women);[21] but an *increased* risk of breast cancer.[22] Women with other risk factors for breast cancer may be wise to keep alcohol intake to a minimum. For other women, especially women with an increased risk of cardiovascular disease, a moderate intake of red wine (one to two standard glasses every second or third day) seems to be beneficial.

Liver clearance of oestrogens

Natural therapists treat symptoms related to 'liver congestion' with bitter herbs or foods (known collectively as 'bitters'). Bitters increase bile production and dilute the bile salts; they also increase the clearance of cholesterol and perhaps, oestrogen. Bitters are Cooling and are prescribed for symptoms which indicate excess Heat such as irritability, acid regurgitation, headaches, excessive bright-red menstrual flow, dry stool, and facial acne.

The exact mechanism whereby bitter herbs affect the menstrual cycle is unknown. Hepatic conversion of oestrogen may be accelerated, perhaps in conjunction with the increased rate of bile flow known to occur when bitter herbs are taken. Their primary site of action might be to alter the bowel flora. The effects are likely to be quite complex, however, since bitter herbs are a large and diverse group with many different actions. Some are known to have separate effects on the uterus which may act in tandem with any oestrogen-clearing effects. The important bitters for gynaecological complaints are discussed in Chapter 19, 'Herbs'.

Foods high in methionine assist with the methylation of oestrogen, the chemical reaction the liver uses to break down oestrogen (oestradiol) into the less potent form (oestriol). Beans, legumes, onions and garlic are high in methionine.

Exercise

Exercise helps with oestrogen clearance, and women who exercise tend to have lighter and less frequent periods.[23] See also pages 168–70.

TOO LITTLE OESTROGEN

A *relative* oestrogen deficiency occurs when too much oestrogen is removed from the body, too little is recycled via the enterohepatic (entero—bowel, hepatic—liver) circulation, and/or too little of the non-ovarian oestrogen is made in the fat cells. An *actual* oestrogen deficiency occurs after menopause.

Low bone density, poor fertility and libido, irregular periods, and premature ageing or excessive dryness and brittleness of tissues including vagina, bones and skin, can all occur when oestrogen levels are too low.

CASE STUDY

Kate's story is a good example of how a relative oestrogen deficiency might occur and what could happen. She was 24 when she first visited the clinic and had problems associated with vaginal irritation and itching, as well as irregular periods. She had been to a variety of doctors and naturopaths and had been told that she had chronic thrush and that her irregular menstrual pattern was caused by cysts on her ovaries.

She had never responded to any of the medical or natural treatments for thrush, but had never had a swab taken to identify the actual cause of the problem. The origin of her ovarian cysts was also mysterious since she had never had an ultrasound. It seemed like a good idea to suggest that Kate have a thorough gynaecological check-up to identify the causes of her mysterious and stubborn complaints.

The gynaecologist found that Kate didn't have thrush, but had the type of vaginal inflammation seen in menopausal women (sometimes called senile vaginitis). Her irregular menstrual periods were associated with erratic ovulation and low oestrogen levels, not cysts on her ovaries. In fact all of Kate's problems stemmed from a low body weight which was causing signs of relative oestrogen deficiency.

The gynaecologist sent her back to the clinic for some appropriate dietary advice. Within two months of being on a sensible diet and gaining some weight, Kate's vaginal irritation had disappeared and her periods showed signs of becoming more regular.

Factors which reduce availability of oestrogen

Body weight

Body weight 15–20 per cent below the ideal body weight can often cause menstruation to stop and oestrogen levels to fall below normal.[24]

The cycle can also become erratic, and fertility and bone density tend to be reduced.

Diet

Fibre

Eating too much fibre, particularly too many wheat bran cereals, lowers oestrogen levels and may increase a woman's chances of developing osteoporosis.[25] Fibre taken as part of whole food does not seem to cause this problem.

Vitamin A deficiency

Vitamin A deficiency causes low oestrogen because of decreased activity of the enzyme, 3 beta-dehydrogenase which is vital to the production of oestrogen (oestradiol) in the ovary. Dietary beta-carotene from orange, yellow and green vegetables or fruits is converted to vitamin A. (Vitamin A supplements are not safe during pregnancy.)

Antibiotics

Antibiotics reduce substantial numbers of the intestinal bacteria necessary to convert oestrogen to the more active form for recirculation. Phyto-oestrogens also need bowel bacteria for their conversion into the active, oestrogenic form. Women who are relying on natural oestrogens from these sources may find that antibiotics decrease their effectiveness. Yoghurt and cultured milks can eventually improve bowel colonies, but trying to avoid antibiotics, except in severe infection, is an even better idea.

Excessive exercise

Over-exercising reduces the levels of circulating oestrogens, and can cause amenorrhoea and low bone density.[26]

Smoking

Smoking alters the metabolism of oestrogen so that more of the inactive oestrogen is produced. Women who smoke are relatively oestrogen deficient,[27] and tend to have an earlier natural menopause and an increased risk of osteoporotic fractures.

Plants can reduce low oestrogen symptoms

Phyto-oestrogens can significantly reduce the low oestrogen symptoms of menopausal women and women with a relative oestrogen deficiency. The isoflavones, coumestrol and lignans can bind to oestrogen receptor sites and are capable of eliciting oestrogen-like effects such as a reduction in hot flushes and oestrogenic changes in the vaginal mucosa. Steroidal and triterpenoid saponins also seem to have 'oestrogenic' and hormone-balancing effects, and many important women's tonic herbs contain high levels of these saponins. Included in this group are *Chamaelirium luteum*, *Trillium erectum*, *Dioscorea villosa*, *Aletris farinosa*, *Panax ginseng* and *Glycyrrhiza glabra*. These effects are discussed in Chapter 18. Phyto-oestrogens can improve bone density. So far researchers have identified positive effects from Chinese herbal formulas,[28] soya products,[29] and coumesterol (a phyto-oestrogen).[30] Research is also currently under way to determine whether *Trifolium pratense* improves bone density.

Saponins in foods and herbs have additional benefits. They seem to improve mineral uptake by causing a mild irritation on the bowel wall, thus making it easier for minerals to pass into the circulation,[31] and they can lower blood cholesterol levels.[32] Dietary sources of saponins include soya products, legumes and potatoes with skins.

PROGESTERONE IMBALANCES

Changes in the availability or synthesis of progesterone seem to be implicated in a number of common gynaecological complaints including premenstrual syndrome, dysfunctional bleeding patterns, cyclic breast disorders and some types of infertility. These conditions are thought to be caused by too little progesterone—known as a relative progesterone deficiency—or arise because of faulty progesterone receptors.

Ovulatory failure

When ovulation fails, no progesterone is produced in the luteal phase. Ovulatory failure is a normal, but transient state after childbirth, miscarriage, a termination, stopping the Pill, and while breast-feeding. It is also seen in dysfunctional bleeding patterns, after stressful events, and around the menopause and menarche.

Luteal phase defects

Progesterone production is altered possibly due to one of three main problems: the corpus luteum is faulty, rupture of the ovarian follicle does not occur, or the messages from the hypothalamic-pituitary unit are faulty or inappropriate.

These disorders are believed to contribute to conditions such as premenstrual tension, benign breast changes and endometriosis. A luteal phase defect is also estimated to affect 3–4 per cent of women who have unexplained infertility and up to 63 per cent of women who repeatedly miscarry.[33]

- Corpus luteum insufficiency: For unknown reasons, the corpus luteum is unable to produce enough progesterone, or to produce progesterone for long enough. The incidence in the general population is difficult to establish because, although many women develop premenstrual tension, the luteal phase often lasts for the usual two weeks. Alternatively the luteal phase may be too short (eleven days or shorter).
- Luteinised unruptured follicle syndrome: This condition is thought to cause infertility, and may particularly effect women with endometriosis. The follicle develops, but the ovum is not expelled, and although progesterone is produced, levels are often lower than normal.
- Abnormal hypothalamic-pituitary function: The problems may originate from faulty FSH secretion which causes abnormal follicular development, or from inappropriate LH surges which adversely affect the function of the corpus luteum. Excessive prolactin production can also prevent ovulation. The causes are unknown, but may be related to stress or an interplay with other hormones.

Abnormal target tissue response to hormones

Progesterone levels are low because of abnormal hormone receptivity in the developing follicle, the endometrium, or other progesterone-sensitive tissues.

The corpus luteum can fail to develop because the follicular tissue lacks normal responsiveness to either FSH or LH; in the endometrium, progesterone receptor-binding might be faulty causing delayed development of the endometrium; in other tissues, such as the breast, a lack of progesterone receptivity might cause cyclic breast pain. Prolactin seems to be implicated in this abnormal tissue response to progesterone.

Infertility, premenstrual syndrome and benign breast disease are believed to be associated with this phenomenon.

Making a diagnosis

Progesterone deficiency can be diagnosed clinically or by tests. These range from simply keeping a menstrual diary to taking the basal body temperature, determining the length of the luteal phase and, for infertile women, blood tests for progesterone levels and/or an endometrial biopsy.

A menstrual symptom questionnaire can be filled out daily for one or more months to ascertain the type, severity and timing of symptoms. Symptoms associated with a progesterone deficiency or lack of availability only occur during the luteal phase of the cycle and include tension, irritability, anxiety or other mood changes.

Basal body temperature (taken by mouth) can be used to determine the availability of progesterone in the luteal phase. The temperature is taken first thing in the morning before any activity at all (including talking or rolling over in bed), and represents the temperature when the body is at rest. An old-fashioned mercury thermometer gives the most accurate reading. The slight, but detectable rise in the temperature associated with progesterone is reliable 77 per cent of the time.[34]

The length of the luteal phase can be measured. The exact date of ovulation is needed and fewer than eleven days from ovulation to the period are highly suggestive of luteal phase defects. Ovulation can be detected using the basal body temperature, a mid-cycle blood or urine test to check for the mid-cycle surge in LH, or an ultrasound scan to view the developing follicle. A scan is the most accurate way of detecting the ovulation date—the least effective way is to subtract fourteen days from the onset of bleeding.

Blood levels of progesterone are usually taken between seven and nine days after ovulation, and readings consistently below 10 nanamol/millilitre are indicative of an abnormally low progesterone. However, blood tests to determine progesterone levels are not 100 per cent reliable because progesterone readings fluctuate widely and can range from normal to very low within a short time span.[35]

An endometrial biopsy might also be suggested if women have undiagnosed infertility to evaluate endometrial development—luteal phase defects are associated with slow endometrial maturation. About one-third of all women have abnormal endometrial development, and the abnormality needs to occur in two or more consecutive cycles before it is considered a cause of infertility.

Treatment

Vitex agnus castus, Paeonia lactiflora and herbs containing steroidal saponins are used to regulate ovulation, and therefore progesterone production. Secondary causes of anovulation and/or relative progesterone deficiency also need to be addressed—stress with nervine tonics, sedatives and adaptogens; low body weight with appropriate diet; excessive exercise with a reduction; and other metabolic or hormonal conditions (for example, thyroid disorders) with medical, herbal or dietary intervention.

Vitamin B_6, E, evening primrose oil and magnesium are also used for the symptoms associated with relative progesterone deficiency.

Premenstrual syndrome, benign breast disease, dysfunctional uterine bleeding and endometrial hyperplasia are discussed fully in the appropriate sections.

6

Prostaglandins

Key words

alpha-linolenic acid
arachidonic acid
dihomogamma-linolenic
   acid (DGLA)
docosahexaenoic acid
   (DHA)
eicosanoids
eicosapentaenoic acid
   (EPA)
essential fatty acid

fatty acid
gamma-linolenic acid
hydrogenated fat
leukotrienes
linoleic acid
omega-3 pathway
omega-6 pathway
prostaglandins
thromboxanes
trans fatty acid

MAINTAINING THE ORDERLY FUNCTION OF THE REPRODUCTIVE ORGANS

The prostaglandins, leukotrienes and thromboxanes—the eicosanoids—are a large family of hormone-like substances involved in the regulation of ovulation, menstruation and labour,[1] as well as many other non-gynaecological events. Usually the production of eicosanoid family members ensures orderly function—when one group causes muscle spasm, another balances that effect by initiating relaxation; when blood clotting is triggered, a balancing anti-clotting response is also initiated.

Sometimes, however, a variety of factors such as infection, inflammation, allergy, hormone variations or poor diet cause production to favour one or more of the family members over the others. These imbalances may be temporary, or continue indefinitely, and are believed to contribute to common gynaecological complaints such as period pain, heavy periods, PMS and endometriosis.

The prostaglandins family can be likened to an extended clan, composed of smaller family groupings like a nuclear family. These families include the prostacyclins and the thromboxanes as well as a group of single individual prostaglandins. Each member of the extended family has a broad role to play. For example, the prostaglandins influence blood clotting, the activity of muscles and the inflammatory responses throughout the body; while the thromboxanes are involved with blood clotting and blood vessel activity.

Members of each of the extended eicosanoid clan are identified by a letter of the alphabet. So for example, one member of the thromboxane family which is responsible for the clumping together of platelets is known as TX A—part of the A branch of the thromboxane family. The leukotriene from the B branch of its family, responsible for attracting white blood cells to inflamed tissues, is abbreviated to LT B. One of the prostaglandins is known as PG E, but there are many others.

Within the thromboxane, prostaglandins and leukotriene families, each member has its own more detailed role. As with all families, some of the members tend to be nuisances, others are more useful. For example, one of the leukotrienes will start some of the processes associated with inflammation, and another one, either a close or distant clan relative, will have the role of calming everything down.

Finally, to help identify what each clan member does, what they are made from, and what they look like, series numbers are added to the names of the different prostaglandins, thromboxanes and leukotrienes.

- Series 1 are anti-inflammatory, relax muscles and are derived from two fatty acids known as linoleic acid and gamma-linolenic acid.
- Series 2 and 4 come from arachidonic acid, found in the cell membranes of animals, and are largely pro-inflammatory.
- Series 3 and 5 reduce abnormal blood clotting and are anti-inflammatory, and are made from eicosapentaenoic acid (EPA).

The key players in the menstrual cycle

Prostaglandins E, series 2 (PGE 2)

PGE 2 is produced by most tissues in the body and is found in large quantities in the ovarian follicle, the uterus and the brain. In the endometrium, PGE 2 stops platelets from clumping together and dilates blood vessels, leading to heavier menstrual blood loss.[2] In the uterine muscle, PGE 2 strongly increases muscle contraction, while in the Fallopian tube, it causes relaxation.

Prostaglandins F, series 2 (PGF 2 α)

PGF 2α (the alpha describes the structure of this prostaglandin to a biochemist) increases as the menstrual cycle progresses, possibly because its production is affected by oestrogen and progesterone. PGF 2α has the opposite effect to PGE 2 in the endometrium where it causes blood vessels to constrict. In the myometrium, both PGF 2α and PGE 2 cause muscle spasm and both are elevated when women have dysmenorrhoea.[3]

Prostaglandins E, series 1 (PGE 1)

PGE 1 is known as the 'good' prostaglandin. Amongst other important functions it stops platelets from clumping; improves sodium excretion, relaxes blood vessels, decreases inflammation, improves the action of insulin and regulates calcium metabolism. The exact role of PGE 1 in the reproductive tract has not yet been determined. It is believed to have a hormone-regulating effect which is most apparent in the luteal phase. It may also reduce tissue sensitivity to prolactin.[4]

Prostacyclin, series 2 (PGI 2)

Prostacyclin (PGI 2) is produced in the walls of arteries, the uterus, the ovarian follicle and the corpus luteum. It stops platelets from clumping together, dilates blood vessels and relaxes uterine muscle. Thromboxane 2 (TXA 2) has the opposite effect on blood vessels and platelets. It induces platelets to clump and blood vessel constriction. PGF 2α which causes uterine muscle to contract, has the opposite effect to PGI 2 on uterine muscle.

Leukotrienes

Leukotrienes in general stimulate uterine contraction and the leukotriene families C, and D are elevated when women have dysmenorrhoea.[5] Leukotriene B (LTB 4) attracts white cells to inflamed tissues and is elevated when women have endometriosis[6] and may also be involved in breast cancer.[7]

The omega-6 and omega-3 pathways

The stimulus for production of the different prostaglandins, thromboxanes and leukotrienes is complex. The ratio of each of the different series produced is not solely dependent on the essential fatty acid building blocks. Tissues produce eicosanoids in response to a stimulus—inflammation, for example—and a number of other biochemical and organ-specific events such as menstruation, also influences the series of prostaglandins, etc. to be produced.

The two pathways by which the fatty acids from foods are converted into fatty acids which serve as substrates for eicosanoids are called the omega-6 and omega-3 pathways. (See Figure 6.1.)

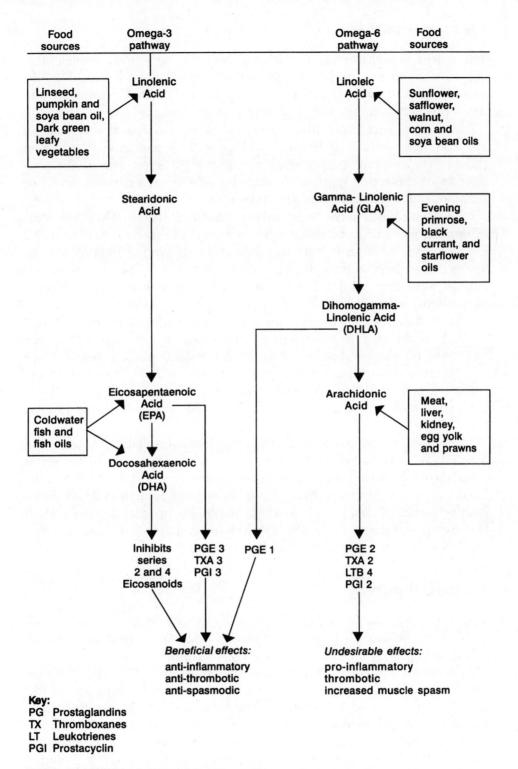

Food sources — **Omega-3 pathway**

Linseed, pumpkin and soya bean oil, Dark green leafy vegetables → **Linolenic Acid**

↓

Stearidonic Acid

↓

Coldwater fish and fish oils → **Eicosapentaenoic Acid (EPA)**

Docosahexaenoic Acid (DHA)

↓

Inihibits series 2 and 4 Eicosanoids

PGE 3 / TXA 3 / PGI 3

PGE 1

Beneficial effects:
anti-inflammatory
anti-thrombotic
anti-spasmodic

Omega-6 pathway — **Food sources**

Linoleic Acid ← Sunflower, safflower, walnut, corn and soya bean oils

↓

Gamma- Linolenic Acid (GLA) ← Evening primrose, black currant, and starflower oils

↓

Dihomogamma-Linolenic Acid (DHLA)

↓

Arachidonic Acid ← Meat, liver, kidney, egg yolk and prawns

↓

PGE 2 / TXA 2 / LTB 4 / PGI 2

Undesirable effects:
pro-inflammatory
thrombotic
increased muscle spasm

Key:
PG Prostaglandins
TX Thromboxanes
LT Leukotrienes
PGI Prostacyclin

Figure 6.1 Essential fatty acid pathways

The omega-6 pathway

The omega-6 pathway starts with the essential fatty acid, linoleic acid which is found as a major component of many seed and vegetable oils, as well as most nuts, organ meats, and human milk. Coconut oil and dairy products contain very low levels of linoleic acid.

Evening primrose oil, blackcurrant seed oil and star flower seed oil are also rich sources of linoleic acid as well as gamma-linolenic acid (GLA). These useful supplements can provide a short cut to the production of the series 1 prostaglandins by selectively increasing levels of dihomogamma-linolenic acid (DGLA).

These seed oils have a number of useful features. They are anti-inflammatory and can reduce the severity of eczema, asthma and allergies; they have an important modulatory role in the immune system and seem to be involved in the activity of the T helper lymphocytes; and as well, they inhibit blood clotting, lower cholesterol and have a vasodilatory effect.[8]

Arachidonic acid, which is converted from linoleic acid or consumed as part of the diet, is also part of the omega-6 pathway and is the precursor for the production of series 2 prostaglandins, thromboxanes and series 4 leukotrienes. This fatty acid is found in animal products including meat and eggs, as well as in human breast milk. Arachidonic acid is not an essential fatty acid since it can be synthesised from linoleic acid.

Changing the amounts of starting materials (linoleic acid, GLA and arachidonic acid) is believed to be able to change the ratio of the series 1 to series 2 prostaglandins. If food sources are primarily from the linoleic acid end of the pathway, both the anti-inflammatory and inflammatory series (series 1 and series 2) might be produced. However, if the dietary emphasis is on the arachidonic-containing foods, the pro-inflammatory series 2 effects will be favoured.[9]

The omega-3 pathway

The first step in the omega-3 pathway is the essential fatty acid, alpha-linolenic acid. It is found in linseed and canola seed oils, walnut oil, soya bean oil, and dark green leafy vegetables.

The same sequence of enzymatic reactions found in the omega-6 pathway transform alpha-linolenic acid into eicosapentaenoic acid (EPA) and docosahexaenoic acid (DHA). The formation of EPA preferentially increases the production of the series 3 prostaglandins and thromboxanes and the series 5 leukotrienes. EPA acts as a competitive inhibitor in the conversion of arachidonic acid to the series 2 and 4 eicosanoids because both compete for the same enzyme to produce their respective end products. For example, when both arachidonic acid and EPA are available, a balance of pro-inflammatory and anti-inflammatory, anti-thrombotic and blood-clotting, muscle relaxing and muscle contracting eicosanoids are produced.

The last member of the omega-3 pathway is DHA which also influences eicosanoid production by inhibiting the series 2 and 4 eicosanoids, but, unlike EPA, does not serve as a substrate for eicosanoid production.

EPA and DHA have a long list of therapeutic effects which includes the reduction of platelet stickiness and the risk of cardiovascular disease; the reduction of inflammation in conditions like arthritis; and an improvement in conditions associated with allergic responses such as asthma and eczema.[10] These oils also have therapeutic potential in gynaecological complaints.

The conversion of alpha-linolenic acid found in seeds and seed oils into EPA to serve as a substrate for the beneficial series 3 prostaglandins does not seem to proceed efficiently in humans. When volunteers ate a low fat diet and took supplements of either linseed oil or fish oils, the levels of EPA increased more in the fish oil group.[11] The conversion of alpha-linolenic acid from seeds is influenced by the amount of linoleic acid in the diet and better conversion rates are seen when the omega-6 fatty acids, especially linoleic acid, are reduced.[12] Oily, cold water fish oils seem to be the most beneficial oils for those trying to prevent or treat cardiovascular disease,[13] and may also prove to be more therapeutically beneficial for gynaecological complaints which respond to improved levels of EPA.

Fish oils provide an alternative source of the EPA for the production of the prostaglandins, thromboxanes and leukotrienes. The best dietary sources are the cold water and oilier fish and shell fish. Fish oils are also available in capsule form to be taken as dietary supplements.

Fatty acids for gynaecological complaints

GLA

A number of gynaecological complaints seem to respond favourably to the fish oils and to the GLA in evening primrose and other seed oils. To gain the best therapeutic effects, however, those foods which selectively increase the series 2 prostaglandins should be avoided where possible. The dietary advice included in Chapter 17, 'Food for health', outlines some possible changes that can achieve this.

Menorrhagia

Women with menorrhagia have altered prostaglandin synthesis which includes higher than normal levels of available arachidonic acid and an increased prostaglandins E2 synthesis (PGE 2).[15] This leads to reduced blood clotting, dilated blood vessels, and contributes to abnormal bleeding. Normally, a percentage of PGE 2 is converted into prostaglandins F2α (PGF 2α), which constricts blood vessels and improves clotting, but this conversion is reduced when women have menorrhagia.

These women also have higher than normal levels of prostacyclin 2 (PGI 2). PGI 2 is another potent dilator of blood vessels and also inhibits blood clotting, leading to increased menstrual bleeding.[16] Prostaglandin-inhibiting drugs, such as Naprogesic and Ponstan, block the conversion of prostaglandins into PGI 2 and can reduce bleeding.[17]

It may be possible to reduce menstrual bleeding by decreasing the dietary fat intake, increasing intake of foods containing the omega-3 oils, and by taking supplements of fish oils[18] or GLA.[19] Both of these oils can reduce the PGE 2 levels in some tissues. Reducing dietary fat lowers oestrogen[20] and perhaps, arachidonic acid which is the dietary precursor to PGE 2 production. A relative excess of oestrogen may also be a stimulus for PGE 2 and PGI 2 production. Women on a low fat diet often claim that their periods are lighter, but so far there is not enough research to establish which factors are primarily involved in this change.

Dysmenorrhoea

Higher levels of both PGE 2 and PGF 2α have been found when women have dysmenorrhoea, and these changes in prostaglandins production can explain the major symptoms of primary dysmenorrhoea, including the increased uterine muscle contractility, the lack of blood flow through the uterus (uterine ischaemia) and the lowering of the pain threshold.[21]

Dysmenorrhoea is more pronounced during ovulatory cycles and is reduced by the Pill, suggesting a relationship between a relative oestrogen to progesterone imbalance and the synthesis of those eicosanoids responsible for muscle spasm. The action of prostaglandins on the uterus is dependent on progesterone levels, and high levels render the uterus resistant to prostaglandins-induced uterine spasm. Dysmenorrhoea occurs when progesterone levels fall just prior to the period.

Leukotrienes also seem to be involved in primary dysmenorrhoea. Women with severe dysmenorrhoea have increased levels of those leukotrienes which increase uterine muscle spasm (C4 and D4)[22]—a diet of oily fish and avoidance of foods rich in arachidonic acid (meat, liver and kidney), reduces the severity of dysmenorrhoea, and improves the synthesis of the series 3 prostaglandins and leukotrienes.[23]

Fish oils seem to be particularly beneficial when dysmenorrhoea has not responded well to the conventional prostaglandin-inhibiting drugs (which do not inhibit the production of leukotrienes). Women taking fish oils (for example, Bioglan MaxEPA) at doses between 2000 and 3000 mg per day report a reduction in their dysmenorrhoea.

Many women also take evening primrose oil for dysmenorrhoea and report a reduction in their pain. The reasons for this are unclear, but may be related to the observed improvement in series 1 prostaglandins levels and a reduction of the series 2 prostaglandins. No studies have specifically looked at these changes in relation to dysmenorrhoea. Improvements in pain are reported from doses ranging from 1000 mg daily for ten days premenstrually to 3000 mg daily all month.

Hormonal imbalance

One theory of the causes of PMS suggests that when abnormal levels of prostaglandins are produced in the brain, breast, gastrointestinal tract, kidney and reproductive tract, the symptoms of PMS develop. A relationship between the hormones oestrogen and progesterone (relative oestrogen excess) may be one of the factors contributing to this imbalance. Drugs that successfully manipulate or inhibit prostaglandins have been shown to relieve PMS,[24] but have a number of undesirable side effects and cautions discussed in Chapter 20 'Drugs and Surgery'.

Dietary supplements containing GLA such as evening primrose oil and star flower oil can improve PMS[25] and have far fewer side effects. They are believed to improve the levels of PGE 1 which reduces the exaggerated effects of prolactin,[26] however, they have not always lived up to expectations and a number of trials failed to show any benefit in relieving the symptoms of PMS.[27]

Suggested doses of between 3000 and 4000 mg of evening primrose oil per day for the entire cycle are often beneficial for PMS, but should be combined with a low animal (saturated) fat diet and an increase in omega-3 oils for best results. In many cases, supplements need to be taken for more than three months before positive results are observed.

Endometriosis

Women with endometriosis have a prostaglandin and leukotriene imbalance which adversely affects ovulation, fertilisation, embryo development, and the motility of the Fallopian tube. The levels of prostaglandins and leukotrienes also influence the degree of dysmenorrhoea.[28]

Women with endometriosis have higher than normal levels of PGF 2α, but lower levels of PGE 2.[29] The elevated PGF 2α may contribute to pain. Leukotriene B (LTB 4) attracts white cells to areas of inflammation and is elevated when women have endometriosis.[30] The increased activity of these white cells is thought to contribute to infertility by interfering with either sperm, ovum or the developing embryo.[31]

Rabbits suffering from endometriosis were given fish oils to examine the effects of DHA and EPA on endometriosis. Neither PGE 2 nor PGF 2α levels increased and the amount of endometriosis was smaller, suggesting that fish oils are useful in treating both the inflammation and the severity of endometriosis.[32]

Both GLA[33] and fish oils[34] reduce the production of LTB 4 and may help with infertility. Star flower, fish and evening primrose oil also improve the ratio of PGE 1 to PGE 2 in white cells[35] which may contribute to a reduction in inflammation and also improve fertility.

Women with endometriosis who have dysmenorrhoea or problems with fertility will probably benefit more from fish oils than evening primrose oils (or similar). Doses from 2000 and 4000 mg daily are recommended.

Benign and malignant breast changes

Animal studies have shown that the leukotriene LTB 4, may be involved in the development of tumours of the breast,[36] and that supplements containing linseed oil or fish oils can inhibit both the growth of tumours and the formation of metastasis.[37] Whether this is of practical significance for women is yet to be proved.

Benign breast changes such as premenstrual pain, swelling and increased nodularity, are thought to be related to the inflammatory changes brought about by prostaglandins. The PGE 2 have been shown to increase heat and inflammation in the breast and cause vasodilation. Again an imbalance between oestrogen and progesterone (higher than desirable oestrogen, lower progesterone) has been postulated to cause an oestrogen-directed increase in the synthesis of the inflammatory prostaglandins. A second effect, brought about by inadequate synthesis of PGE 1, is thought to amplify the effects of prolactin on breast tissue, and aggravate swelling and pain.[38]

Oils containing GLA, which selectively enhance the production of the series 1 anti-inflammatory prostaglandins are prescribed to moderate the effects of prolactin on breast tissue.

Section D

Hormonal lifestages

7

Adolescence

Key words

androgens
anxiety depression
beta-carotene
chromium
functional
   hypoglycaemia

menarche
menorrhagia
PMS
premenstrual

In the years when they are beginning to menstruate, young women experience a range of physical and emotional changes. Some take these changes in their stride and appear not to be affected by them; others have a difficult time coping. Generally, it is not the period itself that causes the problems: the mood swings and physical changes associated with fluctuating hormones have the biggest impact.

The majority of these changes are normal and transitory. Others can be overcome with treatment or altering the lifestyle. This chapter is about signs and symptoms that occur at adolescence; what can be remedied by appropriate self care and which problems may require the assistance of a professional.

BODY AND MIND: THE CHANGES

Menstruation usually begins between twelve and thirteen years, but anywhere between nine and eighteen is considered normal. This is called menarche. Menarche is influenced by inherited factors, but a good diet, plenty of rest and ample exercise are also necessary.

Maintaining a normal body weight is a critical factor. Menstruation starts after a weight of about 47.5 kilograms has been attained, and when the body weight is made up of between 26 and 28 per cent fat.[1]

For menstruation to continue, the weight must be slightly higher than the level at which menstruation commenced. Most women do not drop below this weight unless they become anorexic or seriously ill.

About nine to eleven years

Physical changes usually start somewhere between nine and eleven years (but between fourteen or fifteen is quite normal).

- Rapid increase in height: The height and consequently weight increase rapidly—often accompanied by clumsiness and alternating bouts of energy and exhaustion. Growth rates are different for all young women and almost all adolescents find these extremely rapid changes awkward and embarrassing. This phase can lead to over- or underweight (not necessarily associated with eating disorders— discussed later in this chapter).
- Changes in body shape: The nipples enlarge, but there is no increase in the size of the breasts; the waist becomes more defined and the hips rounder.
- Growth of pubic hair: Sparse pubic hair appears, which can be a paler colour at first. About two years elapse between the first signs of pubic hair and beginning to menstruate.
- Mood changes: Sudden changes in mood are common such as feeling happy one minute and then sad or grumpy the next (adults have these feelings too, but have had more practice in disguising them). These new feelings might make some young women think that they are going crazy. This entirely normal process is associated with becoming more intensely involved with the world and other people rather than having the more limited focus of a child.

About twelve to fourteen years

- Changes in body shape: The hips and waist continue to change and the breasts start to develop. The nipples increase in size and become more prominent. The increasing levels of oestrogen cause other changes including enlargement of the labia (vaginal 'lips') and the production of vaginal secretions which are clear or slightly whitish.
- Body hair: The pubic hair thickens, becomes darker and coarser. Underarm hair grows about two years after the first pubic hairs became apparent. These changes are related to the normal production of weak androgens (male hormones) by the adrenal glands and the ovaries.
- Skin changes: The skin becomes much oilier, particularly over the

chin, nose and forehead, and this sometimes causes pimples. There is a tendency to blush more easily (which passes).

- Changes in moods: It is usual for young women to experience big changes in their moods when they are about to start, or have just started, to menstruate.
- Menstruation: Menstruation starts on average at the age of twelve and a half. Over approximately the first 40 cycles, ovulation and menstruation gradually become more regular. Ovulation does not occur in about 90 per cent of the cycles during the first year after the period starts, and even after four or five years of menstruation, ovulation may not occur during around 20 per cent of the menstrual cycles. The changes associated with menstruation—the cycle, hormones and other physical changes—are described in Chapter 3 'Menstruation and the Menstrual Cycle'.

About fifteen to eighteen years

- Establishing a regular cycle: Typically the period becomes more regular and predictable, however, there is usually a wide range of variation in the regularity, heaviness and frequency of menstruation at this age. Some young women have light periods which last for a few days, others might menstruate heavily for more than a week and as a result, can become anaemic.

WHAT WOMEN NEED TO KNOW

The menstrual chart

Keeping a record of menstrual patterns can be useful to help a young woman get to know her own cycle. (A menstrual symptom diary is included on page 116, but an ordinary calendar will do just as well.) Day one of the menstrual cycle is counted from the first day of the period, and the last day of a cycle is the day before the *proper* commencement of the next period, not counting any spotting.

Charting helps to predict the mood changes which can occur premenstrually, and can also help to predict the first day of the next period, although initially this will often be quite erratic. If supplements or medication have been suggested to offset menstrual or premenstrual symptoms, keeping good records helps pinpoint the best time to take them, and can also indicate whether they were effective.

It is also useful to chart the number of menstrual days, especially when the period is lasting for more than a week. This is helpful to doctors and natural therapists who can use these records to prescribe accordingly.

Exercise

Young women are sometimes told that they should not perform a whole range of activities while menstruating including playing sport, having a bath or washing their hair. This advice originates from the idea that women have to take special care of themselves while menstruating because having a period means being sick. Essentially, though, women should do exactly as they please and whatever feels comfortable when they have their period.

There are two cautions, however. Firstly, getting cold (which may be what the advice to not wash hair while menstruating was all about) can aggravate period pain, and so women who swim may need to be careful about the temperature of the water or the changing rooms. Secondly, some women experience significantly more pain if they undertake vigorous exercise while they are menstruating. In these instances, exercise is counterproductive and should be stopped. It is certainly not the case that *all* exercise is good for *all* menstruating women.

Pads or tampons?

When all is said and done this decision comes down to a personal choice. Historically, both pads and tampons have been used as forms of protection—the tampon was written about extensively in history and used to consist of either wool, linen or, in Egypt, rolled papyrus. Both pads and tampons have advantages and disadvantages.

These days pads are thin, absorbent and easy to wear because they have an adhesive strip which attaches them to underwear. They come in a variety of sizes and shapes for heavy days, night-time use, light days and so on, and it is best to experiment with the different shapes and types until a favourite is found.

Some women don't like pads because pads are messy, they think the pad might be visible through their clothes, and they are worried about the odour of their menstrual blood. (Menstrual blood changes in odour when it comes in contact with air.) Odour can be avoided by changing the pad frequently and it is not possible to see the thinner pads through clothing. Some women who have heavy periods find pads much more convenient, and sometimes period pain seems to be aggravated by tampons, making pads a more suitable choice.

Tampons are popular because they are invisible and greatly reduce the possibility of menstrual blood odour. They also make swimming possible during menstruation, which is a distinct advantage if swimming is a favourite sport or if it relieves period pain. For a variety of cultural reasons, some parents do not want their young daughters to use tampons. It can also take some practice to insert tampons correctly.

A tampon *cannot* get lost somewhere inside a woman's body (it is impossible for a tampon to pass through the opening in the cervix), and tampons do not make a woman lose her virginity. The hymen (the membrane which partially covers the vaginal opening until a woman has had sexual intercourse) is not intact when women start to menstruate—otherwise the menstrual flow would not be able to pass through the vagina. The hymen is elastic and stretches to allow a tampon to be inserted. Very slim tampons are also available.

The biggest problem experienced with tampons is inserting them properly. Once in the correct position, a tampon should be hardly noticeable. If discomfort is felt, the tampon should be inserted more deeply in the vagina. The other rare complication from using tampons is toxic shock syndrome.

Toxic shock syndrome

Toxic shock syndrome (TSS) is a rare condition, but it can have fatal effects which are caused by the release of a toxin from the *Staphylococcus aureus* bacteria ('golden staph'). The toxin attacks various organs in the body and causes characteristic symptoms including a rash and a high fever. 'Toxic shock' can affect anyone who is infected by golden staph, but the term is most commonly associated with tampon use.

Risk factors

The exact reasons why some women develop toxic shock syndrome are unknown, although a number of risk factors have been identified.

- Tampon use is strongly associated with the development of toxic shock syndrome, although a few women who have not used tampons have developed the condition, and men and young children can also develop toxic shock syndrome if they have a 'golden staph' infection.
- The absorbency of the tampon may be a factor, but this may be because 'super-absorbent' tampons tend to be left in place for longer which allows time for the bacterial numbers to develop and enough of the toxin to be produced to cause symptoms.
- The type of material used in tampons may encourage bacterial growth. Some researchers believe the absorbent synthetic fibres change the vaginal secretions and allow more bacteria to multiply.
- Women who use tampons for their entire period seem to be at an increased risk of developing toxic shock syndrome. The cause for this is unknown, but again may be related to a vaginal environment which is conducive to bacterial growth.

Signs and symptoms

- Headaches, sore throat and aches in the joints and limbs, and 'flu-like' symptoms are usually the first signs of toxic shock. Typically these start several days after the beginning of the period.
- This is followed by a sudden onset in fever (temperature usually in excess of 39°C) accompanied by vomiting and diarrhoea.
- After about 48 hours, there may be a dramatic drop in blood pressure which causes the symptoms of shock. These are sweating, paleness, dizziness, collapse and sometimes disorientation or loss of consciousness.
- A skin rash often accompanies these symptoms. The skin becomes red and then peels as though it is sunburned.
- Sometimes the kidneys are affected and fail to produce urine.

Prevention

- Not using tampons will dramatically reduce the chances of developing toxic shock syndrome, but since it is a very rare condition, this is hardly necessary.
- Changing tampons regularly—at least every four hours—may help to reduce the incidence.
- Using the smallest size of tampon that will absorb all menstrual loss in a four-hour time span will reduce the tendency to leave a tampon for long periods of time before changing it.
- The super-absorbent tampons are associated with the highest risk, possibly because of their composition.
- Don't leave tampons in overnight. A whole night is too long to leave a tampon in place and women who use tampons during the day and pads at night have a lower incidence of toxic shock.
- Toxic shock syndrome became much more prevalent when synthetic fibres were used in tampons and so there is a possibility that natural fibres, such as cotton, may reduce risk. Tampons made from organic and untreated fibres are now sold, but there is not yet proof that they are any better.

Treatment

Toxic shock syndrome is an acute medical emergency, and women who develop these symptoms should go immediately to a hospital for evaluation. Any tampon should be removed immediately. Toxic shock syndrome is treated with antibiotics and is likely to require admission to hospital. This is *not* a condition to be treated by natural medicine.

Getting to know what is normal

One of the difficulties about getting periods is knowing what is normal. It's no use comparing stories with friends because everyone is so different. Help or advice should be sought if any of the following symptoms are noticed:

- Any sudden changes in the menstrual cycle such as the period becoming erratic when it was once regular; periods becoming suddenly very heavy or very light;
- Excessive pain during or before each period or new and unusual pain associated with the period.
- Abnormally heavy or long periods. An abnormally heavy period means needing to change pads or tampons every two hours; abnormally long is longer than seven days.
- Any unusual spotting between the periods.
- A yellowish or smelly vaginal discharge, or if there is any vaginal itch or soreness.

Diet during puberty

Diet during puberty is a vexed issue. On the one hand there is the tendency for young women to want to 'go on a diet' because of body image concerns, while on the other, there is the dramatic increase in the nutrient requirement during this time of rapid physical maturation. It is often a time when girls cut back on sport. The dual aims of maintaining normal weight and getting enough of the vital nutrients can only be achieved by that oldest of combinations—regular exercise and a balanced diet.

The rapid growth rate during this time means a young woman's mineral requirements escalate dramatically. Zinc, iron, magnesium and calcium are in especially high demand. (An information page on zinc can be found on page 104, iron on page 189, magnesium on page 272 and calcium on page 150.)

Surveys have shown that up to 85 per cent of women do not get enough zinc.[2] Zinc helps to prevent against the development of acne, and may be especially useful when acne is excessively inflamed. It is an important component of collagen and plays a vital role in the metabolism of hormones linked to sexual maturation.[3] It is necessary for the formation of insulin and tends to help prevent sugar cravings and blood sugar fluctuations.

Calcium is essential during puberty because of the rapid growth of bones. A young woman's calcium requirements increase by 50 per cent (from 800 mg per day to 1200 mg) during these years. Calcium is better absorbed and maintained in bone when magnesium intake is normal. Researchers found that around 40 per cent of women do not get enough magnesium from their diets[4] and about 30 per cent of young women (between 18 and 29) do not get enough calcium either.[5]

Iron deficiency is also common and is associated with anaemia, fatigue, reduced resistance to infection, dizziness, faintness and poor concentration. Iron requirements increase during adolescence because of the increase in muscle mass and blood volume; and because of the increased requirements associated with menstruation—during a period between 15–30 mg of iron are lost. In general the iron absorption from animal sources is twice that of vegetable sources.

The physical changes can be very taxing on the body and result in episodes of exhaustion. When these occur, it is a good idea to get more rest by going to bed by 10 p.m. Energy drinks after school, plenty of vegetables, and, of course, limiting junk food, will also help. Follow the diet in Chapter 17, 'Food for Health', for a balanced eating regime.

COMMON PROBLEMS DURING PUBERTY

Mood changes

Depression and anxiety are the most common mood changes experienced during the years when the menstrual cycle and hormones are becoming established and regular. This can be related to the hormonal fluctuations (somewhat like being premenstrual all the time), or to other factors which become harder to deal with because of the additional stresses of puberty.

Often other people recognise that someone is depressed before the depressed person does. Sometimes the person just feels out of sorts or doesn't want to do anything, and because of their depression, they find it difficult to understand their own behaviour. Always seek professional advice for the treatment of anxiety or depression. The symptoms of depression might be:[6]

- Feeling sad, tearful or crying easily or crying at things that would not normally cause tears or sadness while watching TV for example.
- Finding less or no pleasure in activities that used to be fun or feeling as though these things are boring, too hard, or silly.
- Feeling irritable or agitated most of the time with everyone, including the cat.
- Feeling unwell more than usual, for example, suffering from head-aches or stomach-aches that are not usual or increasing in frequency.
- Not coping with school work, or being absent from school more than usual.
- Having difficulty with concentration, daydreaming or fantasising excessively about better things/times.
- Feeling bored, tired or sleepy all the time.
- Sleeping poorly, dreaming excessively or having nightmares, being tired during the day and wide awake at night, wanting to sleep all the time or not wanting to get out of bed.

- Not eating properly, tending to miss meals, binge eating, unusual appetite or lack of appetite.

Feeling depressed is the usual response to stress, changes, disappointment or loss. A list of the common causes of depression is included below.

Feelings of anxiety can sometimes be hard to identify. It is common for young women to think that they are being silly, boring, that they're going crazy or 'losing the plot' when in fact they are suffering from anxiety. Most of the time, when the major changes in their lives are put into perspective, they realise that a little anxiety is normal under the circumstances. Some of the common symptoms of anxiety are:[7]

- Feelings of losing control, going crazy, that something traumatic is going to happen, such as someone close may die.
- Fear of unusual things that have never been worrying before such as going shopping, driving in the car, going out with friends, having to talk in front of the class at school.
- Anxiety attacks with symptoms like rapid heart beat (palpitations) which may be accompanied by dizziness and extreme fear. This might start suddenly and for no apparent reason, such as when trying to get to sleep.
- Experiencing shortness of breath, difficulty taking a deep breath or sighing a lot.
- Trembling and shaking, feeling faint and dizzy.

Like depression, anxiety is a physical and emotional response people can develop, especially when confronted by a succession of new events. It is also fairly common to experience episodes of 'floating anxiety' or 'non-specific dread' that don't seem to be related to any specific event. These feelings can sometimes be associated with physical changes like premenstrual syndrome (see below), but might also be related to the memory of an anxious event.

Sometimes the symptoms of anxiety and depression occur together and the person then has what is called anxiety depression. Depression, anxiety and anxiety depression during puberty are all usually 'reactive', meaning that they occur as a reaction to too many stresses, changes and unsettling events occurring together.

Following is a checklist of the common events that can trigger any of these symptoms. Experiencing even one of these can lead to anxiety and/or depression around puberty.

- A persistently heavy workload at school, especially when there is difficulty keeping up with the work.
- A relationship break-up, or a severe disappointment concerning a close friendship or relationship.
- Failing an exam or getting low marks after working hard on a project.

- Being teased or otherwise targeted at school.
- Death of someone close.
- Continual tension between parents, or between one/both of parents and the adolescent.
- Major family changes or problems, such as separation, divorce, a much-loved brother or sister leaving home, a family member ill or with a drug problem, family financial problems, or unemployment.
- Other upsetting tensions at home.
- Moving house and/or moving to a new school.
- Being unwell or needing an operation.
- A difficult personal crisis.

Sometimes depression can become very serious and the individual might even become suicidal. If this happens, they are less likely to be able to have a reasonable and objective understanding of what is happening, and family members or friends are often the ones who will need to coax the person into getting some professional help. Symptoms might be:[8]

- An obvious personality change, being difficult to get along with or rebellious, or being withdrawn and introverted.
- Severe changes in eating or sleeping patterns.
- Not caring about personal appearance, dressing sloppily and being careless about hygiene.
- Saying or feeling they're a horrible person, that they're not worth having around, that they're poisonous or rotten inside, or that they are the cause of someone else's problems.
- Having an unreasonably low self-esteem, being unable to take praise or feel as though they can achieve anything worthwhile.
- Using/abusing drugs or alcohol, getting 'out of it' to feel better.
- Saying that no one cares about them, that they wish they were dead, that nothing matters any more, generally having a bleak outlook on the world.
- Giving away their treasured possessions, getting their affairs in order.
- Suddenly becoming unreasonably and unrealistically happy after having been depressed for a long time.

■ ■
■ ■ The medical approach

Some doctors may suggest counselling or may arrange long consultations so they can counsel the patient themselves. Sometimes drugs are necessary, but should only be used as a last resort. The prescription of drugs for depression and psychiatric disorders is a specialty area and it is wise to consult a psychiatrist who is likely to be able to make the best decision about the suitability of drugs for each case. Psychiatrist's fees are covered under the Medicare system.

The natural therapist's approach

It is not advisable to treat severe depression, anxiety and suicidal feelings with herbs or supplements alone. Referral to a doctor, psychiatrist or counsellor should also be arranged.

The nervines are the group of herbs used and of these the best herb for depression is *Hypericum perforatum*. This herb is known as a nervine tonic and tends to work well in combination with other herbs that have a calming effect.

Piper methysticum is excellent for anxiety, and is available through practitioners. Other anti-anxiety herbs are *Verbena officinalis, Scutellaria laterifolia, Matricaria recutita, Passiflora incarnata, Zizyphus spinosa, Valeriana officinalis* and *Eschscholtzia californica*.

Vitamin B complex is a general nerve tonic especially where stress, overwork or too much study are causing the nervousness. Vitamin B complex is a good idea before exams to maintain mental clarity, especially if exams fall on premenstrual days.

 Self care

Depression and anxiety are very rarely related to just one thing like physical problems or stress, and so it is wise to look at all of the possible contributing causes and not target only one area. Sometimes the stresses aren't going to go away for a long time and it may be necessary to consult a counsellor or therapist for some practical suggestions for coping with the problem.

Sometimes mood swings can be aggravated by, or related to physical problems like PMS (see Chapter 8); or sometimes the physical problems arise as a result of the effects of stress on the body—getting an ulcer is an obvious example. Some of the common physical causes for anxiety or depression might be related to hormonal imbalance, 'burn out' or hypoglycaemia. If this is the case, these will need to be treated as well so that there is an 'all-round' improvement.

Exercise

LSD—not the well-known hallucinogenic drug, but long, slow distance exercise—is very useful for improving the response to stress. It is described on page 169.

Eating well

Eliminate junk food and any foods or drinks which contain caffeine. Follow the hypoglycaemic diet (pages 129–30) if blood sugar problems are contributing to the symptoms.

Reducing tension and improving sleep

The section on stress in Chapter 10 is well worth reading in conjunction with this chapter. It outlines some self-help advice on reducing tension, improving concentration and how to get better quality sleep.

Talk it over

Encouraging the person to talk about problems with friends and family is usually a good idea. If friends and family are unhelpful or seem inappropriate, the school counsellor, a trusted teacher, or their health-care practitioner may either be able to help or suggest someone who can.

Hormonal imbalance

The types of feelings women experience when they are premenstrual are very similar to those of anxiety or depression. These are known as PMS. A woman with PMS is likely to have one or more of the following:

- Symptoms which disappear as soon as menstruation commences.
- Symptoms which are only evident in the last part of the menstrual cycle, that is, in the week or ten days before the period starts. Physical symptoms which most women experience when they are premenstrual include breast tenderness, bloated lower abdomen, pelvic discomfort or pain, clumsiness or headaches.

Hypoglycaemia

Hypoglycaemia, or inappropriate fluctuations in the blood sugar can lead to feelings of depression and anxiety. Following the hypoglycaemic diet for several weeks will lead to a rapid improvement in symptoms if the mood swings are related to abnormal blood sugar fluctuations.

Acne

About 50 per cent of young women between the ages of fourteen and seventeen (and about 75 per cent of young men) develop acne. Usually by twenty the problem has cleared up, but sometimes acne continues into later life. Acne is embarrassing and can severely diminish self-esteem so it is advisable to try to prevent it and to treat any sign as quickly as possible.

Acne is not caused by 'dirty' skin, poor hygiene or oily hair on the face. The real causes of acne are related to the increased levels of androgens (male hormones) around puberty, thickening of the tissue around the openings of pores in the skin, bacteria which grows on the surface of the skin, and inflammation which occurs as a result of the bacterial infection.

The curious thing about acne is that some people have hormonal imbalances, but don't get any pimples. When researchers look at the levels of androgens in the blood if someone has acne and compares these to someone who does not, the levels are the same. This may be related to the individual's sensitivity to androgens—some people's skin just seems to be more likely to respond adversely to androgens.

Another reason that androgens may cause acne is because weak androgens can be converted into stronger ones in the hair follicle. This does not result in large amounts of androgens in the blood—the effect is much more localised—but the increased levels in the skin can cause an increase in sebum production, and acne. This seems to be an inherited trait.

■ ■
■ ■ The medical approach

Topical applications include retinoic acid (tretinoin or Retin A) for non-inflamed lesions; or lotions containing antibiotics such as clindamycin, for inflamed lesions. An older preparation, benzoyl peroxide, which comes as a cream, gel or wash, is still suggested by some doctors. Newer preparations which contain glycolic acid (often called fruit acid) are gentle skin 'peels' to remove dead skin and keep the pores open.

Sometimes these lotions or creams can cause inflammation of the skin (contact dermatitis) and they should be stopped until the reaction settles down. Reducing the frequency of applications sometimes solves this problem.

Oral treatments for acne include antibiotics or isotretinoin (Roaccutane). The common antibiotics used include tetracycline (Mysteclin, Tetrex, Vibra-Tabs, Minomycin) or occasionally erythromycin if pregnancy is a possibility or the patient is allergic to tetracycline. The most common reasons that antibiotics do not work is because they are not given for long enough or are not given at high enough doses. To be effective antibiotics need to be given for at least six to eight months and doses may need to be adjusted if an adequate improvement does not occur. They should be taken half an hour before food to increase their efficacy.

Isotretinoin (Roaccutane) can only be prescribed by a specialist dermatologist: it has a number of common side effects including cracked lips, facial dermatitis, severely irritated conjunctiva and eyelids, nose bleeds from dry and sore nasal passages and certain forms of eczema. Some people also develop photosensitivity and sun block must be used to reduce risk of sunburn. Muscle and joint pains can sometimes occur and rarely, bony outgrowths can develop throughout the skeleton. The blood lipids usually become abnormal, and occasionally the liver enzymes are also affected, but return to normal after stopping the medication. Women taking Roaccutane must be on the Pill or use another suitable contraceptive, such as a diaphragm because of the certainty of foetal abnormalities if pregnancy occurs.

Although there are very severe side effects from this drug, it has made the treatment of serious acne much more reliable. Prior to this drug, scarring and cystic acne were difficult to treat with antibiotics alone and adolescents were faced with prolonged and serious acne that could not be treated effectively.

 ## The natural therapist's approach

The natural therapist's approach combines diet, supplements, hygiene, hormone regulation, skin healing and bacterial control. Different combinations of treatments seem to be effective for some people, but not others, so getting it right can be complex.

Eliminating one supposedly problematic food group, like chocolate or sugar, from the diet has been shown time and again to be ineffective in the treatment of acne. But comprehensive diet changes are not a waste of time—they do, however, have to take several factors into consideration.

The diet should include plenty of fresh fruit, vegetables and fibre, but be low in fat and refined sugar. Foods which have high levels of beta-carotene, such as yellow and orange fruit and vegetables and dark green leafy vegetables; and zinc should be included to reduce inflammation, assist with healing and to help regulate hormone levels.

Zinc seems to be very useful in acne, especially where the lesions are excessively inflamed. This is assumed to be related to the general wound-healing properties of zinc, but this mineral also has diverse effects on hormone levels including normalising oestrogen production and reducing excessive androgen levels.[9]

Chromium, from brewer's yeast, improves acne.[10] Yeast products can aggravate, or occasionally cause problems with vaginal candida (thrush) and gut disturbance from yeast overgrowth, especially if antibiotics or the Pill are taken at the same time. Giving brewer's yeast with yoghurt prevents these problems from developing.

Acne that worsens just prior to the period is often helped by vitamin B_6, either alone, or better still with B complex or zinc. Some women take 50–100 mg of vitamin B_6 with 1 teaspoon of brewer's yeast in the week or ten days prior to their period and find this regime very useful.

A number of herbs are routinely prescribed by herbalists for acne. These include *Echinacea angustifolia*, *Calendula officinalis* and *Arctium lappa. Vitex agnus castus* is also useful when there is severe acne associated with hormonal irregularities, but should only be professionally prescribed.

Antibacterial face washes containing tea tree oil (such as Blackmores' Tea Tree Face Wash) are useful. Some people develop a contact dermatitis from tea tree oil products and will need to stop using them. A good homemade face pack can be made from 2 teaspoons yoghurt, 1 teaspoon honey and 1 teaspoon lemon or orange juice. For skin that is very dry, add a drop of olive oil. Apply to the face for 30 minutes, and then wash off with warm water.

Stress can aggravate acne, perhaps because stress can disrupt the normal hormonal balance (see Chapter 10). Following the ideas for stress relief may help to improve acne that worsens during difficult times.

Menstrual problems

Heavy bleeding and erratic cycles

Very heavy periods (menorrhagia) which occur for many months can lead to anaemia. The cause of the problem should be established before any treatment is started. Usually the history (the signs, symptoms and events that accompany the complaint) are sufficient and a physical examination is not needed.

Menorrhagia and erratic cycles are usually caused by hormonal fluctuations and erratic ovulation. Very rarely, a congenital blood-clotting disorder—von Willebrand's disease—is diagnosed for the first time during adolescence because it causes menorrhagia.

After a few years, when hormone production is more reliable, the cycle will develop its own rhythm without any external interference. It is rarely necessary to interfere with ovulation—either to make it more regular with herbs, or to stop it altogether with the Pill (although doctors often suggest the Pill for heavy bleeding). Because stress can delay ovulation, measures to reduce stress might also be appropriate (see Chapter 10).

The sorts of natural remedies outlined in the section on functional menorrhagia (Chapter 11) can be used to control symptoms when needed. *Vitex agnus castus* is not appropriate for adolescent menorrhagia, except in a very limited number of cases. *Never* self-prescribe this herb because it requires a lot of skill and knowledge to get the dose and timing right.

Period pain

Ginger tablets, commonly sold for travel sickness, can help with period pain. They are easy to take and are available in blister packs

(Blackmore's Travel Calm Ginger™). Some young women find two tablets (400 mg) 3–4 hourly are as effective as conventional pain-killers.

Period pain is discussed in Chapter 14.

ZINC FOR GROWTH AND DEVELOPMENT

Sources

Oysters, fresh	45.0–75.0	Peanuts	3.0
Clams	21.0	Chicken, dark meat	2.85
Wheat bran	16.0	Walnuts	2.25
Wheatgerm	13.0	Bread, wholewheat	1.65
Brazil nuts	7.0	Shrimp or prawns	1.15
Ginger root, dried	7.0	Egg, whole	1.10
Meats, muscle	4.5–8.5	Milk, low-fat	0.75
Parmesan cheese	4.0	Oatmeal, cooked	0.5
Peas, dried	4.0	Carrots, raw	0.5
Hazelnuts	3.5	Sardines	3.0

Deficiency signs and symptoms

- Slow growth
- Infertility/delayed sexual maturation
- Hair loss
- Skin conditions of various kinds
- Diarrhoea
- Immune deficiencies
- Behavioural and sleep disturbances
- Night blindness
- Impaired taste and smell
- Impaired wound healing
- White spots on fingernails

Conditions which may be caused by zinc deficiency

- Frequent or severe infections
- Many skin problems
- Delayed wound healing
- Post-operative complications
- Congenital malformations
- Psychiatric disorders
- Dandruff, hair loss
- Impaired glucose tolerance
- Connective tissue disease
- Reduced appetite

Inadequate dietary intake of zinc may be due to

- Anorexia nervosa, fad diets, weight-reducing diets
- Exclusion diets for food allergies

- Strict vegetarianism
- A restricted protein diet
- Long term intra-venous therapy or naso-gastric tube feeding
- Alcoholism

Zinc absorption may be impaired because of

- High fibre diets
- Iron tablets
- Coeliac disease
- Low or absent gastric acid levels
- Alcoholic cirrhosis
- Pancreatic insufficiency
- Advanced age when zinc absorption is diminished

Zinc requirements are increased in the following conditions

- Burns, starvation, diabetes mellitus
- Diuretic use
- Use of penicillamine
- Chronic blood loss or renal dialysis
- Exfoliative dermatitis, excess sweating
- Irritable bowel syndrome, intestinal parasites and hookworm
- Alcoholism
- Liver disease including viral hepatitis
- Chronic diarrhoea and ileostomy fluid loss
- Surgery and trauma

Specific conditions with an increased need

- Cancers
- Growth spurts and puberty
- Pregnancy and lactation
- Psoriasis

8

The menstruating years

THE PREMENSTRUAL SYNDROMES (PMS)

PMS and PMT (premenstrual tension) are really interchangeable terms. However, some people use the term PMT to describe only those symptoms which indicate emotional difficulties—tension, irritability and tearfulness for example. To avoid confusion, I use the term PMS to describe both the emotional and physical symptoms suffered by women when they are premenstrual.

Physical discomfort and changes in mood and behaviour have been associated with menstruation since ancient times. Originally, these sorts of symptoms were thought to have bizarre origins. One of the more colourful was the theory of the wandering womb, which was believed to wander through the body looking for a baby. While on its journey, it might cause symptoms of 'hysteria' (*hystera* is Greek for uterus) and suffocation if it occupied the chest, or a choking sensation if it lodged in the throat. Of course, when back in its rightful position, the symptoms would resolve and menstruation would start which added further fuel to the 'wandering womb' theory.

While it was a strange idea, this explanation at least gave the women who developed PMS some credibility for their symptoms. Not so during the 1950s, 1960s and 1970s when conventional medical wisdom decided that PMS was a problem associated with 'nerves' or failure to cope. Sedation might be suggested to relieve the symptoms, but because science could not discover a cause, the condition was given little credence.

Today we are no closer to an answer. Symptoms are only seen during those cycles when ovulation has occurred, are 'cured' by menstruation, and also stop following surgically or medically induced menopause. One or several hormonal factors occurring together have been suggested as the cause, however, tests have not been developed to identify which group of hormones create the symptoms and many of the explanations remain speculative.

The symptoms

Despite a lack of understanding of the causes of PMS, a great deal is known about how it makes a woman feel. A staggering 150 different symptoms have been recorded in association with PMS. Luckily, no-one gets all of them at once. Most women have a group of complaints that recur, but sometimes a new symptom might be apparent. Symptoms might also change after a major biological event—such as the birth of a child—and women tend to develop different types of symptoms as they approach menopause. For example, headaches can become more prevalent.

But it is the timing, rather than the exact nature of symptoms, that is the most important indicator of PMS. In the classical presentation, symptoms are absent for the week following the period, but can appear at any time in the two weeks preceding menstruation, and then decline at the beginning or in the first days of the period. The most common and recurring physical and emotional symptoms are shown below.

THE COMMON SYMPTOMS OF PMS

Physical

- Abdominal distension, bloating and discomfort
- Breast swelling, pain, discomfort and/or lumpy breasts
- Headaches
- Abnormal appetite, craving sweet foods, alcohol and/or fatty foods
- Fatigue and weakness
- Weight gain of more than 2 kg
- Fluid retention
- Premenstrual acne

- Joint pains and/or backache
- Pelvic discomfort or pain
- Increased incidence of upper respiratory tract infections, including sinusitis and recurrent colds
- Premenstrual genital herpes outbreaks, recurrent vaginal thrush and/or other infections
- Change in bowel habit
- Palpitations
- Dizziness or fainting
- Altered libido

Emotional and mental

- Nervous tension
- Mood swings
- Irritability
- Anxiety
- Depression
- Tearfulness
- Confusion
- Aggression
- Lack of concentration
- Forgetfulness
- Insomnia

Five different PMS sub-groups have been suggested to refine the treatment of PMS, each having a different hormonal, biochemical and/or nutritional cause[1]. PMS-A (A = anxiety) where nervousness and irritability predominate; PMS-C (C = cravings) which is associated with premenstrual sugar cravings and hypoglycaemic symptoms; PMS-D (D = depression) which is accompanied by depression and withdrawal; PMS H (H = hyper-hydration) where fluid retention is the main symptom; and PMS-P (P = pain). Women with PMS may develop more than one of the sub-groups.

Incidence

The estimated incidence of PMS varies widely, but the real number of women with PMS is likely to remain unknown. Many women do not consult practitioners, often believing that there is little to be done. Cross-cultural studies have indicated changes in the frequency of symptoms, but not in the type: Japanese women rarely complain of breast symptoms; Nigerian women often complain of headaches;[2] Anglo-Australian women have more psychological symptoms, but Greek, Vietnamese and Turkish women living in Australia have more physical symptoms.[3]

Theories about the causes of PMS

Despite the commitment to discover the cause/s of PMS, we are no closer to any real understanding. A medical saying states that 'in absence of cure, treatments multiply'. In relation to PMS, we could say 'in absence of a cause, theories multiply' as well.

The theories include abnormal hormone levels, discrepancies in other biochemical pathways, nutrient deficiencies or inappropriate diet. Psychological factors have been suggested and recently, a multi-factorial model has been proposed which incorporates hormonal, dietary, lifestyle and emotional factors as co-factors in the development of the symptoms.

Hormonal factors

Oestrogen/progesterone ratio imbalance

This theory proposes that oestrogen is too high in relation to progesterone. Oestrogen excess is thought to increase feelings of irritability, aggressiveness and anxiety by increasing the availability of norepineph-rine (noradrenaline) in the brain.[4] When oestrogen is produced *without* progesterone, these symptoms do not occur, for example, in non-ovulating cycles, and when women take oestrogen without progesterone for menopausal symptoms.

The fluid retention of PMS is thought to be caused by a relative progesterone deficiency. Progesterone inhibits the activity of another hormone (aldosterone) which promotes the retention of sodium and water. When progesterone levels are low fluid retention worsens.

This has remained one of the favoured theories even though studies of hormonal profiles when women have PMS have been conflicting, showing either lower progesterone,[5] higher oestrogen;[6] or that both oestrogen and progesterone levels were normal.[7]

Progesterone receptors

Another theory is that PMS is not caused by abnormal hormone levels, but by an abnormal *response* to normal hormone levels.[8] In particular, the sites where progesterone 'docks' to the cells, the progesterone receptors, may be faulty and unable to transport the progesterone into the cell.[9] The adrenal hormones, norepinephrine and epinephrine, which are elevated during stress, also block these receptors and make them even less responsive to progesterone.[10]

Progesterone receptors are found in all areas susceptible to the symptoms of PMS including the brain, nose and respiratory passages, uterus, skin, eyes and breasts and many of the progesterone receptors are dependent on oestrogen for their initial activation, suggesting a receptor 'priming' problem. PMS also tends to worsen around times of hormonal chaos (puberty, amenorrhoea associated with hormonal imbalances, and following pregnancy) when the oestrogenic activation of the progesterone receptors is likely to be inadequate.[11]

The adrenal hormones

Abnormal communication between the adrenal gland, the hypothalamus and pituitary glands may be the cause of PMS. The adrenal glands secrete the hormones cortisol and aldosterone which seem to be implicated in some of the common symptoms.

Cortisol is often elevated during depression and anorexia nervosa, but depressed women with PMS have a *lower* than normal level of this hormone. It has been suggested that this is related to the intermittent and cyclical nature of PMS—when the hypothalamic-pituitary unit sends continual messages to the adrenal gland as occurs in depression, for example, the level of cortisol increases; but when the messages only occur some of the time during the menstrual cycle, the levels of cortisol remains lower than normal.[12]

The hormone aldosterone maintains normal levels of sodium and water in the body and plays an important role in the regulation of blood pressure and fluid balance. It has been implicated in the fluid retention of PMS.

Stress can affect aldosterone secretion by triggering the pituitary secretion of adrenocorticotrophic hormone (ACTH) which stimulates an increased secretion of hormones from the adrenal gland. Stress (and severe blood loss) also trigger a chain of events (known as the 'renin-angiotensin system') which start with the production of an enzyme in the kidney (renin) and also culminate in an increased production of aldosterone.

Magnesium deficiency (to be discussed later), and low progesterone (already discussed), also influence the activity of aldosterone. Oestrogen also has an effect—when oestrogen levels are high, aldosterone levels also increase—adding to the theory that an oestrogen: progesterone ratio imbalance causes fluid retention because of changes in aldosterone levels.

Despite the apparent validity of the aldosterone theory, it has been difficult to verify by testing aldosterone levels. Some women were shown to have increased urinary excretion of aldosterone premenstrually, but their blood levels were no different from control women.[13]

Prolactin

The hormone prolactin is thought to cause some of the symptoms of PMS, particularly breast soreness and swelling. Prolactin is secreted by the pituitary gland and is normally elevated in breast-feeding women. Women with PMS are believed to develop an excessive sensitivity to

normal or mildly elevated prolactin levels. The term 'latent hyperprolactinaemia' has been coined to describe this state.

Again, the picture is unclear, however, and although some of the
drugs and herbs used for the symptoms of PMS work by reducing
elevated prolactin levels, no studies have conclusively shown that the
prolactin levels of women with PMS are dramatically higher than other
women.[14]

Brain chemistry

Endorphins

Endorphins are natural opiates produced in the brain which can elicit
a sense of well-being, but when too low, may cause PMS. Opiate and
endorphin withdrawal cause similar symptoms to PMS and provide an
attractive explanation for some of the seemingly diverse and unrelated
symptoms seen when women are premenstrual.[15]

Endorphins may also regulate the release of pituitary hormones.[16]
When endorphin levels are high, the levels of luteinising hormone are
low, but when a drug like the opiate antagonist naloxone is given, LH
levels increase,[17], suggesting an opioid chemical in the pituitary is
effecting the production of gonadotrophins.

Adrenalin, noradrenaline, serotonin and dopamine

Adrenalin is said to trigger anxiety; noradrenaline to induce hostility
and irritability; serotonin to cause nervous tension, inability to concentrate and fluid retention, while dopamine is believed to play a
complementary role by inducing feelings of relaxation and mental
alertness.[18]

Oestrogen is believed to inhibit the deactivation of adrenalin, noradrenaline, and serotonin,[19] but enhance the deactivation of dopamine.[20]
If dopamine levels are low, anxiety, irritability, tension and mood swings
are likely to result. Dopamine is also the 'prolactin-inhibiting factor'
and low levels may lead to elevated prolactin levels. Magnesium deficiency has also been linked to low dopamine levels.

Other factors

Prostaglandins

The symptoms of PMS occur in many parts of the body and are similar
to the symptoms caused by prostaglandins. As a result, prostaglandins
have become guilty by association without a mechanism of action having

ever been proven.[21] Therapies that successfully manipulate[22] or inhibit[23] prostaglandins can relieve PMS, adding more fuel to the theory.

Candida

Candida overgrowth (also known as systemic candida or candidiasis) is believed to cause the symptoms of PMS because of the toxins that the yeasts produce in the bowel. This is a very popular theory amongst some natural therapists, but is difficult to prove, and a mechanism for the purely cyclic nature of PMS has never been adequately explained. Yeast overgrowth could occur, however, because of the hormonal imbalance associated with a relative excess of oestrogen. If so, then candida is only one of many syndromes that can arise as a result of these imbalances.

Nutrients

The popular theory that nutrient deficiencies cause PMS has not been substantiated. Deficiencies of vitamin B_6,[24], vitamin E[25], and vitamin A[26] were not found amongst women sufferers. This does not necessarily imply a lack of effect—nutrients taken at larger than dietary doses are capable of improving symptoms of disease and seem to improve PMS, and some nutrients may work to moderate imbalances in hormone levels or rectify other problems.

Vitamin B_6

Vitamin B_6, or pyridoxine, is one of the most popular treatments for PMS and is believed to improve many of the abnormal hormone levels that are associated with PMS.

Vitamin B_6 improves depression and anxiety associated with the use of the Pill,[27] and because of this a role was assumed for depression in PMS. It is also necessary for the formation of serotonin and dopamine which reduce levels of the hormones prolactin and aldosterone which are associated with breast pain and fluid retention.[28] Low B_6 levels may be associated with a relative deficiency of dopamine, which may lead to feelings of anxiety and irritability.[29]

Vitamin B_6 is also a co-factor in the production of essential fatty acids and the series 1 prostaglandins, and is also known to normalise low intracellular magnesium levels in women[30]. Finally, a B_6 deficiency increases the responsiveness of oestrogen-sensitive tissues making them more sensitive to the proliferative effects of oestrogen.[31]

Despite these hypotheses, numerous studies have failed to show a 'better than placebo' result from administration of vitamin B_6. The ambiguous results may result from questionable trial designs which fail to include enough women, which do not give B_6 at large enough doses or for long enough, or which do not differentiate between women who have PMS and those who have other mood changes.

Vitamin B[6] given at high doses (2–6 g per day for more than twelve months[32]) can cause sensory neuropathy (a type of reversible nerve damage associated with vitamin B[6] overdose) which has also dampened enthusiasm for its use.

On the positive side, some larger studies have shown a positive effect with B[6] in doses ranging from 40–200 mg daily[33] or when B[6] (300 mg) is given in conjunction with other nutrients and a healthy diet.[34] At these doses and for short periods of six months or less, sensory neuropathy has not been seen.[35]

Magnesium

Magnesium deficiency has been associated with depression[36] and depleted levels of dopamine.[37] Magnesium deficiency can also cause increased aldosterone secretion and fluid retention, but in a strange twist, aldosterone increases magnesium excretion via the kidneys. As a result, bigger and bigger losses of magnesium lead to increased aldosterone production and so on.

Magnesium is also necessary for normal sugar metabolism. A deficiency leads to increased insulin secretion[38] and may cause blood sugar instability premenstrually.

Low magnesium may be related to the diet. Magnesium absorption may be reduced by excessive consumption of dairy products, and excretion is increased by refined sugars. Some women with PMS were found to eat more dairy products and refined sugars than non-sufferers.[39]

PMS sufferers have pronounced premenstrual fluctuations in their magnesium levels,[40] and magnesium supplements reduce PMS symptoms such as aches and pains, depression, irritability, mood swings and fluid retention.[41] In fact, magnesium is one of the unsung heroes in the treatment of PMS. Its use is scientifically verifiable and it invariably helps with symptoms. (See the information on magnesium included in Chapter 16, 'Ovarian cysts'.)

Magnesium levels are best reflected by testing cellular rather than serum levels.[42]

Vitamin E

Vitamin E improves benign breast disorders and pain,[43] and also improves tension, irritability, incoordination and other physical symptoms associated with PMS.[44] Doses between 150–600 IU are beneficial. The mechanisms of action are not known, however vitamin E can modulate the production of prostaglandins and reduce inflammation. Vitamin E was also shown to improve the oestrogen:progesterone ratio in women with premenstrual breast changes.[45]

Vitamin A

Vitamin A megadosage has been linked with improved PMS symptoms since at least 1937.[46] Vitamin A might help to improve the symptoms of PMS by assisting with the inactivation of thyroxine and oestrogen in the liver, or might exert a direct anti-oestrogenic effect.[47] Large doses can quickly result in vitamin A toxicity and are toxic during pregnancy. They should only be taken under strict supervision. Recent trials have included vitamin A as a component of treatment and in much smaller (and safer) doses.[48]

Evening primrose and star flower oil

Evening primrose and star flower oil have been the subject of numerous clinical trials which have yielded ambiguous results. Successful outcomes are more likely following long-term administration. These nutrients do not seem to work in isolation and require adequate levels of zinc, magnesium, and vitamins C, B_3 and B_6.[49] In fact, many of the reported successes of evening primrose oil occurred when women took either B_6 or a multivitamin at the same time.[50]

Diet

Blood sugar levels

PMS is often associated with hypoglycaemia symptoms, such as sugar cravings; and faintness, weakness and irritability when meals are delayed. Early research showed that women with PMS frequently had an abnormal glucose tolerance test (GTT) premenstrually and a normal GTT after the period.[51] These researchers suggested that the change in glucose tolerance may be linked with the luteal rise in oestrogen levels and may cause the sugar cravings associated with PMS.

Psychological factors

The biopsychosocial model of PMS

The theory of the biopsychosocial (biological, psychological and social) model proposes that biochemical defects are the essential first step in the development of PMS, but both social and psychological factors also have an impact.[52] Therefore, women with biochemical changes will only become symptomatic if the appropriate social or psychological stressors 'tip the scales'.

Depression

Depression has been described as the most commonly encountered women's health problem in the Western World.[53] Women who are anxious and/or depressed report more PMS symptoms, and large numbers of women with PMS have been found to be moderately or severely depressed.[54]

Diagnosis

There are no blood tests that can diagnose PMS. The best diagnostic method is to use a menstrual symptom diary which outlines the classical symptoms. The diary should show the typical variations in timing which suggest PMS—a complete cessation of symptoms after the period; and an increase in symptoms in the second half of the cycle.

Mistaken identity

Functional hypoglycaemia

Functional hypoglycaemia can be easily confused with PMS because of the similarity of the symptoms. A simple way to differentiate between these two closely related groups of symptoms is to use the Hypoglycaemic Questionnaire (page 118). Fill in the left-hand column on the days immediately after the period, and the right-hand column during the worst premenstrual days. If functional hypoglycaemia is the problem, the symptoms will not vary dramatically during the month.

Menstrual distress syndrome

Many women seek treatment for PMS, genuinely believing that their mood swings are 'hormonal', however, they are more correctly suffering from the menstrual distress syndrome. Their symptoms are present all month, but worsen premenstrually and these women benefit more when the anxiety or depressive state is treated properly.

■ ■
■ ■ The medical approach

The medical treatment of PMS either concentrates on symptom relief with diuretics, prostaglandins-inhibiting drugs or anti-depressants; or on the manipulation of the hormonal axis with drugs that either disrupt ovulation—the Pill, danazol, GnRH agonists; or selectively targets one of the abnormal hormones—bromocriptine. These drugs are discussed in Chapter 20 'Drugs and surgery'.

Table 8.1 Menstrual symptom diary

NAME: _____ AGE: _____ HEIGHT: _____ WEIGHT: _____

GRADING OF MENSES

0–none	3–heavy
1–slight	4–heavy and clots
2–moderate	

GRADING OF SYMPTOMS (COMPLAINTS)

0–none
1–mild–present but does not interfere with activities
2–moderate–present and interfere with activities but not disabling
3–severe–disabling; unable to function

Day of cycle	1	2	3	4	5	6	7	8	9	10	11	12	13	14	15	16	17	18	19	20	21	22	23	24	25	26	27	28	29	30	31	32	33	34	35	36
Date																																				
Menses																																				
PMS–A																																				
Nervous tension																																				
Mood swings																																				
Irritability																																				
Anxiety																																				
PMS–H																																				
Weight gain																																				
Swelling of extremities																																				
Breast tenderness																																				
Abdominal bloating																																				
PMS–C																																				
Headache																																				
Craving for sweets																																				
Increased appetite																																				
Heart pounding																																				
Fatigue																																				
Dizziness or faintness																																				
PMS–D																																				
Depression																																				
Forgetfulness																																				
Crying																																				
Confusion																																				
Insomnia																																				
DYSMENORRHOEA–PAIN																																				
Cramps																																				
Backache																																				
General aches/pain																																				

Source: From Abraham G.E., 'Nutritional Factors in the Etiology of the Premenstrual Tension Syndromes', J. Reprod. Med. **28**: 446–64, 1983

Day of cycle	1	2	3	4	5	6	7	8	9	10	11	12	13	14	15	16	17	18	19	20	21	22	23	24	25	26	27	28	29	30	31	32	33	34	35	36
37.5																																				
37																																				
36.5																																				
36																																				
35.5																																				

**Basal
Body
Temperature
Graph**

As symptom relief is not an acceptable option for many women and hormonal manipulation frequently carries many unwanted risks, many medical practitioners adopt a conservative approach which comprises some or a number of the recommendations listed below in the section 'a more natural approach', and suggest drug therapy only for those women who do not respond to these safer methods.

 ## A more natural approach

Treatments for PMS are based on the five different sub-categories of PMS, devised by G.E. Abraham in 1983, and are comprised of a mixture of supplements and dietary advice, herbal remedies and lifestyle changes.

PMS-A (A = anxiety)

This type of PMS is thought to be associated with a relative oestrogen/progesterone imbalance, with a relative excess of oestrogen and a relative deficiency of progesterone, possibly related to poor liver clearance of oestrogens, abnormal progesterone production or faulty progesterone receptors.

Symptoms
- Nervous tension
- Mood swings
- Irritability
- Anxiety

Treatment
- *Vitex agnus castus* berries extract, 1:2, 40 drops every morning, starting on the first day of the cycle and continued for between three and six months. This herb must be taken under supervision. It is specifically indicated for a relative progesterone deficiency and for latent hyperprolactinaemia.
- Vitamin B₆ 100–200 mg, or vitamin B complex containing 50 mg vitamin B₆ for ten to fourteen days before the period.
- Magnesium 200–800 mg daily of elemental magnesium in the form of magnesium phosphate, aspartate, orotate or chelate.
- Nervines such as *Valeriana officinalis, Scutellaria laterifolia, Matricaria recutita* for anxiety.
- *Withania somnifera* for anxiety with exhaustion.
- *Anemone pulsatilla* tincture is especially useful for tension headache with nervousness, especially when combined with *Passiflora incarnata*.
- *Stachys betonica* is used for headache, anxiety states, hysteria, especially in combination with *Scutellaria laterifolia*.
- *Bupleurum falcatum, Paeonia lactiflora* and *Angelica sinensis* is a common combination used in Chinese medicine for menstrual irregularity accompanied by premenstrual anxiety and irritability.

- Phyto-oestrogens in foods and herbs (see Chapter 18, 'Phyto-oestrogens').
- Bitters to aid liver clearance of oestrogens (see page 257).
- Restriction of full-fat dairy products and refined carbohydrate.
- 'Natural' progesterone creams, allegedly made from plants such as *Dioscorea villosa* (wild yam) are also advocated for the treatment of PMS. Their use is controversial and they are discussed in Chapter 18.

Table 8.2 Questionnaire for suspected functional hypoglycaemia
Score symptoms from 0–3 depending on severity or frequency

1	___	Common desire for sweets and quick energy foods	___
2	___	Fatigue relieved by eating or drinking	___
3	___	Irritability before meals	___
4	___	Get shaky if hungry	___
5	___	Feel better after breakfast or early morning coffee etc.	___
6	___	Need to eat often	___
7	___	Faintness when meals delayed	___
8	___	Headaches or heavy head relieved by eating or drinking	___
9	___	Sleepy during the day and after meals	___
10	___	Heart palpitations if meals missed or late	___
11	___	Number of cups of tea/coffee: Score 1 for 2–3 cups, 2 for 3–5 cups and 3 for more than 5 cups daily	___
12	___	Number of teaspoons of sugar in beverages: Score 1 for 1 teaspoon, 2 for 2 teaspoons and 3 for 3 or more teaspoons	___
13	___	Low energy	___
14	___	Reduced stamina, tire easily and quickly on exertion	___
15	___	Sluggish or lethargic in the morning	___
16	___	Tiredness in mid or late afternoon	___
17	___	Sleep disturbances or dream disturbed sleep	___
18	___	Hot flushes and/or night sweats	___
19	___	Difficulty concentrating	___
20	___	Cannot decide easily	___
21	___	Fluctuating emotions	___
22	___	Frequent anxiety	___
23	___	Become tearful easily for insufficient reason	___
24	___	Bouts of anger or unreasonable behaviour	___
25	___	Magnify insignificant events	___
26	___	Periods of depression or melancholy	___
27	___	Above symptoms worse premenstrually	___
28	___	Cigarette smoking Score 1 for 1–10/day, 2 for 10–20/day, 3 for more than 20 per day	___
29	___	Alcohol consumption Score 1 for average 1 glass daily, 2 for 2 glasses daily, and 3 for more than 3/day	___

PMS-C (C = cravings)

PMS-C rarely exists as a form of PMS in isolation and often accompanies PMS-A. It is associated with functional hypoglycaemia which may be caused by a magnesium deficiency, a sugar-induced sensitivity to insulin, or an imbalance in prostaglandins.

Symptoms
- Headache
- Craving for sweets

- Increased appetite
- Palpitations
- Fatigue
- Dizziness or fainting

Treatment
- Magnesium 200–800 mg daily of elemental magnesium in the form of magnesium phosphate, aspartate, orotate or chelate.
- Small, frequent meals.
- Restricted sugar and salt intake.
- Dietary and herbal bitters to regulate blood sugar metabolism.
- Essential fatty acid supplements, such as evening primrose oil or star flower oil. Doses of 3 g evening primrose oil containing 216 mg of linoleic acid and 27 mg of gamma-linolenic acid or the equivalent taken from mid-cycle until menstruation may be useful in the treatment of the proposed deficiency of PGE1.[55]. Vitamin B_6 and zinc are necessary co-factors in the production of the series 1 prostaglandins.
- Vitamin E between 100 and 600 IU per day can also positively influence the symptoms of prostaglandins imbalance.
- Restricted animal fats, but increased intake of raw vegetable and seed oils selectively decrease the dietary precursors of series 2 prostaglandins and increase the series 1 prostaglandins.

PMS-H (H = hyper-hydration)

PMS-H is related to fluid retention thought to be brought about by an increase in circulating aldosterone levels. Aldosterone may be elevated in response to the lower progesterone secretion, elevated oestrogens, magnesium deficiency, serotonin and dopamine irregularities, or stress. Prolactin may be implicated when breast soreness predominates.

Symptoms
- Breast tenderness
- Abdominal bloating
- Weight gain
- Swelling lower body, and eyelids

Treatment
- All treatments for PMS-A plus
- Vitamin E 400–800 IU per day is specifically indicated for breast tenderness.
- *Taraxacum officinale* leaf as a tea is a mild diuretic and reduces fluid retention.

PMS-D (D = depression)

This form of PMS is accompanied by depression and withdrawal and is thought to be associated with relative oestrogen deficiency. The causes are thought to be associated with the lower oestrogen secretion of peri-menopausal women; depleted oestrogen pool which occurs when women are too thin or eating too much fibre; or blocked oestrogen receptors caused by lead intoxication.

Symptoms
- Depression
- Forgetfulness
- Crying
- Confusion
- Insomnia

Treatment
- Magnesium as for PMS-C to decrease lead absorption and retention.[56]
- Phyto-oestrogens from dietary sources (see Chapter 18 'Phyto-oestrogens').
- The 'oestrogenic' herbs which contain steroidal saponins such as *Chamaelirium luteum*, *Aletris farinosa*, *Dioscorea villosa* and *Glycyrrhiza glabra*. Glycyrrhiza is contraindicated when fluid retention accompanies symptoms.
- *Cimicifuga racemosa* especially where premenstrual headaches accompany the symptoms of depression.
- *Hypericum perforatum* and *Withania somnifera* for symptomatic treatment of depression.

PMS-P (P = pain)

In this category of PMS, the major problem is an increased sensitivity to pain which is believed to be associated with prostaglandins imbalance. Causes are thought to be associated with elevated oestrogen levels, and excessive dietary intake of animal fats which both increase production of the series 2 prostaglandins.

Symptoms
- Aches and pains
- Reduced pain threshold
- Dysmenorrhoea

Treatment
- Magnesium reduces sensitivity to pain in doses of 200–800 mg.
- Essential fatty acids such as evening primrose oil, 3 g per day, with vitamin B$_6$ and zinc.
- *Tanacetum parthenium* is a prostaglandins inhibitor and is useful for the symptomatic treatment of dysmenorrhoea and migraine headaches.

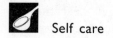 Self care

Diet

An effective way to control PMS is to increase the intake of complex carbohydrates and to eat more frequently—a 'grazing' or hypoglycaemic diet (see page 129). The positive effects may be related to stabilisation of blood sugars as well as to indirect influences on progesterone. One theory is that progesterone cannot be transported into cells which do not contain sugar, and that progesterone levels drop because breakdown speeds up after a large meal.[57]

When fluid retention, bloating and weight gain are prominent symptoms, salt intake should be restricted and dietary potassium in the form of vegetables, grapefruit juice and bananas increased. Many processed foods are high in sodium and should also be restricted.

Women who experience breast soreness, muscle or joint pains or period pain respond well to reducing animal fats, vegetable oils, foods containing hydrogenated fats, coconut oil; and increasing the intake of essential fatty acids and vitamin E.

Coffee, alcohol, and chocolate aggravate feelings of depression, irritability and anxiety, as well as worsening many breast symptoms. Restriction or complete avoidance is warranted during the premenstrual phase.

Many of the symptoms of PMS have been attributed to magnesium deficiency. Where this is the case, it may be beneficial to eat more magnesium-containing foods and restrict dairy products in the diet during the premenstrual phase. A relative oestrogen excess is believed to enhance the retention of calcium in the body to the detriment of magnesium levels, leading to a relative ratio imbalance between calcium and magnesium.

Phyto-oestrogens are indicated for PMS associated with relative oestrogen excess because they act as competitive inhibitors to endogenous oestrogens. Phyto-oestrogens also improve symptoms thought to be associated with a rapid decline of oestrogens just before the period such as headaches, migraines and depression.

Exercise and stress management

Women with PMS, who use long slow distance exercise—such as walking—or yoga seem to be able to handle the physical changes much more capably than women who do not incorporate these lifestyle activities in their daily life. Suitable stress management techniques, such as meditation, and even counselling are also useful.

CYCLICAL BREAST COMPLAINTS

Cyclical breast changes and pain are common complaints. Half of all women complaining of PMS have breast pain unless they come from Asian countries like Japan where the incidence is very much lower.[58] The pain can be associated with lumps, breast enlargement, nipple soreness, a sense of warmth or burning, increased 'ropiness' when the breast is palpated, and soreness or congestion into the armpit. The symptoms may effect one or both breasts. Lumpiness or structural changes can also occur without any pain, however, the most common symptoms are pain and lumpiness in the upper, outer quadrant of both breasts, which occurs in the luteal phase of the cycle.

Disease or normal changes?

When examined, individual women's breasts show a wide variation in nodularity and other structural changes which occur as a result of *normal* cyclical effects of oestrogen and progesterone. Oestrogen is 'proliferative', or makes cells in the breast grow in size and number. Progesterone changes the cells which line the ducts so that they become 'secretory' and able to produce milk if pregnancy occurs. The blood supply to the breast is also enhanced by progesterone.

During the period, there is a time of relative cellular dormancy when the proliferative glandular tissue stimulated by both oestrogen and progesterone involutes. For reasons which are not entirely clear, this process of involution can be incomplete, leading to breast changes which range from palpable breast lumps to microscopic changes in the breast tissue.

Fibrocystic breast disease was once the term used to describe these findings and is sometimes still used as a diagnosis.[59] Fibrocystic breast disease technically means fibrous and cystic breast changes, but many women who have been given this diagnosis have breast changes which fall within the normal range of cyclic proliferation and involution already described. Additionally, some women with breast pain have neither of these changes, while women who *do* have fibrous and cystic changes might have little or no pain.

Terms such as benign mammary hyperplasia, mammary dysplasia and benign cystic hyperplasia, which technically only apply to those changes detected microscopically, are also sometimes used.

Understandably, this leads to a lot of confusion and concern as many women equate these types of diagnoses with malignancy. Medically, the *favoured* term is 'aberrations of normal development and involution' (ANDI), however, to avoid confusion and unnecessary concern, many practitioners will use simple terms such as cyclical breast pain, mastalgia or non-specific breast lumpiness to describe *to a woman* the benign changes which occur before her period.

Diagnosis

A woman might visit her practitioner after discovering a discrete lump or generalised breast lumpiness; with a complaint of cyclic or persistent breast pain; or a combination of these problems. The possibility of cancer can be a major concern for a woman who discovers breast lumps, but many women simply want some sort of treatment for bothersome pain and are convinced that their problem is 'just hormonal'. For a diagnosis of a purely cyclic and benign complaint to be given, however, all other possible causes of the symptoms must be first excluded.

Diagnosis usually proceeds down a fairly well-worn path. When a woman has a symptom of breast pain only, her breasts should be examined *after* the period to rule out the possibility of breast lumps. Many women will palpate their breasts when they experience discomfort—before the period—precisely the time when non-cyclical changes are most difficult to find.

When women have breast lumpiness, referral for a breast examination should be arranged after the period *if the problem has not been resolved.* All breast changes which persist after the period—even if they have the characteristic 'hormonal' pattern of worsening premenstrually—need thorough evaluation. The current myth that lumps that are painful, or symptoms that worsen premenstrually, will not be cancerous is incorrect. Up to ten per cent of women with cyclical breast changes may also have cancer.

There is absolutely no problem in waiting until after the period to re-examine breasts, even when breast cancer is a distinct possibility, because all changes take many months to develop. It is much easier to find breast changes when palpating breasts in the post-menstrual phase, and there is less likelihood of making an inaccurate diagnosis.

When a woman or practitioner feels a woman's breasts, they might find either generalised lumpiness, a dominant lump, or an area of thickening which is quite different to the rest of the breast tissue.

A dominant lump or area of thickening might be:

- Cancer which is often an immobile, hardened, non-discrete area.
- A well-defined breast lump which might be a fibroadenoma, a cyst or a lipoma.
- A less well-defined area of thickening or lumpiness.

The discovery of a dominant lump suggests the need for referral to a breast clinic or specialist to rule out the possibility of breast cancer. On average, one in every five breast lumps discovered is malignant, and the incidence of malignancy increases with age.

Investigations for these findings are fairly routine:

- mammogram and/or ultrasound
- needle aspiration and histology
- lumpectomy and biopsy.

More commonly, breast changes will be cyclical and present as a *generalised* lumpiness of the breast, which represents a normal variation of hormonal activity in the breast. These changes may require no further investigation apart from regular monitoring.

Causes

As with PMS, oestrogen excess with progesterone deficiency is widely accepted as being in part responsible,[60] but there is also a strong possibility of additional factors. An oestrogen-induced increase in the pro-inflammatory (series 2) prostaglandins has been suggested.[61] PGE 2s have been shown to increase blood vessel dilation and thereby contribute to engorgement and pain. Diets high in omega-6 polyunsaturated fatty acids may also be responsible for or aggravate the increase in PGE 2 and breast pain.

Prolactin stimulates glandular breast tissue and may also be involved. Suggested mechanisms are a mild increase in prolactin secondary to elevated oestrogen and depressed progesterone (latent hyperprolactinaemia),[62] or an increased sensitivity to prolactin brought about by low levels of series 1 prostaglandins relative to series 2.[63]

Cyclic breast pain also seems to be affected by lifestyle factors. One Australian study found that women who developed mastalgia exercised less than other women, and had either not breastfed or had done so for less than two months.[64] Taking hormone preparations which contain oestrogens or progestogens can also cause breast pain and stopping these medications can result in markedly reduced symptoms.[65] Coffee consumption has also been linked to breast pain and breast changes,[66] as has a high fat intake.[67]

When pain is severe enough to warrant treatment, it is wise to wait and monitor the symptoms with a menstrual chart (see page 116) for two cycles first. This not only provides a record of the type, frequency and severity of the symptoms, it can also help to monitor the effectiveness of subsequent treatment. As many cases of mastalgia are short-lived, expensive or unnecessary treatments may also be avoided.

■ ■ The medical approach

Bromocriptine reduces prolactin levels and breast soreness; Danazol also has a high success rate (around 70 per cent), but both drugs are accompanied by many unwanted side effects. GnRH agonists and tamoxifen, an anti-oestrogen, are also effective in reducing cyclic breast pain, however, research is still in preliminary stages and neither of these drugs are currently approved for this use. Progestogens were once commonly prescribed, but have now gone out of favour, and the Pill improves the symptoms of some women with breast pain and lumpiness. These drugs are discussed in Chapter 20, 'Drugs and surgery'.

There seems to be a correlation between hypothyroidism and the development of cyclical breast disorders and women with these complaints improve when they are given thyroid hormone or iodine-containing drugs.[68] Diuretics,[69] antibiotics[70] and 'natural' progesterone[71] have also been used, but their effectiveness is questionable.

The natural therapist's approach

Natural therapists believe that cyclical breast disorders are caused by a number of inter-related hormonal factors which culminate in pain, swelling and tissue changes. Principal among these are relative oestrogen excess, progesterone deficiency and a prostaglandins-induced sensitivity to prolactin.

Improving oestrogen–progesterone balance is achieved by restricting fats and increasing fibre; using herbs such as *Paeonia lactiflora* and *Vitex agnus castus* to improve progesterone levels (discussed in Chapter 19 'Herbs'); increasing phyto-oestrogens to compete with the more active endogenous oestrogens, especially linseeds (which additionally improve the oestrogen–progesterone ratio); and using bitter foods and herbs for oestrogen clearance.

Vitamin E is useful and reduces pain and nodularity, possibly by inhibiting the release of arachidonic acid from its storage pool and decreasing the availability of the pro-inflammatory prostaglandins precursors. Vitamin E also improves the oestrogen–progesterone ratio at doses between 500 and 1000 IU daily.[72]

Vitamin B_1 (thiamine) has also been used for breast pain since World War II, when prisoners of war who developed gynaecomastia (excessive development of the breast in males) responded to treatment with vitamin B_1. This vitamin is necessary for the hepatic metabolism of oestrogens, and since relative oestrogen excess may be responsible for cyclic breast disorders, the use of vitamin B_1 has continued. Although improvement has been reported, no double-blind studies have ever been published. Doses of between 60 and 100 mg per day are usually recommended.

Prostaglandins imbalance is addressed by increasing the intake of the precursors of the series 1 prostaglandins with evening primrose, star flower or black currant seed oils. These seed oils must be taken for a minimum of three months for effects to become evident, although even then only about 45 per cent of women responded favourably in one study.[73] The recommended dose of evening primrose oil is from 3000 to 4000 mg per day.[74] Dietary fats should also be reduced (see following).

A French trial showed that a standardised extract of *Gingko biloba* (containing 24 per cent *Gingko* flavone glycosides and 6 per cent terpenoids) was an effective treatment for breast pain. The double-blind study monitored 165 women over two menstrual cycles who took 160 mg per day of the standardised extract or placebo from day 16 of the menstrual cycle through to day 5 of the following cycle.[75] *Gingko biloba* decreases abnormal capillary permeability, increases capillary resistance and reduces oedema. The terpenoids also counter the effects of the pro-inflammatory platelet-activating factor (PAF) which may also contribute to tissue swelling.

Some women may develop breast lumps because of an underactive thyroid gland. This may be 'sub-clinical' (not detected with blood tests) and manifest as a low basal body temperature, increased sensitivity to cold and erratic menstrual cycles. Hypothyroidism causes levels of SHBG to fall, which may contribute to a greater availability of oestrogen. These women often respond to iodine-containing herbs such as *Fucus vesiculosis*, or the addition of seaweeds to the diet.

Additional benefits are also seen when herbs which improve lymphatic drainage are prescribed. These include *Calendula officinalis*, *Viola odorata*, *Phytolacca decandra*, *Galium aparine*, *Stillingia sylvatica* and *Trifolium pratense* (which has the additional benefit of containing phyto-oestrogens). These herbs are believed to improve the removal of lymphatic debris and to reduce the incidence and severity of breast lumps.

Topical applications of creams containing *Zingiber officinale* 15 per cent and *Phytolacca decandra* 10 per cent (as tinctures), applied twice daily, also improves pain and breast lumpiness.

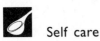 Self care

The self-care message is simple—avoid saturated fats and excessive consumption of vegetable oils. Some of the best results, clinically and experimentally,[76] have been associated with dietary change involving reduced fats and increased complex carbohydrate consumption. Saturated fats include animal fats such as those found in full-cream dairy products and meat, and those from coconut and palm oils. A diet which contains very little saturated fat, reasonable amounts of vegetable oil, is high in fibre, contains large amounts of phyto-oestrogens, vegetables, grains and legumes is recommended.

Avoiding methylxanthines (caffeine, theobromine and theophylline) in tea, coffee, cocoa and cola drinks also leads to dramatic improvements in many cases. Exercising regularly seems to be beneficial.

FUNCTIONAL HYPOGLYCAEMIA

Hypoglycaemia means low blood sugar and the term 'functional' refers to an inability of the blood sugar stabilising mechanisms to function in an appropriate manner.

Functional hypoglycaemia often accompanies other complaints, especially those associated with prolonged periods of stress or anxiety, including chronic fatigue syndrome and post-viral fatigue syndrome sufferers. PMS has many symptoms which are similar to those of functional hypoglycaemia, and is often improved by a hypoglycaemic diet.

A diverse group of symptoms can be associated with hypoglycaemia—having one or a few symptoms is not necessarily diagnostic of hypoglycaemia because these symptoms could accompany other complaints. True hypoglycaemia should respond to adequate dietary change within a week. If this does not occur, other reasons for the symptoms should be sought.

The main symptoms

- Tiredness, vagueness or shakiness which is alleviated by eating.
- Tiredness or irritability if meals are late, or first thing in the morning.
- Sugar cravings.
- Hungry all the time or soon after eating.
- Headaches when meals are delayed.
- Inappropriate feelings of anxiety or inadequacy which disappear after eating.
- Waking in the middle of the night feeling abnormally hungry.

Causes

- Prolonged stress
  Prolonged periods of stress trigger the 'fight or flight' mechanism which causes a series of changes in hormone levels and fluctuations in the blood sugar levels.
- Diet
  A number of dietary factors adversely affect blood sugar levels including an over consumption of refined carbohydrates and sugars,[77] and an inappropriate alcohol intake (alcohol without eating, or alcohol with sugar-based mixers).[78]

Dieters often develop hypoglycaemia because of their low energy diets. This causes them to 'break out' and eat large amounts of starchy or sugary foods. The rapid drop in blood sugar initiates a very counterproductive cycle of sugar craving, hypoglycaemic symptoms,[79] and no doubt, weight gain. Following the diet for hypoglycaemia (below) is a successful way to lose weight slowly and progressively because it breaks the cycle of 'fast and feast'. Short term 'crash' diets are asking for trouble.

Chromium;[80] niacinamide,[81], and magnesium supplements[82] improve functional hypoglycaemia.

Diet

The most effective treatment for functional hypoglycaemia is dietary change. Usually strict adherence to the diet is required for about three weeks and then a slightly more relaxed routine can be adopted. This will depend on each individual's response to the regime and the severity of both the complaint and the underlying causes.

Some general guidelines

- Eat small amounts of protein regularly at meals and with snacks.
- Eat small, frequent meals.
- Avoid all sugar, honey and dried fruit.
- Consume only small quantities of unsweetened, dilute fruit juice.
- Avoid all stimulants such as tea, coffee, chocolate, and cola drinks.
- Avoid alcohol and cigarettes.
- Eat only whole grain foods. Avoid white flour and refined cereals.
- *Always* eat breakfast.

Complementary proteins

All animal protein is 'complete', and therefore meals containing milk products, eggs, meat or fish provide first class protein. Incomplete (plant) protein foods, however, need to be combined to provide the same quality protein as animal protein.

Beans with grains: tofu and rice, lentils and rice, corn and beans, buckwheat and tempeh, muesli and soya milk, kidney beans and barley.

Beans and seeds: tahina and beans, tofu and sesame seeds.

Grains and nuts: nut butters on bread, rice and cashews, rice and peanut sauce.

Suggested menus

Breakfast
- Fruit with yoghurt, seeds and ground almonds.
- Whole grain bread toast with nut butters, hoummos or egg.

- Homemade muesli: oats, rolled barley, triticale, rice flakes, rice bran, seeds, coconut, and crushed almonds or cashews. Add fresh fruit and soya milk, low-fat milk or yoghurt as desired.
- Cooked cereal e.g. oats, rice or buckwheat, with a selection of seeds.

Morning, afternoon or supper snack

- Mixed seeds and nuts.
- ½ banana and almonds.
- Soya milk with seeds and nuts.
- Small container of low-fat yoghurt.
- Whole grain dry biscuits with nut butters or hoummos.
- Energy drink: Blend together: ½ cup fresh fruit or juice, ½ cup low fat yoghurt, and seeds with almonds, and/or wheatgerm and lecithin.

Lunch

- Mixed vegetable salad with protein—either fish, cheese, hoummos, meat or other appropriately combined vegetable proteins.
- Salad sandwich with protein as above.
- Vegetable soup with yoghurt, cheese, or a combination of beans and grains.
- One of the dinner choices.

Dinner

- Bean and grain dish: e.g. stir-fry vegetables with rice and tofu, dhal with vegetables and rice, tortilla and beans, buckwheat noodles with vegetables and tempeh, vegetable soup with barley and red kidney beans.
- Grain and nut meal: e.g. steamed vegetables with rice and peanut sauce, stir-fry vegetables with cashew nuts, pasta and pesto sauce (wheat and pine nuts).
- Beans and seeds: many of the Middle Eastern vegetarian meals are based on this principle. e.g. felafel and hoummos.
- Meat or fish with plenty of vegetables.

Meal sizes should be reduced so that the overall food intake does not increase above normal: six snack-size meals should be substituted for three normal-size meals.

9

Menopause

Key words

androgen
androstenedione
climacteric
endometrium
follicle-stimulating
   hormone
GnRH agonist
gonadotrophin-releasing
   hormone
HRT
luteinising hormone

menopause
menorrhagia
oestradiol
oestrone
peri-menopause
phyto-oestrogen
post-menopause
pre-menopause
SHBG
testosterone

Imprinted in the collective psyche of mid-life women is the picture of the 'typical' menopausal woman they might become. Anxious, nerves jangled through lack of sleep, she struggles through her day forgetting everything and being constantly overwhelmed by debilitating hot flushes. Well on her way to becoming incontinent, she neither looks for nor gains any sexual pleasure. Her life over, depressed and forgotten, she might just as well curl up in the corner with her aches and pains and dowager's hump, and let the world pass her by.

This so-called 'typical' menopausal woman rarely comes through my clinic door. The menopausal woman we usually see may have some problems with menopausal complaints, but by and large, they don't stop her from getting on with her life. Instead, she might be running her own business, or occupy a senior position in a company, school or the public service. She might be an active member of her church group; or looking after her grandchildren; she could be a painter, photographer or sculptor; she might be studying, taking a degree in something she's always been interested in; she could have a new lover. Whatever she's doing, she's usually busy, organised, out there and achieving. Often, she has an exercise program: swimming laps, walking, dancing.

Far from becoming an old crone overnight, the menopausal woman is often more financially secure, and is energetic and ready for the challenges this new phase can bring.

Being fifty-something isn't old, but for all sorts of complex reasons, women have somehow confused ageing and menopause. Many lump together the years between menopause and 80 with the tag 'post-meno-pausal woman'; and it's not the energetic 50-year-old, it's the 80-year-old they visualise.

Menopause *is* a time of change. And making it a time of positive change is not just pot-luck! There is now plenty of evidence to suggest that preparing sensibly for mid-life with a good diet, lifestyle and an exercise program will greatly influence the way a woman experiences her menopause—and beyond.

Definition

Menopause literally means stopping menstruation. The word is made up of Greek: *meno* (monthly) and *pausis* (to stop). Women won't know menopause has occurred until a whole year has passed since the date of the last period—the actual date can only be decided retrospectively, by counting backwards. Menopause then, occurs on one distinct date and is not what most people mean when they describe themselves, or the women who consult them, as 'menopausal'.

The more correct term, the 'climacteric' is rarely used; peri-meno-pausal is now the favoured lay and medical term. The peri-menopause is analogous to puberty and the years when the menstrual cycle starts to become established; both are characterised by hormonal and some-times emotional fluctuations, and menstrual irregularity.

Age and menopause

Menopause which occurs between the ages of 45 and 55 is considered normal. For most women in Australia, menopause occurs between 48 and 53. Body weight tends to influence the age of menopause: thinner women are much more likely to have an earlier menopause than women who are heavier. Being very overweight may delay the onset of meno-pause until well into the fifties.

Premature menopause

Premature menopause is when the last period occurs before the age of 40. The ovaries may stop working prematurely, menopause can be deliberately induced for medical reasons, or prematurely brought on by surgery, drugs and certain illnesses.

Premature ovarian failure

The reasons for premature ovarian failure are largely unknown. Some women associate the onset with a period of extreme stress. One theory is an error in the way the body recognises its own tissue causes antibodies to be produced to ovarian tissue. This causes premature ovarian failure and menopause.

Some other illnesses are associated with an earlier menopausal onset. These include auto-immune diseases, and rarely, mumps.

Medically-induced menopause

Medically-induced menopause is more frequent now that drugs can be used to induce a temporary menopausal state to treat conditions such as endometriosis and uterine fibroids. These drugs are called gonadotrophin-releasing-hormone agonists (GnRH agonists), commonly Zoladex. The menopausal state is reversible.

Nevertheless, the changes are the same as would be experienced by any naturally menopausal woman for the time that the drug is taken: bone density loss, vaginal dryness, hot flushes and mood changes are common. Although each of the symptoms is reversible when drug use is discontinued, bone thinning may occur at an age when regaining the bone density is very difficult.

Menopause can also occur after radiation therapy for cancer, particularly of the pelvic region. Sometimes this is not deliberate, but the changes can be permanent. The ovarian tissue degenerates and fails to produce follicles in the usual way, and menopause is the result. The herb *Angelica sinensis* (Dang gui) may help to protect the ovary from the effects of irradiation when destruction of ovarian tissue is not desirable.[1]

Some drugs used in the treatment of cancer, such as cyclophosphamide, chlorambucil, mechlorethamine and vincristine, can cause menopausal symptoms and permanent infertility. Tamoxifen, used as an anti-oestrogen in the treatment of breast cancer, can also cause menopause-like symptoms. Hot flushes, vaginal dryness and itch, and vaginal bleeding have been reported.[2]

Surgically-induced menopause

Although much less frequent because of the efficiency of GnRH agonists and anti-oestrogen drugs like Tamoxifen, menopause may be deliberately induced by removing the ovaries. A complete hysterectomy and bi-lateral salphingo-oopherectomy where the ovaries and uterus are both removed, or removal of the ovaries only (but not the uterus) will immediately lead to menopause. This type of surgery may be performed for endo-metriosis, oestrogen-responsive breast cancer, ovarian tumours or ovarian cancer.

A hysterectomy which leaves the ovaries intact should not be associated with an interruption in ovarian activity. Up to one-third of women having this type of hysterectomy, however, experience symptoms that indicate they have become menopausal.[3]

If menopause does not occur immediately after a hysterectomy, on average, it will occur five years earlier than women who still have their uterus.[4] Ovarian failure is thought to occur prematurely because of the alteration in ovarian blood supply which occurs after the surgery. A controversial theory holds that tubal ligation may also be associated with premature menopause for much the same reasons,[5] but this is a hotly debated issue which requires more research to be resolved.

Normal transition or disease?

Some doctors believe menopause is a deficiency disease, characterised by a lack of oestrogen, and comparable to other (medical) conditions caused by hormone deficiency such as diabetes, Cushing's disease and hypothyroidism. At the Sixth International Congress on Menopause held in Bangkok in 1990, doctors explained (to each other) how every woman is a hormonal tragedy waiting to occur.

Hormone deficiency diseases, they claimed, are defined as states where the administration of the deficient hormone can reverse or prevent adverse effects in the body. Naturally, say the proponents of this theory, medication is needed to treat the menopause and return the body to normal. They vigorously endorse the use of Hormone Replacement Therapy (HRT) and believe that all post-menopausal women, having outlived the functional lives of their ovaries, are diseased and in need of continued medical attention until they die.

Some doctors have introduced an air of vagueness into this debate. In an apparent attempt to have a bet each way, Dr Miriam Stoppard in her book for the mid-life woman, writes 'While I believe that the menopause is a normal stage in a woman's life, I also believe that it is a true deficiency state . . .'[6] She also endorses HRT.

For these doctors, menopause is just like other hormonal disorders, such as diabetes, but has the peculiarity of affecting *all* women at about the same time in their lives. Something seems very wrong with reasoning which suggests all women are biologically faulty and in need of treatment and medication.

Natural therapists view menopause as a normal transition. Menarche, menstruation and menopause are seen as normal phases which effect women in their passage through life, and which may need supportive treatment. Rather than encouraging mid-life women to believe they have a disease, most natural therapists (and many like-minded doctors) encourage menopausal women to adopt positive lifestyle changes, good eating patterns and a positive attitude to this phase.

A positive lifestyle

Researchers in one study found that the well-being of mid-life women was related to being physically well, exercising moderately, having a positive attitude to menopause and feeling happy. Exercising, even once per week, was associated with fewer symptoms, as were positive relationships and friendships. Hormonal status was not the relevant feature of a positive menopausal experience.[7]

Diet has a direct influence on menopausal symptoms and is believed to contribute to the marked differences in symptoms experienced by women from other cultures, especially hot flushes.[8] Changing dietary intake of various foods containing natural oestrogens (phyto-oestrogens) reduces hot flushes and symptoms associated with vaginal dryness.[9] The positive effects of phyto-oestrogens are discussed in Chapter 18, 'Phyto-oestrogens'.

The changes at menopause

When to contact the doctor
- Bleeding, no matter how light, which occurs one year after the last menstrual period.
- Bleeding after sex.
- Persistently heavy periods.
- Mid-cycle bleeding or bleeding between periods.
- Pain, if never experienced before.

Hormone levels

Peri-menopausal hormonal changes start slowly; some two to three years before ovulation stops. The output of both oestrogen and progesterone declines gradually, sometimes in association with irregular menstrual patterns. When hormone production changes gradually, fewer menopausal symptoms may be the result. This may be one reason why 'naturally' menopausal women tend to suffer fewer symptoms than women with premature menopause or women whose menopause is induced surgically or with drugs.

During the menstrual cycle, oestrogen usually inhibits the levels of follicle-stimulating hormone (FSH), but as oestrogen declines, FSH increases because of the lack of feed-back inhibition. FSH levels in blood are sometimes used as a biochemical indicator of menopause.

Luteinising hormone (LH) also increases, but more slowly than FSH. Both LH and FSH are released about every 60–90 minutes in small bursts, and the release of LH has been shown to coincide with hot flushes. LH also stimulates ovarian production of small amounts of an androgen (androstenedione) which is converted into a type of oestrogen, known as oestrone.

Oestrone is the dominant oestrogen of post-menopausal women, but its production has little to do with the ovary. While both the ovary and the adrenal gland produce the starting hormone, androstenedione, the adrenal gland is responsible for the far greater volume. The androstenedione is then released into the circulation and finally converted into oestrone in the fat, liver and kidneys.

This is referred to as 'extraglandular' (not in a gland) or sometimes 'peripheral' oestrogen conversion. Its production levels are greater in women who are in the average to high ranges for body weight, and lower in thin women. The presence and amount of oestrone may partially account for the increased bone density and lack of peri-menopausal symptoms experienced by heavier women.

Oestrone is about twelve times weaker than the ovarian oestrogen, oestradiol. Overall, total post-menopausal oestrone production is about two-thirds of the usual pre-ovulatory levels in menstruating women and with only minute amounts of the most active oestrogen, oestradiol, oestrogen effect is greatly diminished.

Testosterone production by the ovary continues after menopause at almost the same rate as menstruating women. Testosterone is an androgen (male hormone) and is usually thought to be responsible for some of the hair pattern changes, like facial hair and male pattern baldness, that some post-menopausal women develop. Its effects in the body are more apparent because oestrogen would normally balance its androgenic effects.

Testosterone (but not oestrone) is normally carried by a protein called sex hormone-binding globulin (SHBG) and the amount of SHBG determines whether testosterone will be freely available or bound and unable to interact with cells. In general, increasing the amount of SHBG decreases the amount of freely available and active testosterone, which reduces its unwanted masculinising effects. Vegetarian diets[10] and diets with a high phyto-oestrogen content[11] increase SHBG.

Progesterone production is erratic around the menopause because ovulation occurs less frequently and follicle development is less predictable. Once a woman is menopausal, the production of progesterone ceases because follicular development and ovulation are necessary for progesterone to be produced by the corpus luteum. This can cause a number of the common problems of menopause including mood changes and heavy periods.

All of the hormonal variations, and not just declining oestrogen, orchestrate the physical and biochemical changes which accompany menopause. The most common symptoms caused by these fluctuations are the change in the menstrual cycle, hot flushes and premenstrual mood changes.

Menstrual cycle changes

The hormonal fluctuations are mirrored in menstrual changes and are usually the earliest sign of menopause. Some women stop menstruating suddenly, but there is a usual pattern of menstrual change associated with the onset of the peri-menopausal phase. These usually begin some time in the fourth decade.

Gradually, changes become apparent in either the menstrual flow or the regularity of the cycle. The period may become more frequent; but more often, less frequent ovulation causes the cycle length to increase. This stage may last for a few months or for many years. Women can still become pregnant during this time.

Other symptoms can include vaginal dryness, insomnia, hot flushes and night sweats. These are related to changes in the oestrogen levels. As mentioned, some women also experience symptoms which are similar to premenstrual syndrome. If this occurs, they should be treated with the appropriate remedies for PMS.

The next phase is quite variable. Some women stop menstruating all of a sudden; others may have increasingly infrequent, but normal periods; still others, infrequent 'flooding'. This is sometimes referred to as the 'transitional phase' because it represents the stage immediately before menopause. Eventually the periods stop altogether and the woman becomes menopausal.

Diagnosis

Common tests

There are a number of ways to tell whether menopause is approaching. Single tests are not very reliable and are generally used in conjunction with symptoms. Sometimes symptoms are the most reliable indicators of all.

Blood tests for levels of FSH are not infallible, but are often used to diagnose menopause. Elevated levels reflect the declining levels of oestrogen. (Table 9.1 shows the normal range for FSH.) FSH levels often fluctuate during the peri-menopause and can give misleading results, but will remain consistently high once a woman has become menopausal. By then, however, she won't need a blood test to tell her.

Sometimes the blood levels of oestrogen and progesterone are measured to see whether they are within the normal limits, but this is an even more unreliable test than the FSH level and in most cases this test will only be a waste of time and money.

The vaginal walls can show early changes which are caused by the declining oestrogen levels. They might look thinner and drier, and sometimes bleed. These signs are generally quite late, but women who have evidence of chronically low oestrogen (low body weight, undertake strenuous exercise, and women on a poor diet) might develop symptoms early in their menopausal transition.

It can be quite difficult to tell, even with tests, if a woman is menopausal. Symptoms are important and a menstrual diary will be a great help. (The menstrual diary is on page 116 and can be photocopied for regular use.) In many cases, and with all of the best intentions, a woman will still only know she is menopausal once she hasn't had a period for a whole year.

Menopausal symptom index

The menopausal symptom index (See Table 9.2) is used to monitor the severity of menopausal symptoms and their response to treatment. The most common symptoms are graded according to their severity (very strong = 3, moderate = 2, slight = 1, not present = 0) and multiplied by a 'constant factor' (column two). Scores of >35 indicate severe symptoms; 20–35 moderate symptoms; and 15–20 slight symptoms. The chart can be filled out every month to assess the efficacy of treatment. Medication (but not dietary or lifestyle changes) is usually stopped once the score is below 15.

The management of common menopausal symptoms

Changes in the period

The menstrual changes characteristic of the peri-menopausal years are

Table 9.2 Menopausal symptom index (after Kupperman)

Symptoms	constant factor	prior to treatment	after 1 month	2 months	3 months	4 months	5 months	6 months
		variable factor of severity ▶						
Hot flushes	4							
Sweating	2							
Insomnia	2							
Nervousness irritability	2							
Depression	1							
Lack in concentration	1							
Joint pain	1							
Headache	1							
Palpitation	1							
Total								

very strong = 3,   moderate = 2,   slight = 1,   not present = 0 associated with three major changes: the frequency of ovulation; the levels of oestrogens; and the production of progesterone.

When the frequency of ovulation is altered, the cycle length and regularity of the period also change. This can be normal and many women will experience erratic ovulation and menstruation as the only features of their approaching menopause. No treatment is necessary unless the erratic cycles are accompanied by menorrhagia (heavy periods) or spotting.

Erratic ovulation also means that the cells of the endometrium tend to be exposed to lower levels of oestrogen for longer periods of time, but to little if any progesterone (which is only produced once ovulation occurs). This is sometimes referred to as the 'unopposed effect'—oestrogen continues to stimulate the endometrium 'unopposed' by progesterone.

As a result, the endometrium looks and behaves differently from endometrium exposed to both oestrogen *and* progesterone. It tends to be fragile, to bleed more readily, and the periods can become excessively heavy. Spotting is common and, if prolonged, the endometrial cells can undergo cancerous changes. Abnormal bleeding of this nature is discussed in the section on dysfunctional uterine bleeding in Chapter 12 'Erratic bleeding'.

Hot flushes

The symptom that consistently correlates with being menopausal is hot flushes. About three-quarters of all menopausal women experience some form of hot flushes;[12] and about one-third of these women will find them debilitating enough to seek treatment. Two studies indicate that almost 40 per cent of menopausal women experienced 'troubling' hot flushes,[13] but not all women took medication or sought help for their symptoms.

Flushes are likely to be as different as the women who have them. Some have transient episodes of feeling a bit hot or sweaty; others might be drenched with perspiration, feel uncomfortably hot, go red in the face and be troubled by palpitations. Sometimes headaches, a sense of increased pressure in the head, vagueness, transient chills, fatigue, dizziness and nausea follow or accompany a hot flush. The body usually adjusts to the changing hormones after about one year and the hot flushes disappear completely. Rarely, they will last for five to ten years after the period has stopped.

Many women feel embarrassed and uncomfortable when they have a flush. They feel as though they lose concentration, or that they won't be taken seriously. Some women do obviously perspire and flush in the face, but most of the time, other people don't notice hot flushes.

Flushing is definitely related to oestrogen decline—women who have never menstruated do not flush unless they have been given oestrogen and then it is withdrawn. Hot flushes are more severe when a woman is very thin, probably because body fat is an alternative source of oestrogen (oestrone). Women who become menopausal suddenly or at a younger age than usual, often experience hot flushes that are more severe, perhaps because the body is not prepared for the abrupt decline in oestrogen status.

Even so, it is not the oestrogen itself that fluctuates when a woman has a hot flush. Instead, luteinising hormone increases because of a flurry of activity in the hypothalamus and the release of gonadotrophin-releasing hormone. This leads to the usual symptoms associated with flushing. Afterwards, there is often a slight drop in temperature caused by loss of body heat from sweating. Temperature fluctuations can cause the on again, off again problem with clothing and lead to a serious disturbance in sleep patterns.

Some women seem to flush more, or only flush, when they are tired or over-worked. Natural therapists believe that exhaustion is related to unhealthy function of adrenal glands. Certainly, post-menopausal women rely on the production of androgens from the adrenal glands which are converted into oestrone, once the ovaries stop producing oestrogen. These types of symptoms have historically been treated with a group of remedies called the adrenal adaptogens.

Some menopausal women can find that even apparently mild emotional response will trigger disproportionately severe flushes. Being 'flushed with excitement' takes on a whole new meaning for a menopausal woman. As does being 'hot and flustered', 'hot-headed' or any number of other idioms that indicate the relationship between the nervous system, body heat and the emotions. A number of common medicinal herbs are used for menopausal symptoms aggravated by stress or anxiety.

Lately, there has been speculation that hot flushes are not just a nuisance and that they may serve a positive role. One theory is that the increase in body temperature sets the stage for a healthier old age by burning up toxins and stimulating the immune response (similar to the increase in immune activity when we have a temperature caused by a cold or the flu). Another is that they represent surges of creative and positive energy.

■ ■ The medical approach

Almost without exception, the medical treatment of any menopausal symptom is hormone replacement therapy (HRT)—and hot flushes respond well to this medication. Somewhere between 60 and 90 per cent of women with hot flushes who are treated with HRT improve dramatically. It is a useful medication, but in view of the concerns raised about its use, natural remedies may be more appropriate unless there are compelling reasons why HRT should be considered.

 ## The natural therapist's approach

Natural remedies are prescribed according to the factors that contribute to the menopausal symptoms.

CASE STUDY

Anna's case is a good example of how this is done and why it is necessary. She was 38 when she had a total hysterectomy for severe endometriosis. Prior to her operation, she had run her own extremely taxing business and was suffering from a complete physical and emotional collapse.

On the first day after her hysterectomy, she started to suffer from extreme hot flushes and was immediately put on HRT. There was no change in her symptoms, so the dose was increased, and then increased again. By the time she was discharged from hospital, she was on an extremely high dose of HRT, but was still experiencing severe flushing. Her doctor told her to just alter the dose of oestrogen until she experienced relief from her symptoms.

Because of Anna's previous history, it was important to also treat the exhaustion and debility that had preceded her operation. She was put onto some herbal adaptogens and nervine tonics. Her HRT dose is now substantially reduced and her hot flushes are almost entirely gone.

The need to differentiate between the differing triggers for hot flushes has long been accepted in herbal medicine. Treatments for menopause were and are categorised according to the system they are to target. It makes the treatment more complex, but much more likely to bring relief of the symptom *and* the cause.

Diet

The dietary intake of phyto-oestrogens improves many of the menopausal symptoms. Adding just 100 g tofu and 1 tablespoon of ground linseed to the diet every day can reduce hot flushes and improve vaginal dryness.[14] Researchers have also observed a link between eating foods with high levels of phyto-oestrogens and lower rates of oestrogen-responsive cancers. These foods are so important that a whole chapter is devoted to their positive and therapeutic effects (see Chapter 18).

Some foods seem to aggravate hot flushes and should be avoided.

They include coffee, excessively spicy foods and alcohol. Drinking or eating foods that are extremely hot can also trigger a flush and simply eating foods at a lower temperature can help.

Oestrogenic herbs

Herbs containing plant oestrogens have been used for centuries for the management of hot flushes and other oestrogen-related symptoms. All plant oestrogens are rather weak and have been estimated to be many times less potent than synthetic oestrogens or the oestrogens made in the body.[15] However, when a woman becomes menopausal and produces virtually no oestrogen of her own, the plant oestrogens become the dominant oestrogen in the system, and can exert some useful effects.

Of particular interest to herbalists is *Cimicifuga racemosa*, long recognised and used by the Europeans, native Americans and Chinese for menopausal symptoms. It has been the subject of a number of open and double-blind trials in Germany where many doctors prescribe it routinely for menopausal symptoms. The results are extremely favourable, especially for hot flushes and vaginal dryness. *Cimicifuga racemosa* is discussed in Chapter 19.

Anxiety
Anxiety or worry can bring on a hot flush and a number of herbs are specifically indicated. They include *Hypericum perforatum*, for flushes associated with anxiety depression states; *Humulus lupulus*, for flushing and insomnia; *Tilia cordata* and *Leonurus cardiaca* for menopausal symptoms which are accompanied by anxiety, insomnia and palpitations; and *Verbena officinalis* for anxiety associated with thyroid dysfunction.

Fatigue and overwork
In cases of fatigue and overwork, the adaptogens are indicated. The most commonly used are *Panax ginseng*, *Eleutherococcus senticosus*, *Codonopsis pilosula*, *Glycyrrhiza glabra*, and *Astragalus membranaceus*. These herbs are usually prescribed as compound herbal formulations as a fluid extract.

Night sweats
Night sweats can cause debility and depression because they disrupt sleep. *Humulus lupulus* regulates LH surges and is specifically indicated for insomnia caused by flushing. In some cases, simply improving the quality of sleep with herbal hypnotics will improve hot flushes. *Valeriana officinalis*, *Scutellaria laterifolia*, *Passiflora incarnata*, *Avena sativa* and *Matricaria recutita* are commonly available either as teas or in tablets.

Severe sweating
The two herbs which are specific for menopausal sweating are *Salvia officinalis* and *Astragalus membranaceus*. They are usually combined with the other remedies for flushing. One common Chinese formula for

sweating associated with weakness contains *Astragalus membranaceus, Codonopsis pilosula, Angelica sinensis, Cimicifuga racemosa, Atractylodes macrocephala* and *Bupleurum falcatum.*

Salvia officinalis is oestrogenic, improves circulation to the head, and is an emmenagogue. A simple home remedy for the treatment of hot flushes and sweating is as follows: Chop about 6 fresh sage leaves and soak overnight in lemon juice. In the morning, strain and drink the juice. Seven to ten days of this mixture will usually control flushing and sweating, and also improves digestion and concentration. It should not be continued for longer than two weeks.

Supplements

Vitamin E
A number of studies in the 1950s validated the effectiveness of vitamin E for menopausal symptoms. In clinical trials, doses ranged from 10–100 mg daily[16] (100 IU is equivalent to 67 mg). My own clinical experience has also demonstrated that Vitamin E reduces the severity of hot flushes and other symptoms associated with menopause. Between 100 and 500 IU is the usual dose required.

Women with blood pressure or heart problems should seek professional advice before using vitamin E.

Vitamin C and the bioflavonoids
In the early 1960s the bioflavonoid hesperidin, derived from citrus fruits, was shown to reduce the severity of hot flushes.[17] Sometimes moderate to high doses of vitamin C seem to help too—perhaps by increasing the bio-availability of oestrogens in the body. Further research is needed.

Evening primrose oil
Many women find that evening primrose oil is useful for a variety of menopausal symptoms, including flushing, mood changes and fluid retention. Even so, studies have shown that it is little better than a placebo[18] and many of the symptoms which are reportedly improved by evening primrose oil seem to be related to PMS rather than menopause. Peri-menopausal PMS is discussed later in this chapter.

Evening primrose oil is also rather expensive and the other herbs and supplements are often more cost effective for menopausal women. The dose range is between 1–3 g daily.

 Self care

Women suffering from hot flushes can dress to reduce the severity of the symptoms. Light and loose-fitting clothing made from natural fibre such as cotton is much less likely to aggravate sweating. A lighter layer underneath a jacket or cardigan that is easily shrugged off helps with rapid temperature fluctuations. Cotton nightwear is also helpful, and some women sleep on a towel or folded sheet so they can throw it out of the bed if it becomes wet rather than having to change the sheets.

Tissue changes

Declining oestrogen levels are associated with changes in the mucus membranes and skin, and can affect the tissues of the vagina, vulva, and urethra, or the eyes and mouth. A range of symptoms might be experienced from none at all, to varying degrees of burning, dryness and irritation. When vaginal, vulval or urinary tract symptoms occur, they can have a serious impact on the quality of life.

Vaginal dryness, thinning of the vaginal walls and urinary symptoms usually occur after menopause, but can affect some peri-menopausal women. Like other menopausal symptoms, there is a large variation in the incidence of symptoms and their severity. Sex might be associated with extreme discomfort or even pain brought about by vaginal dryness and failure to lubricate adequately. Declining oestrogen levels can also lead to increased alkalinity of the vagina which can cause irritation, itch or infections. Surveys of women show that about 40 per cent of women past 55 have some dryness and about half of these report moderate to severe symptoms. The presence of symptoms and their severity seems to be connected to dietary factors, body weight and stress.

When urethral tissue is affected by declining oestrogens, frequency, burning, cystitis, and incontinence can be recurring problems. These complaints require active treatment, and all women who develop urinary tract symptoms around the menopause, or later, should consider mucus membrane change as a potential cause: only treating the urinary tract infection will almost certainly mean that a recurrence can be expected.

The lower levels of oestrogens after menopause lead to changes in collagen metabolism. These changes can cause bone to become more brittle and play a role in pelvic tissue weakness and in other skin and mucous membrane changes associated with ageing.[19]

■ ■
■ ■ The medical approach

Vaginal dryness, soreness, and painful sex are usually treated with oestrogen-containing creams, tablets or pessaries. They should be used at night and their benefits and cautions are described in Chapter 20 'Drugs and surgery'.

Collagen disorders which affect other tissues such as bones, the pelvic organs and the skin, are increasingly being treated with oral oestrogens.

Natural therapists often recommend creams for vaginal dryness. An aqueous cream or vitamin E cream can be used as a base to which herbs and oils are added. This can be made at home: 10 mL infused oil of *Calendula officinalis* (marigold); 30 mL olive oil; 20 mL oil of evening primrose in 75 g of aqueous cream. Apply two or three times daily, or as required.

Oestrogenic herbs can also be used in creams, since oestrogen is well absorbed through the skin. Middle Eastern women reportedly use topical applications of *Trigonella foenum-graecum*,[20] but the pungent odour makes it unpopular with many women. Using a water-based lubricant, such as Wet Stuff, during sex will also help.

Oral prescriptions of *Cimicifuga racemosa* have been shown to reduce dryness and changes of vaginal tissue. In a German study, 80 women were given either *Cimicifuga racemosa*, oestrogen or placebo and were evaluated every four weeks for menopausal symptoms and mood changes. At the end of twelve weeks, a vaginal smear was taken to assess the state of the vaginal mucosa. All three parameters improved in the group of women given *Cimicifuga racemosa*.[21]

For collagen health throughout the whole body, including bones, vitamin C and the bioflavonoids (commonly rutin or hesperidin) are essential. Silicon, zinc and the vitamins B_6, B_{12}, A, K and folic acid are also important. Sometimes supplements are required, but a balanced diet is the best starting point for these nutrients.

Peri-menopausal 'PMS'

Women in their forties with PMS are often told, or believe themselves to be menopausal. Symptoms related to hormone fluctuations are not necessarily indicative of menopause unless they are accompanied by menstrual irregularity, and even then there may be other causes. Some of the commonly associated menopausal symptoms like hot flushes, migraines and palpitations are experienced by women in their twenties and thirties who are not menopausal, and certainly not in need of replacement hormones.

One study of recently menopausal women showed that although hot flushes increased with the cessation of periods, symptoms like breast discomfort, irritability, excitability, depression and poor concentration '. . . improved after the cessation of menstruation, . . . [which] suggests that these symptoms are more likely to be related to menstruation than to the menopause.'[22]

Evening primrose oil capsules are commonly recommended or self-prescribed for so-called peri-menopausal symptoms even though they

Table 9.3 PMS and peri-menopausal treatments and treatment aims

Treatments and treatment aims	Premenstrual	Peri-menopausal
Aim	Regulate hypothalamic–pituitary–ovarian unit	Support declining oestrogen levels
Herbs		
Hormone regulators	*Vitex agnus castus*	*Cimicifuga racemosa*
Nervines	*Verbena*	*Humulus lupulus*
Others	*Avena sativa*	*Hypericum perforatum*
	Bitters	Phyto-oestrogens
Supplements	Vitamin B$_6$	Vitamin C
	Evening primrose oil	Bioflavonoids
	Magnesium	Vitamin E
	Zinc	Calcium
		Magnesium

are no better than placebo for menopausal symptoms when scientifically trialled.[23] Evening primrose *is,* however, useful for PMS and it seems very likely that women who feel better on the capsules do so because it relieves the symptoms associated with an oestrogen to progesterone ratio imbalance rather than symptoms related to declining oestrogen.

As a general rule, women who are forty-something, with fairly regular periods, and no hot flushes or vaginal dryness should consider causes for their complaints other than menopause. And as far as treatment is concerned, many of them will respond better to remedies for PMS rather than those for menopause.

A detailed description of the treatment of all types of PMS is outlined in Chapter 8, 'The menstruating years'.

Mood changes

About one woman in ten experiences depression, anxiety or feelings of inadequacy around menopause, but there is some dispute about why they occur. Some researchers have shown that these symptoms are related to hormone changes, others found these symptoms were more common when women had pre-existing problems, difficulties with coping generally, or menstrual mood changes.[24] We could call these the psycho-social theory and the hormone fluctuation theory.

According to the psycho-social theory, a woman's attitude to menopause and ageing affect her menopausal experience. Women with a negative attitude to either or both, were found to be much more likely to experience problems than women who saw menopause and ageing as positive experiences.[25] Peri-menopausal mood changes are seen to be coincidental to, rather than caused by, the hormone changes at menopause.

Two observations underpin the hormone fluctuation theory. The stress associated with mood changes may cause oestrogen levels to drop further and aggravate menopausal symptoms.[26] In one study, meno-pausal women recovering from depression had higher levels of oestrogen in their urine as they improved.[27] Sleep deprivation is believed to be another cause of peri-menopausal depression. Flushes disrupt sleep and dreaming patterns and prevent deep, refreshing sleep. When oestrogen levels are increased, sleep patterns return to normal.

Treatment

Treatment for mood swings is quite varied because the causes are often correspondingly diverse. When PMS is the cause, symptoms will only occur before the period. For all types of mood changes, simple lifestyle changes, such as exercise, stress management techniques, yoga and meditation are helpful. Sometimes depression, anxiety or self-esteem problems will require the skills of a counsellor. Anti-depressant drugs or sedatives should rarely be needed. Whatever the choice of treatment, vitamin, herb or drug, it is far better that the cause of the depression or mood swings be found rather than prescribing to elevate mood.

HRT does not appear to have a significant effect on mood over and above placebo effects. It does improve flushing and vaginal symptoms and alterations in mood may occur as a result of this.[28] Even so, doctors commonly prescribe HRT in the belief that it alleviates the mood changes associated with menopause.

Hypericum perforatum, a herb which has been compared to tricyclic anti-depressants in efficacy, has a long history of use for menopausal complaints which are associated with anxiety or depression. Herbalists refer to this plant as a nervine tonic, specific to the management of menopausal complaints.

B vitamins, particularly vitamin B_6, or any of the other remedies used for PMS, are helpful for mood changes in the peri-menopause. In fact, a lot of mood changes at this time are really PMS.

Fatigue

Women with insufficient stamina to meet their daily needs often think that their symptoms must be due to menopause. In reality, they may be due to any of the usual causes of fatigue including hypoglycaemia, iron deficiency, adrenal exhaustion or depression. Assessment of the meno-pausal woman must first exclude these non-hormonal causes.

Women who are well, but fatigued, respond to combinations of the appropriate herbs for the nervous system, adaptogens and Vitamin B complex, along with appropriate dietary changes and increase in exercise. *Eleutherococcus senticosus* 500 mg–1 g twice daily, combined with Vitamin B complex 1 twice daily, is often effective. Other adaptogens are discussed in the herbal section.

Migraines

The frequency and severity of premenstrual symptoms can increase as a woman approaches menopause. Premenstrual migraines are often related to the dual effects of rapid fluctuations in the blood sugar levels, in association with the rapid decline in oestrogens just before menstruation. The rapid fall triggers a vascular response, usually blood vessel spasm, which causes pain.

The regime described for premenstrual migraines, almost always in conjunction with the herb *Cimicifuga racemosa*, helps to regulate the oestrogen levels. Increasing the amount of phyto-oestrogens in the diet is also useful. *Lavandula angustifolia* in the form of an extract taken orally is also useful for menopausal migraines.

CHECK LIST FOR THE MID-LIFE WOMAN

- Breast self-examination monthly. Most doctors also recommend a mammogram every two years for women between 50 and 70, especially for women with significant risk for breast cancer.
- Internal gynaecological examination *yearly.*
- Pap smear at least every second year, at the same time as the internal examination, or as recommended by medical practitioner.
- Weight bearing exercise for 30 minutes at least every second day.
- Calcium intake: 1500 mg daily.
- Magnesium intake: 800 mg daily.
- Body weight maintained at middle to upper level of ideal weight.
- Blood pressure check annually, more frequently if elevated.
- Bone density check if there's a strong family history of osteoporosis or many risk factors. Re-check in two–five years, depending on result.
- Cholesterol check for high density lipoprotein (HDL) and low density lipoprotein (LDL) ratio in mid-fifties. Repeat if there's a family history of heart disease or if advised by doctor.

CALCIUM—ESSENTIAL FOR BONES

It is essential to maintain bone density to prevent osteoporosis by continuing a high calcium intake before, during and after menopause. The following table gives quantities of foods to be eaten to obtain 300 mg of calcium. Post-menopausal women should consume 4–5 serves of these foods each day in order to obtain enough dietary calcium, preferably from different sources.

High calcium, low kilojoule foods	Calcium (mg)	kJ
1¼ cups cooked spinach or other greens	300	252
2 cups cooked broccoli	300	336
⅔ cup plain low-fat yoghurt	300	420
1 cup buttermilk	300	420
¼ cup grated Parmesan cheese	300	483
50g Swiss or Cheddar cheese	300	630
1½ cups full cream milk	300	630
1¼ cups plain yoghurt	300	700
200 g tofu	300	840
1 small standard can sardines	300	970
300 g can salmon	300	1050
2 cups low-fat cottage cheese	300	1772

Recommended Daily Allowance (RDA)

The RDA for calcium varies with age	mg
Infants:	350–550
Children aged 1–10 yrs:	800
Teenagers:	1200
Young women 20–35 years:	800–1000
Pregnant/breastfeeding women:	1500
Pre-menopausal women 35 years and over:	1000
Post-menopausal women:	1500

How to check on calcium intake

It is easy for anyone to check that their dietary intake is adequate. I recommend they keep a diet diary of everything they have eaten and drunk over a one-week period. They can calculate their daily calcium intake for each day by using Table 9.4. By adding up the totals from every day they can calculate an average daily intake by dividing the total figure by the number of days recorded. If they are not getting enough calcium, they can either increase the number of serves of calcium-rich foods, or take a supplement.

Table 9.4 Sources of calcium (mg of calcium per 100 g of food)

Dairy products		Seeds	
Skim milk powder (dry)	1190	Unhulled sesame seeds	1160
Whole milk powder (dry)	900	Linseeds	271
Whey powder	645	Hulled sesame seeds	110
Physical milk™ 100 mL	205	Sunflower seeds	98
Yoghurt-cow's	180	Pumpkin seeds	52
REV milk™ 100 mL	150	**Grains and cereals**	
Goat's milk	130	White SR flour	350
Skimmed cow's milk	123	Muesli (depends on brand)	200
Buttermilk	115	Wheat flour (white or brown)	150
Cow's milk, whole	115	Wheat bran	110
Human milk	30	Bread (brown or white)	100
Cheese		All Bran™	75
Parmesan	1091	Rice bran	69
Gruyère	1000	Wheatgerm	69
Mozzarella	817	Wheat crispbread	60
Cheddar	810	Oatmeal	55
Gouda	810	Rye crispbread	50
Edam (30% fat)	800	Brown Rice	33
Edam (45% fat)	678	Weetbix™	33
Gorgonzola	612	**Meats**	
Camembert (30% fat)	600	All meat has <20mg/100 g	<20
Danish Blue	580	**Legumes** (cooked)	
Blue (50% fat)	540	Navy beans	95
Camembert (60% fat)	400	Chickpeas	70
Fetta	353	Kidney beans	70
Ricotta	223	Lentils	50
Cottage (low fat)	77	Black eyed beans	40
Cottage	67	Split peas	22
Eggs		**Sprouts**	
Duck (whole)	63	Alfalfa sprouts	28
Chicken (whole)	56	Mung bean sprouts	20
Fish		Lentil sprouts	12
Whitebait	860	**Vegetables**	
Sardines (canned)	550	Parsley	260
Scallops	120	Watercress	190
Salmon (canned)	100	Dandelion greens	185
Lobster	60	Spring onions	140
Soya products		Onions	135
Soya milk (dry)	330	Spinach	135
Soya grits	255	Broccoli	125
Dried soya beans	225	Silverbeet	115
Soya flour, full fat	210	**Fruits**	
Tofu	170	Dried figs	260
So Good™	116	Lemons	110
Vita Soy™	32	Lemon juice (100 mL)	8
Nuts		Rhubarb (stewed)	93
Almonds	250	Orange juice (100 mL)	60
Brazil	180	Blackberries	60
Pistachio	136	Other fruit except dried fruit	<50
Pecan	75		
Peanuts (fresh)	60	**Other**	
Walnuts	60	Kelp	1095
Macadamia	50	Crude molasses	654
Hazelnuts	45	Torula yeast	425
Peanut butter	35	Carob powder	355
Cashews	30	Brewer's yeast	210

Section E

When things go wrong

WHEN THINGS GO WRONG

Problems with periods are all too common. More than half of all women have period pain, about three-quarters have PMS, and it's usual for women to experience episodes of heavy periods or to miss a period from time to time. Some of these problems are just minor irritations and represent a deviation from the normal functioning of an organ or a hormonal imbalance; at other times, these symptoms are severe enough to disrupt the woman's life. They may even represent conditions that require immediate attention or prolonged treatment.

The difficulty with menstrual problems is because they occur so frequently, it is sometimes difficult to know which symptoms might represent the need for investigation and treatment. This is particularly so for abnormal bleeding patterns. While almost everyone will consult their health-care provider if they experience pain; abnormal bleeding, especially 'nuisance' or slight bleeding, is often ignored in the hope that it will 'just go away'.

Abnormal bleeding

Bleeding is abnormal if the period is too heavy, prolonged, too light or does not occur often enough.

The other type of abnormal bleeding is bleeding between periods. This is always a cause for concern and should be investigated, especially when it occurs after sexual activity. Bleeding at ovulation is normal for some women and is usually related to minor hormonal variations, but it should always be reported straight away to exclude other possible causes.

Too heavy, too often

There are two ways of defining 'too heavy' and 'too often': by the quantity of menstrual blood loss, *or* as a deviation from the woman's own usual menstrual pattern.

Medical textbooks (and some doctors) tend to use the first definition and describe excessive bleeding in terms of the quantity of blood lost and the frequency of menstruation or bleeding episodes. Using this definition, the bleeding will:

- continue for more than seven days
- occur more often than every 21 days, and/or
- exceed 80 mL in volume (about $\frac{1}{2}$ cup)

Trying to determine what a greater than 80 mL menstrual loss will look like, or how many pads or tampons will be used when bleeding is this heavy, is almost impossible. It is much more useful to define excessive menstruation as a change in the usual pattern. Using this definition, the period:

- lasts for three days longer than expected
- requires two or more pads or tampons per day than is usual, and/or
- arrives five days or more earlier than usual

The second definition is a much simpler and more practical way to define abnormal bleeding. It identifies deviations from the usual and expected pattern for a particular woman, and because of the huge range of normal (as discussed in Chapter 3) it is much more likely to alert an individual to changes.

One heavy period is not an indication for investigation (or treatment) unless the bleeding is severe. It is usual for women to have an uncharacteristic period every now and then, especially after stress or overseas travel.

Too little or too infrequent

A period is considered to be abnormal when it:

- continues for less than three days
- occurs less often than every 35 days
- is very slight or almost absent, and/or
- requires two or less pads or tampons per day

156

Missing a period occasionally is not a major concern (unless unexpected pregnancy is the cause). Many women will miss a period after travel or major upheavals; sometimes a period can be missed for no apparent reason at all. It is a good idea to seek medical advice if there is persistent change in the menstrual cycle, and if menstruation has ceased for three months or more.

Spotting or bleeding between periods

For some women, spotting just before or after their period is a usual part of their cycle, but if the symptom is new, it should be investigated. Bleeding between periods is usually slight, often painless, and frequently inconvenient. From a practitioner's point of view, it is also the most troubling. The cause is usually hormonal, but spotting after sexual activity can be highly suggestive of lesions of the uterus or cervix, such as polyps or cancer. This sort of bleeding should always be investigated, especially when:

- it is not part of a woman's usual cycle (some women always 'spot' a few days before their period or mid-cycle)
- the woman is 40 or older
- it occurs after sexual activity of any kind

Any bleeding experienced by a post-menopausal woman must be investigated immediately by a medical practitioner, no matter how scant or transient. It is vital to exclude uterine cancer as the cause of bleeding after the menopause. Other causes of post-menopausal bleeding might be polyps or lesions on the cervix.

Abnormal bleeding patterns

Abnormal bleeding patterns are not in themselves a disease or condition. For example heavy bleeding, called menorrhagia, is a *symptom* of a condition such as fibroids or endometriosis; amenorrhoea (no periods) can be caused by polycystic ovarian disease.

Menorrhagia

An abnormally heavy period with a normal cycle length is called menorrhagia. Menorrhagia may be related to either the hypothalamic-pituitary unit; the ovary; excessive stimulation of the endometrium by oestrogen; failure to produce progesterone; or an imbalance in prostaglandins levels. Systemic factors such as hypothyroidism, low iron stores, and clotting abnormalities can also be causes. Problems with the uterus such as lack of uterine tone, intra-uterine devices, uterine infections and fibroids may also be implicated.

157

Metrorrhagia

Bleeding which occurs at times other than at the period is called metrorrhagia. Sometimes it is also referred to as inter-menstrual bleeding or threshold bleeding. The bleeding commonly occurs at ovulation, although it may happen at any time during the cycle. Many conditions can cause metrorrhagia: hormonal factors are common as are cervical lesions. Cancer of the uterus is another possible reason for this type of bleeding.

Polymenorrhoea

The bleeding pattern associated with periods which occur too frequently (less than every 21 days), but are otherwise normal is called poly-menorrhoea. Causes may originate in the hypothalamic-pituitary unit or the ovary. Frequently the origin of the problem is ovulation: either it does not occur, or it is too early.

Polymenorrhagia

Periods can be too early (polymenorrhoea) and too heavy (menorrhagia). In combination, this is called polymenorrhagia. Any of the factors which cause polymenorrhoea or menorrhagia may be responsible.

Amenorrhoea

Amenorrhoea is the absence of the period. There are two types—primary, where the menarche does not start at the usual time; and secondary, where the period starts but stops again at some time during the woman's usual menstruating years. The causes are discussed in Chapter 13, 'Amenorrhoea'.

Oligomenorrhoea

Menstruation that is markedly diminished in amount is called oligomenorrhoea. *Oligo* is Greek meaning too little, few or scanty. Heavy but infrequent periods are termed oligohypermenorrhoea (*hyper*—too much). Light and infrequent periods are referred to as oligohypomenorrhoea (*hypo*—not enough).

10

The usual suspects

Key words

adaptogen

aldosterone

amenorrhoea

anorexia nervosa

beta-carotene

bioflavonoid

body mass index

bone density

bulimia nervosa

dysmenorrhoea

epinephrine

hyperprolactinaemia

menorrhagia

scoliosis

Stress

'Stress' can be defined as any event or series of events, physical or emotional in a person's life that leads to physiological and biochemical changes. These changes, either pleasant or unpleasant, include exams; travelling overseas; moving away from home; relationship break-ups; serious illnesses or extreme physical exertion. Stress can interfere with the menstrual cycle and cause a temporary cessation of menstruation, heavier than usual periods, erratic cycles, or increased menstrual pain.

Stress affects the whole body

The body's first reaction to stress is an 'alarm' response (see Figure 10.1). Messages from the hypothalamus stimulate the (sympathetic) nervous system which in turn stimulates the adrenal gland to produce epinephrine (commonly known as adrenaline). This leads to a faster heart rate; increased production of sweat; contraction of the spleen to return blood to the circulation; dilation of the pupils, and of the bronchioles in the lungs; and release of stored sugars. Some functions slow down, including digestion and the production of urine.

This response is known as the 'fight or flight mechanism' and was much more in demand when a quick getaway was needed or when it was necessary to fight bears (or something else furry and dangerous). A rapid heart rate and contraction of the spleen mean that more blood is available for muscles, sugar is at hand for instant energy, the person can see better, breathe faster and is more alert.

These responses occur irrespective of the type of stress. In an office or in many other modern-day situations, they are quite inappropriate. There is no need to run, fight or physically protect oneself. The excess adrenaline/epinephrine, with no appropriate avenue of discharge, circulates around the system leaving the person with a sense of being 'on edge' and unable to relax. On top of that, digestion is slowed for the duration of the stressful event.

In times of prolonged stress such as occurs in chronic illness, pain, emotional trauma or just being 'stressed' all the time, the 'alarm' response changes into the 'resistance' response. During this phase, there is a need for an inexhaustible supply of glycogen as an energy source. To achieve this, the liver increases the conversion rate of fats; corticosteroids accelerate the conversion of both proteins and fats; and the thyroid increases the conversion of carbohydrates.

The kidneys conserve more water and sodium because of the action of another hormone from the adrenal gland, aldosterone. Aldosterone conserves sodium, but increases the excretion of potassium, one of the minerals essential to the normal function of muscles, including heart muscle, and the normal activity of the nervous system.

During this phase, the body is under enormous physical strain and the nutritional requirements are very high. But the digestive functions are impaired by the effects of stress on the digestive organs, and the production of digestive enzymes remains low. Just when a constant supply of good quality nutrients is required, the person is likely to suffer from loss of appetite, indigestion and poor assimilation.

The combination of excessive output of epinephrine, thyroxine and the fluctuating blood sugar create a sense of irritability and sometimes, anxiety attacks. Disturbed sleep is common, especially waking after a few hours of sleep. Night sweats are also common and may result from inappropriate physiological function where the body works day and night in response to the stress.

The menstrual cycle is another casualty of stress. The hypothalamus stops secreting GnRH in the usual pulsatile manner and the stimulus for ovulation (via LH and FSH) can be turned off or down graded. This can cause irregular menstruation and conditions such as dysfunctional uterine bleeding where bleeding is often heavy as well as erratic. Stress affects fertility by causing a temporary cessation of ovulation or by disrupting the luteal phase of the cycle.

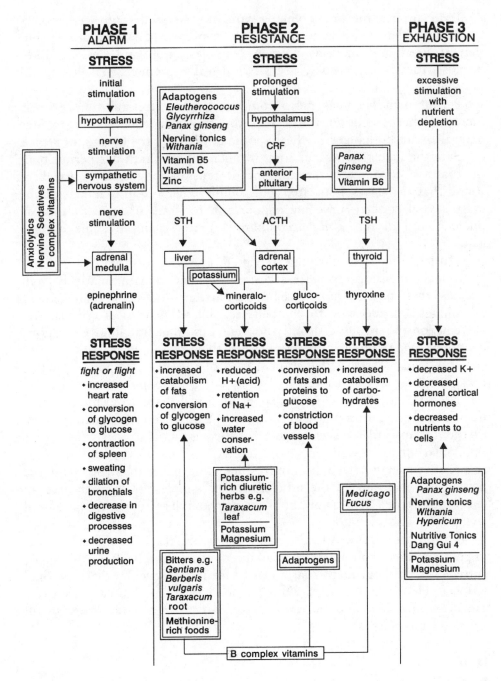

Figure 10.1 The three phases of stress

PMS can become worse when a woman is stressed—some researchers even think that most women have some premenstrual symptoms, but that stressed and anxious women cope less well and develop PMS because they are unusually sensitive to the premenstrual hormonal fluctuations.

Period pain becomes more common during stressful times. Stress increases the perception and lessens the ability to cope with pain, but may also cause changes in the hypothalamic-pituitary hormones which regulate the menstrual cycle. Some women report that their period pain fluctuates according to the amount of tension they feel. Researchers found that the stress associated with family tension, guilt feelings about early sexual contact, or being encouraged to think of menstruation as unclean and disagreeable, accompanied period pain in some adolescents.[1]

Most people live through repeated episodes of the 'alarm' and 'resistance' phase of the stress response. They remain relatively well because their nutrient intake, exercise patterns and stress management techniques are adequate to compensate. But some stresses are just too extreme or too prolonged and the very best diet and lifestyle regime cannot provide enough protection from them.

This leads to the 'exhaustion' phase of the stress response. Unable to keep going at the same rate, many of the organs go into decline. Research in the 1950s showed that protein is utilised from body tissues during the exhaustion phase and that in the absence of adequate protein intake, organs are used as protein substitutes.[2]

Potassium and sodium are excreted in the urine, the immune response weakens, sleep is unrefreshing and often disturbed and the person is exhausted all the time. Even the simplest task seems like an enormous chore. Depression, poor memory, anxiety and irrational mood swings are also common.

During the alarm, resistance or exhaustion responses to stress, the impact on the hypothalamic–pituitary–ovarian feed-back loop can be sufficient to disrupt menstruation or cause interference in the hormonal balance. However, for most women, the changes associated with stress are often transient and the cycle returns to normal after the stressful situation has passed.

■ ■
■ ■ The medical approach

Medicine has only recently embraced non-drug related methods for stress management, and this has by no means been adopted by all medical practitioners. Sedation or drugs to reduce anxiety are not indicated for stress-related menstrual changes and should rarely need to be prescribed. Stress management techniques are the treatments of choice.

The natural therapist's approach

In conjunction with stress management techniques, the herbal and dietary management of stress involves improving the body's capacity to adapt to stress with herbal adaptogens. This group of herbs include the ginsengs, especially *Eleuthrococcus senticosus*, which are discussed in Chapter 19 'Herbs'. Nervine herbs are also indicated when sleep is disrupted, along with B vitamins, magnesium and avoiding stimulants.

Specific herbs are also usually needed to regulate the period. Those herbs which regulate menstruation via the hypothalamic–pituitary–ovarian axis following stressful episodes are *Vitex agnus castus* for erratic menstruation and PMS; *Cimicifuga racemosa* (especially for peri-menopausal women); *Leonurus cardiaca* and *Verbena officinalis* for menstrual irregularities associated with anxiety and palpitations; and *Chamaelirium luteum* if ovulation has ceased.

Herbs with a specific effect on the uterus are *Trillium erectum* for menstruation which is heavy and erratic as is seen in dysfunctional uterine bleeding; *Angelica sinensis* for exhaustion and debility, especially after blood loss or heavy menstruation; and *Alchemilla vulgaris* for menorrhagia of adolescents. The astringent herbs are also indicated when bleeding is heavy.

 Self care

The diet included on pages 129–30 is intended to improve an individual's capacity to cope with long-term stress. Types of stress management could include yoga, 'long slow distance' exercise, using tapes to relax or learning meditation techniques. Having fun, dancing and relaxing with friends may be just as useful if the idea of meditating is unappealing.

Reducing tension

Herbal teas such as chamomile and lime flowers (*Tilia europa*) reduce tension and can be mixed together. Lemon balm is useful for stomach upsets caused by anxiety, especially when combined with chamomile. Oats or porridge are good for the nervous system, and an extract of the green oat seed (to be taken as a herbal mixture) is used by herbalists for depression and exhaustion. Rubbing a drop of oil of ylang ylang or lavender on the temples reduces anxiety and some people find these oils useful for headaches associated with tension. (Do not take essential oils internally.)

Rescue Remedy, a Bach flower essence available from health food shops and most natural therapists, is useful to relieve anxiety associated with worrying events, exams or public speaking, for example. It is usually used short term for isolated events that cause anxiety, but can also be used for sleeplessness associated with worry.

Improving sleep

There are three aspects of sleep that require attention: the ease with which a person gets to sleep, the quality of the sleep and the time that they wake up. Sleep quality generally improves when a person is less tense, and they usually get to sleep much more easily as well. Waking up too early, such as at five o'clock every morning, can be a sign of depression and if this is persistent, may indicate a need for professional help.

General rules for better sleep include not undertaking stimulating activities such as strenuous exercise or watching exciting movies just before bed; reducing or eliminating stimulants such as caffeine and sugar; setting up a relaxing routine around bedtime such as having a bath and a warm drink (soya or cow's milk and honey is a good idea); and trying to establish a regular routine by going to bed at the same time. Many of the Eastern traditions suggest that the two hours before midnight are the two most valuable hours sleep to have.

A hot bath with lavender oil is very relaxing and can be used for insomnia. Kalms (Nutricare) is a good over-the-counter sleeping preparation which contains small amounts of valerian and other herbs which improve relaxation and shorten the length of time it takes to get to sleep. They rarely cause drowsiness or fogginess in the head the next day and are generally well tolerated.

Dreaming excessively or nightmares can be one of the effects of stress and can seriously disrupt sleep patterns. It can also be caused by 'overdosing' on B vitamins, particularly vitamin B_6, so people taking vitamin B should try to take it in the morning. Dreaming more than usual can indicate that the person doesn't get into deep sleep and so the remedies for insomnia can be used to improve sleep quality. If over-the-counter remedies do not work, professional guidance is needed.

Being underweight

Being underweight is defined as having a body-fat composition of less than 22 per cent. Women need about 17 per cent of their total body weight to be made up of fat in order to menstruate at all, and 22 per cent body fat to have periods regularly. On average, women stop having periods once their body-fat composition is below 20 per cent of their total body weight and many underweight women, including sportswomen, gymnasts, ballet dancers and dieters, stop having periods.

Causes

Being underweight has a number of causes. The most troubling are the eating disorders anorexia nervosa, which effects small but increasing numbers of women mostly in their teens, and bulimia nervosa, which seems to affect women who are in their late teens and older. Extreme weight loss can also be associated with a number of serious illnesses such as cancer, malabsorption syndromes and dysentery (particularly when travellers have difficulty getting medical attention quickly). Over-exercising without appropriate kilojoule intake can also lead to abnormal weight loss.

Women who become vegetarian or vegan can sometimes lose too much weight if they are unaware of how to manage these diets correctly.

Diagnosis

One of the ways to tell if body weight is within the normal range is to calculate the body mass index (BMI). This is done by dividing the weight in kilograms by height in centimetres squared. The normal range for BMI is between 20 and 25. Anything below 20 is considered to be underweight; overweight is 26 and 30; and obese is more than 30. See Table 10.1.

Table 10.1 Body mass index (BMI)

The BMI is a guide only, and some variation needs to be taken into account when the body frame is very slight or very large. The calculation is only relevant after full height is attained—that is after eighteen or twenty.

The body mass index (BMI) is a method used to determine whether a person's weight is in the correct range for their height. The BMI is expressed in numbers.

- Less than 20 is considered to be underweight.
- 20–25 is considered to be normal.
- 26–30 is considered to be overweight.
- Over 30 is considered to be obese.

To determine BMI divide weight in kilograms by height in metres squared.

For example, when a woman weighs 52 kg and her height is 1.75 m, her BMI is calculated by dividing 52 by 1.7 x 1.7 (2.89) which equals 17.99. Her BMI is 18 which is considered to be underweight.

Recognising eating disorders

Eating disorders can vary quite dramatically in severity. It is fairly usual for many people to overeat as a result of stress, tension, and extreme fatigue; or to use food to lessen the feelings of disappointment, anger or poor self-esteem. At the other end of the spectrum are those who are constantly on one diet or another, who excessively restrict their intake of certain food groups and who are obsessed with their body size. These sorts of behaviours may indicate that the person has a mild form of eating disorder, but usually they cause little real physical damage. This is quite different from the two most severe eating disorders, anorexia nervosa and bulimia nervosa.

For more information on treatment and support for people with an eating disorder and advice for friends and family, contact your local hospital or the anorexia and bulimia support group in your area.

The common symptoms

These conditions can be very difficult to recognise because people with eating disorders often deny they have a problem and try to hide their behaviour from others. If family or friends have noticed that the person is behaving in a worrying manner, they may need to be quite persistent to get the individual to seek help. Here is a list of symptoms which might indicate either disorder.

- Extreme weight loss with denial that weight gain is necessary (anorexia nervosa).
- An unnatural fear of gaining weight.
- An obsession with food—thinking and talking about food too much, particularly in a negative manner.
- An unrealistic body image—feeling fat all the time and an inability to recognise when body weight is normal.
- Avoiding social situations which involve eating.
- Going to the bathroom after eating, or long stays in the bathroom. Running the tap or flushing the toilet to disguise vomiting.
- Exercising excessively to change body weight and shape.
- Weighing frequently.
- Inability to concentrate or think clearly; depression.

Obviously some of these symptoms might be related to something other than an eating disorder. Someone who always visits the bathroom after eating might have bowel problems such as diarrhoea; not wanting to eat out might be related to low self-esteem or shyness; and not being able to concentrate has multiple causes. However, a number of these behaviours occurring together may be an indication of an eating disorder.

Menstrual changes commonly occur because of low body weight. Hormone levels become low, the stimulus from the hypothalamus and pituitary gland is 'turned off', and ovulation does not occur. Bones and other tissues, such as collagen, which depend on oestrogens for their strength begin to weaken, and some women even develop menopausal symptoms like hot flushes and vaginal dryness.

■ ■
■ ■ The medical approach

Anorexia nervosa and bulimia nervosa require some form of counselling or psychotherapy to help change the person's perception of themselves and their relationship to food. This may take the form of family therapy, individual counselling or group counselling. Very occasionally drug therapy is used for severe and disabling depression. Hospitalisation is necessary if the body weight falls below 35 kilograms.

Doctors often refer sufferers to a dietitian to ensure that a balanced diet is eaten, and so that there is a better understanding of the necessity of some of the food groups. Sometimes a special diet will be needed to rectify specific nutrient deficiencies.

 The natural therapist's approach

Natural therapies such as herbs, homoeopathics or diets, *cannot* correct eating disorders. Sufferers of these conditions need extensive counselling to help them overcome the complaint, and while some natural remedies may help to rectify some of the physical problems, they are best advised as adjunctive treatments.

Despite the weight loss often seen in eating disorders, serum albumin (protein), cholesterol, and betacarotene are usually normal. However, blood levels of trace metals such as zinc and copper are often depleted.[3] Zinc deficiency seems to play a major role in anorexia nervosa, and some preliminary work suggests that correcting zinc levels may improve adaptation to stress in eating disorders.[4]

Herbs such as the bitters and the nervines are useful to assist with digestion, assimilation and stress; and the hormone regulating herbs such as *Vitex agnus castus* may be needed to regulate the period once the appropriate weight has been gained. General tonics and nutritive herbs are also useful such as *Eleutherococcus senticosus* and *Medicago sativa*.

The phyto-oestrogens (discussed in Chapter 18) can assist temporarily with low oestrogen symptoms, but they can never replace the effects of oestrogens produced in the body.

Beware!—fasting, raw food diets and 'elimination' diets

Becoming healthy, some people believe, is a tortuous process, bound to involve at least some restriction in diet, if not a complete fast. Some natural therapists are very fond of these strategies to 'improve' health and a number of popular texts have been written stressing the virtues of a clean diet and correct way to eliminate toxins from the system. These theories of 'purity' and 'internal cleanliness' are often expanded on by those who believe that menstruation is somehow impure or unclean. The arguments—usually implied—are that a woman who has difficulty with menstruation, or who menstruates heavily, or even a woman who menstruates at all, has become in some way 'toxic' and in need of a purifying regime.

This impression is strengthened by the association between the common premenstrual symptoms of constipation, acne, fluid retention and bloating. These are seen as the ultimate proof of the toxicity—after all, they disappear once the 'cleansing' process of menstruation starts. These theories had their recorded genesis in the Ancient Greek medical texts where it was quite strongly held that menstruation was a purifying process, necessary to prevent a great number of unpleasant ills (see Chapter 3). Gradually over the years, this theory has been modified by some to read 'no menstruation means purity'. The proponents of this dotty theory quite happily tell their patients to fast or use extreme elimination diets to reduce or stop menstrual flow!

Restricted diets can reduce or stop menstruation, but not because the body is detoxified. Often the resultant weight loss means that the body mass index is below that needed for ovulation and menstruation to occur. Excess fibre intake can diminish menstrual flow by reducing the availability of oestrogen—and has deleterious effects on bone density as well.

Sometimes prolonged dietary restriction of iron and vitamin B_{12} can cause anaemia and *excessive* menstruation.[5] The same can be said of bioflavonoid and vitamin A deficiency both of which can occur as a result of extreme dietary restrictions.

Unfortunately, even with the increased information available about hormones and the menstrual cycle, it still needs to be stressed that menstruation is a natural and desirable process for a woman. And although various dietary changes can alter or even stop menstruation, this does not necessarily make for improved health—indeed, severely restricted and fad diets often do more harm than good. A sensible diet can, however, alleviate uncomfortably heavy periods and symptoms of PMS.

The benefits of exercise

Exercising regularly and moderately has many health benefits for women. These include improved cardiovascular health, better bone density, maintenance of a healthy body weight, prevention of obesity, and a general reduction in stress. Menstruation is positively affected by moderate exercise as well. The severity of period pain is reduced and in some cases entirely relieved by exercise; PMS improves when women exercise; and exercise can even reduce the volume and duration of menstrual flow.[6]

Regular exercise reduces the incidence of a number of common gynaecological complaints as well. Women who do regular exercise may have a reduced risk of endometriosis because the rate of oestrogen production is lower. The incidence of endometriosis increases amongst women who lead sedentary lives and amongst younger women who stop exercising earlier than their peers.[7] Cyclic breast pain and cystic disease of the breast are also less common amongst women who exercise moderately and regularly.[8]

So what is moderate exercise and how often does it need to be done to achieve these benefits on the menstrual cycle? The answer depends on what needs to be achieved. It might be as little as half an hour a few times a week for some women; dysmenorrhoea and PMS can even improve when women exercise only during the week leading up to the period.

The type of exercise doesn't seem to be important either, except that exercise that increases the heart rate (aerobic exercise) like walking, swimming, cycling, jogging, team sports or aerobics are associated with the most all-round benefits. Although not usually thought of as an aerobic-type of exercise, specific yoga exercises which improve pelvic blood flow can give considerable relief from pelvic pain and discomfort. Yoga often incorporates a relaxation component which is also useful to help cope with pain and can reduce the severity of PMS. These exercises can be taught by a yoga teacher or learned from a text with specific exercises for the pelvic region.

One of the best types of exercise, especially when stress aggravates period pain or PMS, is long, slow, distance exercise. This is when rhythmic and repetitive exercise, usually walking, bike-riding or swimming, is sustained at a moderate pace for about three quarters to one hour. This has the effect of calming the nerves, shutting off the inappropriate adrenal response and improving stamina.

Weight-bearing exercise—literally, bearing your own weight—improves muscle strength and stamina, accelerates weight loss, and most important of all, increases bone density. Not exercising increases the amount of calcium and other minerals lost from bone. Calcium is even lost from bone during a normal night's sleep. The positive effects of calcium, oestrogen and exercise on bone tend to be cumulative and exercise is most beneficial during the years when oestrogen is available, and when the dietary intake of essential nutrients is good. There is more benefit gained from exercise up until menopause, but an exercise-related increase in bone density is seen at all ages, including after the menopause.[9]

Any weight-bearing exercise, but particularly types which stress the large muscles, has the potential to improve bone mass. The best types are walking, running or playing sport. Swimming and cycling are still important even though they are not classically included in the weight-bearing group. For maximum benefit, exercise should be daily or every second day for about 60 minutes.[10]

Staying fit and active is important for older women too. Muscle strength and physical fitness are associated with not only increased bone mineral density, improved agility, and better cardiovascular health, but a reduced incidence of falls and fractures. Even when falls do occur, they are likely to be less awkward or cause serious injury.

For beginners, rapid walking for half to one hour every second day and then every day as stamina improves is an easy way to start. *Instant Vitality*, a book containing a detailed and varied exercise program written by Debbie Flintoff-King,[11] gives some excellent advice for a varied fitness program.

Too much exercise

The effects of rigorous exercise are not all positive. Women who engage in strenuous physical activity *during* menstruation have an increased risk of endometriosis, perhaps related to the increased amount of menstrual blood passing back up the Fallopian tubes,[12] When exercise is prolonged, such as during endurance training, exercise-induced menstrual infrequency or amenorrhoea (no periods) may result. This usually occurs in conjunction with a number of predisposing factors which work together to create the abnormal hormonal environment. These include:[13]

- The age of the woman when she started to train
  Young women who start to exercise excessively before menstruation has commenced and before communication between the hypothalamus, the pituitary and the ovary is established, are inclined to have a much later onset of menstruation. When training starts around the menarche, there is a higher incidence of amenorrhoea.
- Previous menstrual history
  Women who have a prior history of irregular menstrual cycles, light periods or amenorrhoea are more prone to these problems when they undertake strenuous exercise.
- Body weight
  Women with a low body mass index or who lose large amounts of weight during training are more prone to menstrual irregularities.
- Nutritional intake and kilojoule balance
  Energy expenditure during exercise should be replaced by foods containing adequate kilojoules to prevent excessive weight loss. The requirements for most minerals, especially calcium, iron, zinc, magnesium and potassium increase during exercise and may contribute to delayed physical development and menstrual irregularities.
- Distance run during training
  Menstrual disorders increase proportionally with the distance run.

Women who run more than 80 km per week have a higher incidence of amenorrhoea.

- Stress experienced during training
  Women who experience more stress during training may be at greater risk of developing menstrual irregularities.
- Type of training
  Amenorrhoea is much less frequent amongst swimmers than in runners, gymnasts and ballet dancers.

Excessive exercise can cause specific menstrual cycle problems throughout a female athlete's life. During adolescence, not only is the onset of menstruation delayed, but so are other aspects of physical maturity, such as attaining normal height. Infertility is also common because ovulation is either erratic or ceases in tandem with the menstrual irregularities. The major concern associated with these menstrual changes, though, is the possibility of irretrievable changes to bone density. This can lead to a failure to reach peak bone mass, reduced bone density, scoliosis (spinal column curvature) and stress fractures.[14]

Causes of the menstrual changes

When women undertake endurance exercise, a relative oestrogen deficiency can develop. This is probably caused by a (reversible) suppression of the frequency and amplitude of the pulsatile secretion of GnRH from the hypothalamus and leads to low levels of LH, but not of FSH. The decline in LH may be a survival mechanism which was once geared to reducing fertility in times of stress and physical endurance when pregnancy would be undesirable.[15]

Maintaining a regular period and healthy bones

The reduced oestrogen levels are responsible for the irregular cycles, amenorrhoea and low bone density, but at least some of the time, eating disorders also contribute to the picture.[16] It is important for athletes to remember that if the diet is good, body mass index is maintained within a healthy range, menstruation continues, and bone density is maintained.[17]

Additional complex carbohydrates will be needed to meet the kilojoule requirements of endurance training. Calcium in the range of 1000–1500 mg per day is also necessary—the higher range is necessary when menstruation is erratic or absent. Women with prolonged menstrual irregularities or amenorrhoea may need to consider the Pill if their bone density is low. Further advice is included in the section on relative oestrogen deficiency (see page 72).

Prescribed drugs

A number of drugs affect menstruation. Some increase flow while others reduce it; some influence the regularity of the cycle; and some can even cause menstruation to cease temporarily. Not all drug influences are negative—some drugs are deliberately prescribed to re-establish menstrual flow and regularity; to reduce pain or to minimise heavy flow. Some of the common drug effects on the menstrual cycle include:

- Oral contraceptives (the Pill)
  The Pill is used as a therapeutic agent for a number of gynaecological conditions. It has many benefits, including a reduction in menstrual flow and period pain, as well as more regular cycles. It can also cause unwanted side effects. The cautions, side effects and drug interactions, as well as the benefits and complaints which respond well to the Pill are discussed in Chapter 20 'Drugs and surgery'.
- Progestogens
  These drugs are commonly prescribed for endometriosis and abnormal bleeding. They can often cause bloating, fluid retention, weight gain and mood changes.
- GnRH agonists
  These drugs cause a temporary menopausal state which includes cessation of the period, menopausal symptoms and a loss of bone density. They are used for fibroids and endometriosis, and their use for PMS and benign breast disease is under review.
- Corticosteroids
  The corticosteroids can cause a drug-induced Cushing's Syndrome which is associated with menstrual irregularities or amenorrhoea, and androgenising (male hormone-like) effects. Loss of bone density is a common and serious side effect from long-term corticosteroid therapy. The common types of corticosteroids are prednisolone (Solone), hydrocortisone (Hysone), betamethasone (Celestone) and dexamethasone (Decadron).
- Prostaglandins-inhibiting drugs
  The prostaglandin (synthetase) inhibitors, for example, Ponstan and Naprogesic, are used for period pain and occasionally for menorrhagia as well. Sometimes they can delay the onset of the period and their use is associated with an increased risk of gastrointestinal ulcers.
- Anti-coagulant drugs
  Drugs which affect clotting time can occasionally increase menstrual flow. These include Calciparine, Dindevan, heparin and warfarin.
- Cytotoxic drugs
  The cytotoxic drugs which are used in the treatment of cancer, such as cyclophosphamide, chlorambucil, mechlorethamine and vincris-

tine, can lead to infertility, irregular menstruation, amenorrhoea and premature menopause.

- Tamoxifen
  Tamoxifen is an anti-oestrogen in the treatment of breast cancer, and sometimes for benign breast disease. It can cause menopause-like symptoms, and less frequently, abnormal vaginal bleeding and irregular menstruation.
- Drugs which affect prolactin levels
  The drugs which effect prolactin levels can interrupt cyclic regularity. They are discussed in the section on hyperprolactinaemia on page 213.

Recreational drugs

Alcohol, cigarettes, opiates and cocaine can all affect the menstrual cycle. Coffee (more than two cups per day) which is linked to infertility,[18] does not necessarily cause menstrual irregularities, but can increase menstrual pain especially if consumed during the period.

Excessive use of alcohol has been associated with infertility due to ovulatory failure amongst women with endometriosis, and increases the risk of developing endometriosis by about 50 per cent.[19] Alcoholism increases the chance of early menopause,[20] and can also increase prolactin production.[21] These complaints can be associated with erratic cycles, menorrhagia or amenorrhoea.

Cocaine use is associated with higher levels of prolactin and abnormal menstrual cycles.[22] Methadone and possibly other opiates increase prolactin levels, but do not appear to have long-term effects on ovulation.[23] Cigarette smoking lowers oestrogen levels, and is associated with an increased incidence of menstrual irregularity, infertility and earlier menopause.[24]

Recreational drugs which interfere with menstruation usually have an impact on the levels of one or more of the hormones. These effects can translate into more serious problems such as osteoporosis and infertility. It is wise to curtail any activities which negatively affect menstruation.

11

Heavy menstruation

Key words

adenomyosis
androgen
astringent
beta-hydrogenase
Cold
D&C
Dry
emmenagogue
endometrial hyperplasia
endometrium
flavonoid
GnRH agonist
Hot
hyperplasia
hysteroscopy

isoflavonoid
laparoscopy
Moist
myometrium
pathology
pedunculated
phyto-oestrogen
prostacyclin
prostaglandins
saponin
sarcoma
serum ferritin
spiral arterioles
uterine tonic

Heavy periods are the bane of some women's lives. There are a number of reasons why a period might be heavier than normal and each of these should be investigated. The most common causes are 'functional' where nothing is essentially wrong, but there is an abnormality of function; and fibroids. These causes of menorrhagia will be covered in this section.

It cannot be said too many times that treating abnormal menstrual bleeding without knowing its cause is an extremely foolish thing to do. The need for an accurate diagnosis is vital. Sometimes a diagnosis can be made using only the history and routine examinations; sometimes procedures, such as dilatation and curettage (D&C), laparoscopy or hysteroscopy are necessary. Some of these procedures require a general anaesthetic.

The diagnostic techniques used by natural therapists such as iris, tongue or pulse diagnosis, are much less invasive (and therefore much more desirable), but in my opinion, do not give the type of information needed to pinpoint the origin of the abnormal bleeding. They should never be used as an alternative to the appropriate medical examinations.

THE COMMON CAUSES OF HEAVY PERIODS

1. Functional menorrhagia

The term menorrhagia can be used to either describe a bleeding *pattern* or as a term to define a functional disorder which presents as heavy menstruation.

Functional menorrhagia is a condition which presents as abnormally heavy menstruation, and a normal menstrual cycle. There is no demonstrable pathology found either within the uterus or from blood tests.

2. Uterine fibroids

These are non-cancerous (fibrous) tumours of the uterus, usually in the myometrium (muscle wall). Fibroids are common in women over 30 and affect about one in every five women. They may vary in size and number and can be diagnosed with an ultrasound. Fibroids may be symptom free, or exert pressure effects like urinary frequency if the tumours are larger. Heavy bleeding at menstruation is a common symptom that accompanies many, but not all fibroids. Rarely, fibroids can undergo malignant change and develop into sarcoma.

3. Endometriosis

This is caused by the endometrium (normal cells which line the uterine cavity) growing in incorrect places. These cells still have hormonal sensitivity and therefore bleed during menstruation and might grow on the ovaries, tubes, pelvic ligaments, bowel or bladder. Endometriosis is most common amongst 20 to 30 year olds, but women of any age who are ovulating and/or menstruating can develop the complaint. Endometriosis can cause pain, heavy periods, abnormal bleeding patterns and/or infertility.

4. Adenomyosis

Adenomyosis is similar to endometriosis in that normal endometrial cells become displaced and grow in the wrong place, in this case within the uterine wall. The tissue is responsive to hormonal stimulation and the bleeding into the muscle layer causes pain and often heavy menstruation. It is a common cause of menstrual pain in women over 40.

5. Pelvic inflammatory disease (PID)

PID is caused by infection, which may or may not be sexually transmitted. The symptoms include abnormal bleeding and heavy periods in about 30 per cent of women, but typically fever, malaise and pelvic pain are the presenting complaints. A bloody or purulent discharge is common if the PID is caused by gonorrhoea.

6. Contraceptive causes

These are rare for women who use either natural family planning (based on the detection of ovulation); or barrier methods (condoms, diaphragm or cervical cap).

i) IUD

The IUD or 'loop' can cause heavier and more painful periods. Some women experience bleeding between periods, especially in the first three months after insertion. Severe pain and/or bleeding may indicate that the IUD has dislodged or an infection has developed and requires immediate assessment.

ii) Tubal ligation

Tubal ligation has been shown to be associated with altered menstrual patterns including menorrhagia. This may be a result of the procedure or be secondary to having stopped the Pill.

7. Non-gynaecological causes

Disturbance in hormone levels, blood clotting or deficiencies of certain nutrients may result in heavier periods. The more common causes are related to the following systems.

i) The blood

Disorders of blood production or blood clotting can be related to bleeding abnormalities. Causes range from nutritional deficiency to leukaemia. Anaemia and low serum ferritin can cause heavy bleeding. von Willebrands disease, a congenital clotting abnormality, may become obvious for the first time as menorrhagia in adolescence.

ii) The endocrine system

Imbalances of the adrenal hormones, either associated with drug use or adrenal disorders may result in abnormal uterine bleeding.

The thyroid gland controls the general rate of the body's functions, including menstruation.

The hypothalamic–pituitary unit is involved in the control of the entire endocrine system. It is sensitive to the effects of stress, drugs, and variations in the production of all hormones in the body.

iii) *The liver*

The liver metabolises the reproductive hormones and synthesises clotting factors. Poor liver function can lead to menorrhagia.

8. Pregnancy and bleeding

Pregnancy-related conditions are the most common causes of abnormal bleeding amongst women from the age of 20 to 40. Pain may accompany the abnormal bleeding.

i) *Miscarriage*

A late and/or painful, heavy period may be an early miscarriage or a 'blighted ovum' where the foetus fails to develop normally. Bleeding later in an established pregnancy, and before the fourteenth week, might also indicate that a miscarriage is occurring.

HEAVY PERIODS (FUNCTIONAL MENORRHAGIA)

The medical term for a heavy period not related to any other condition (organic pathology) is functional menorrhagia. 'Functional' means that the menorrhagia occurs because of disordered function of an otherwise healthy-looking uterus. The diagnosis implies an absence of diseases in the reproductive tract, normal hormone function, and an absence of other diseases which might cause abnormal bleeding. Women with functional menorrhagia have heavy *periods*, but their menstrual *cycle* is normal.

Cause

Heavy menstruation is almost always in some way related to a prostaglandins imbalance which causes reduced blood clotting, and dilated blood vessels. One of the prostaglandins, prostacyclin 2 is a potent dilator of blood vessels and also inhibits blood clotting, leading to increased menstrual bleeding.[1] Prostaglandins imbalance may be caused by relative oestrogen excess and/or a high intake of saturated fats.

■ ■

■ ■   The medical approach

A diagnosis of functional menorrhagia is a 'diagnosis of exclusion' and is made by eliminating all diseases and 'organic' complaints as the reason for the heavy period. Past and present history, Pap smear results, the findings from an internal examination and blood tests may all be necessary in some cases to differentiate between the different causes of the excessive bleeding.

Depending on the age of the woman, a hysteroscopy or diagnostic D&C is sometimes also suggested if the history of the complaint, the pattern of the bleeding or the age of the woman are suggestive of a pre-cancerous or cancerous condition, or if there is a suspicion of an intra-uterine lesion such as a polyp or fibroid. These procedures are often diagnostic rather than therapeutic, although bleeding patterns sometimes return to normal after a D&C. The reasons for this are not always clear.

If there are no obvious causes of the heavy period, a diagnosis of functional menorrhagia is made. The medical practitioner might suggest the following treatments, usually starting at the top of the list and progressing though until a satisfactory outcome is achieved. More details on each of the drugs and surgical procedures is included in Chapter 20 'Drugs and surgery'.

- The Pill
  The Pill is a common treatment for menorrhagia and is often the most efficient way to establish a regular cycle and a lighter period.
- Prostaglandins inhibitors (Naprogesic, Ponstan)
  Prostaglandins inhibitors such as Naprogesic and Ponstan are sometimes used to treat menorrhagia. They block the conversion of prostaglandins into prostacyclin 2 and reduce bleeding[2] and work best when women are ovulating, or in combination with the Pill or progesterone tablets. Some doctors combine these treatments.[3]
- Progestogens in the second half of the month or continually (often Provera or Primolut)
  Progestogens are used for menorrhagia even though many women who have this problem do not have irregularities in either progesterone production or hormone balance. When the hormone medication is withdrawn after 10 to 20 days, the endometrium is shed completely and the period often goes back to normal. Progestogens can also be given continuously, which causes the endometrium to shrink.
- A hysteroscopic D&C
  This diagnostic procedure allows the gynaecologist to view the uterine cavity, detect any problems and then perform a curette to remove abnormally developed endometrium.
- Temporary medically induced menopause
  The GnRH agonists (Zoladex, Synarel) which create a 'medical menopause', can be suggested for abnormal bleeding which has failed to respond adequately to other methods.

- Uterine endometrial ablation

  The lining of the uterus (endometrium) is destroyed using laser or cauterisation via a hysteroscope which leads to cessation of or reduction in menstruation.

- Hysterectomy

  The removal of the uterus, which may also involve the removal of the ovaries (hysterectomy and bilateral salphingo-oopherectomy), is reserved as the last treatment option for excessive menstrual loss.

 The natural therapist's approach

Many women visit natural therapists for abnormal bleeding because 'nothing else has worked'. Often they have been examined by a doctor and told that they just have heavy periods, and that nothing is wrong. When a physical examination has not been performed, the woman should be referred to a doctor for the appropriate examinations. A complete gynaecological check-up is recommended for all women with menorrhagia who are 40 or older, and for any woman who has symptoms which may indicate other conditions.

Once the possibility of other conditions has been eliminated, the first step in a natural therapist's diagnosis is to determine whether the excessive bleeding is associated with hormonal imbalance. Symptoms such as premenstrual syndrome, an irregular cycle, and spotting or intramenstrual bleeding are suggestive. Taking a basal body temperature reading can also assess whether ovulation is occurring. If there is no evidence of a hormonal irregularity, remedies to regulate hormone levels are not necessary, even though it is common for the medical treatment to include hormones.

Natural therapists can use a variety of clinical assessments to evaluate the causes and the type of treatment they will use for functional menorrhagia. Problems might be confined to the uterus, or be part of a more systemic complaint related to the 'constitutional state' of the woman.

Uterine problems might be associated with:

- abnormal uterine tone
- prostaglandins imbalance
- an excess of Heat, Cold, Dryness or Moistness in the uterus

Or, the bleeding may occur because of an imbalance in the entire system and be caused by:

- nutritional deficiencies
- weakness and lack of vitality leading to a systemic imbalance and (usually) a tendency to become Cold
- liver congestion leading (often) to irritability and headaches, and a tendency to become Hot

In reality, there is considerable overlap in these types of complaints, both in their presentation and treatment. For example, abnormal uterine tissue tone will often occur when there are nutritional deficiencies, particularly iron, and when there is a more generalised lack of vitality. Herbs to nourish blood and improve vitality often also affect uterine tone (for example, *Angelica sinensis*); and iron is believed to improve both anaemia and uterine tone.

Nutritional and dietary aspects of functional menorrhagia

Iron

Anaemia can be the cause as well as the result of abnormal uterine bleeding. In 1964 researchers showed that women who had heavy periods also had depleted iron stores (serum ferritin), but not necessarily anaemia.[4] They speculated that the menorrhagia was caused by a relative weakness of both the uterine muscles and the spiral arterioles of the endometrium which were unable to stop bleeding by contracting. This condition is very similar to the lack of uterine tone described by natural therapists.

Vitamin A

Vitamin A is an important nutrient in the growth and development of adolescents[5] and ensures healthy endometrial growth.[6] Women with normal menstrual loss appear to have significantly better levels of Vitamin A than women with menorrhagia. When the women with heavy menstrual loss were given Vitamin A improvement resulted in more than 92 per cent of cases.[7] Normal oestrogen levels are dependent on Vitamin A, and a deficiency leads to impaired activity of an enzyme called 3 beta-dehydrogenase which is vital to the production of oestrogen (oestradiol).

Vitamin A is only useful for menorrhagia associated with a restricted or inadequate intake. Levels of 10 000 IU for 3 months are safe (but not for women trying to become pregnant), however, doses of up to 25 000 to 30 000 IU daily have been used and were associated with negligible toxicity.[8] These doses should be supervised. Vitamin A is restricted to 5000 IU tablets for over the counter sales and is toxic if taken for prolonged periods.

Vitamin K

Crude chlorophyll has been used historically for excess menstruation,[9] although exactly why it should help has been unclear. One theory is that chlorophyll contains high levels of Vitamin K which is necessary for the normal clotting of blood. Vitamin K was shown to reduce the number of menstruating days when menstrual irregularities were associated with longer than normal periods.[10]

Deficiencies of vitamin K are said to be uncommon because dietary intake is usually assumed to be adequate, and anyway, bacterial colonies can manufacture vitamin K in the absence of a good intake. However, the major food source of Vitamin K, green leafy vegetables, are often lacking in the average diet and altered bowel flora, especially with the administration of antibiotics,[11] can interfere with normal manufacture of vitamin K. Supplements should not be necessary. A balanced diet containing dark green leafy vegetables and yoghurt should improve any deficiency quickly.

The flavonoids

The flavonoids are a diverse group of compounds which naturally occur in food and medicinal plants, and are some of the major physiologically active constituents of herbal medicines.[12] Flavonoids have diverse effects in the body; several of which may affect menorrhagia. They improve capillary fragility; interact with oestrogen receptor sites, reducing the proliferative effect of oestrogens (some phyto-oestrogens are isoflavonoids);[13] and inhibit production of oestrogen due to inhibition of the enzyme responsible for its synthesis.[14] But with over 500 different flavonoids identified, it is likely that many of the effects of flavonoids in gynaecological conditions are yet to be identified.

Flavonoids are commonly found in astringents; plants traditionally used for menorrhagia. This may be related to their affect on capillary fragility. Citrus bioflavonoids reduced the menorrhagia of almost all of the women in one study who were treated with 600 mg of water soluble bioflavonoid compound. The results were thought to be due to improved capillary strength which reduced permeability and bleeding.[15]

Dietary phyto-oestrogens

Phyto-oestrogens are thought to inhibit the effect of oestrogen on the endometrium by binding to the same receptor sites as oestrogen and preventing it from having a stimulatory effect. When menstruating women have a high intake of soya products, studies have shown that they ovulate later, and the period tends to become lighter and shorter.[16]

Prostaglandins and menorrhagia

Prostaglandins play a major role in the initiation of menstruation and are also involved in menorrhagia and dysmenorrhoea. Prostaglandin-inhibitors are used in medicine for the control of bleeding, and it seems likely that some herbs will have similar prostaglandin-inhibiting actions.

Of particular interest are the medicinal plants *Equisetum arvense*, and *Panax notoginseng*, which have been traditionally used for heavy menstruation and which may influence prostaglandin levels. At present, there is not enough research to say whether it is the prostaglandin-inhibiting or other constituents in the herbs which are responsible for regulating the volume of menstrual loss.

Manipulating the diet by reducing saturated fats improves menorrhagia. Benefits may arise from the dual effects of a reduction in relative oestrogen excess and improved prostaglandin ratios.

Herbs for functional menorrhagia

Herbs for functional menorrhagia are chosen from the following categories.

- Herbs which affect uterine tone and regulate uterine bleeding: the astringents, uterine tonics and emmenogogues.
- Herbs which have diverse 'systemic' effects, and which improve the overall vitality or constitutional state of the woman: the female tonic herbs and the Liver herbs which reduce bleeding by clearing Heat and (often) aiding oestrogen clearance.

Astringents

Herbalists refer to astringents as being Drying—in fact one of the ways to tell if a herb has an astringent effect is to see whether it has the typical drying and puckering sensation in the mouth. This 'astringent' effect is caused by tannins, but tannins are not responsible for the effects on the uterus because they are not absorbed from the gut.

The 'uterine astringents' usually contain the tannins characteristic of most herbal astringents, in addition to other (non-tannin) constituents, primarily flavonoids and saponins which regulate bleeding. Some of these effects are quite complex, and not all of them are understood. They are discussed in greater detail in the section on astringent herbs in Chapter 19.

Uterine astringents used to treat menorrhagia include *Trillium erectum*, *Equisetum arvense*, *Achillea millefolium*, *Tienchi ginseng*, *Capsella bursa-pastoris* and *Hydrastis canadensis*. The important astringents for menorrhagia in adolescence are *Achillea millefolium*, *Alchemilla vulgaris*, *Capsella bursa-pastoris* and *Geranium maculatum*.

Uterine tonics

Herbs which affect the muscle tone of the uterus, the uterine tonics, are believed to affect bleeding by normalising the uterine tone. The uterine tonics are accepted as being capable of improving weak muscle activity and relaxing excess spasm and are often combined with the uterine astringents in the treatment of menorrhagia. They include *Angelica sinensis*, *Chamaelirium luteum*, *Rubus idaeus*, *Caulophyllum thalictroides*, *Mitchella repens*, and *Aletris farinosa* and are discussed in the section on uterine tonics in Chapter 19.

Emmenagogues

Emmenagogues are used to treat menorrhagia associated with a lack of uterine tone. This group of herbs increases muscular activity and the resting tone of the uterus and are indicated for heavy bleeding immediately after delivery, when fibroids interfere with the normal muscular activity of the uterus, after a miscarriage or termination, or following frequent full-term pregnancies. They should only be prescribed by a trained herbalist.

Liver herbs

Liver herbs are often used for conditions associated with excess Heat such as irritability, headaches, acne, feeling hot and thirsty. When this is confined to the premenstrual phase of the cycle, it is often thought of as an imbalance in the hormone levels caused by a relative oestrogen excess.

Liver herbs are bitter and Cooling. Dietary changes are usually recommended at the same time.

Tonic herbs

Herbalists recognise a type of uterine bleeding that is associated with a lack of vitality or general body weakness. The usual characteristics are that the woman will be unusually tired, weak and pale. This type of bleeding has been recognised for a long time: it is recorded as a cause of bleeding in the *Medieval Woman's Guide to Health* as 'weakness of the woman who cannot keep the blood inside her'.[17]

The cure was reported to be a good diet of 'plump hens' and 'comforting food'—still good advice. In addition, the uterine and female tonic herbs, of which there are few better than *Aletris farinosa* and *Angelica sinensis*, would also be suggested. These are both Warming herbs.

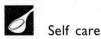 Self care

Lifestyle changes

Exercising and reducing stress levels have many effects on the menstrual patterns of women. These are described in Chapter 10 'The usual suspects'.

Dietary changes

A diet to complement the treatment of functional menorrhagia should reflect the assumed causes. If these are related to iron deficiency, additional iron-containing foods that are also low in fat can be included. A low fat, high fibre diet will reduce menstrual flow by increasing oestrogen clearance and regulating prostaglandin balance. Saturated fats, should be avoided or at least reduced. These include those fats found in full-cream dairy products, meat, eggs and some vegetable products, including peanuts and coconut. Fibre also improves oestrogen clearance. Additional information on the effects of fibre and fat on oestrogen levels is included in Chapter 5.

If bioflavonoid deficiency is the assumed cause of the bleeding, citrus fruits, fruits and vegetables generally, or even buckwheat leaf tea can be taken to correct the problem. But because flavonoids are ubiquitous in the plant world, just increasing the intake of fruit and vegetables will increase flavonoid intake.

UTERINE FIBROIDS

Uterine fibroids, also known as uterine leiomyomas or uterine myomata, are fibrous (and non-cancerous) tumours of the uterus which affect from 20–25 per cent of women past the age of 35.[18] They vary greatly in size, number, and position; some growing to vast sizes and causing pressure symptoms; others remaining small and discrete. A fibroid is comprised of dense muscular fibres arranged in circular layers and encapsulated in a layer of compressed smooth muscle cells. The blood supply reaches the fibroid via vessels which traverse the outer capsule; the tumour itself having relatively few blood vessels within its structure.

Fibroids may cause few symptoms; occasionally quite large ones are discovered because of a routine examination or ultrasound scan for another reason. In fact, fibroids which are not interfering with fertility or causing unwanted symptoms require no surgery or drugs, medical, natural or otherwise to shrink or remove them. Regular monitoring is advisable, and some general measures to moderate the effects of 'relative oestrogen excess' are useful to contain growth and reduce the risk of additional fibroids.

Large fibroids, those that are pedunculated (growing on a stem), and those that grow rapidly should be monitored closely. A rapidly growing fibroid can be associated with an increased risk of sarcoma which is an aggressive type of tumour. Often doctors suggest that they be removed before any abnormalities develop.

Symptoms

The most common symptom associated with fibroids is heavy bleeding. Larger fibroids are also associated with urinary frequency, pressure symptoms, heaviness and congestion in the lower abdomen. Some women have a heavy feeling, sometimes described as a sensation 'as though everything might fall out' before or during the period. Very large fibroids may cause abdominal enlargement and the woman may look like she is in the early stages of pregnancy. Sometimes fibroids will cause a miscarriage or infertility and rarely, pregnant women may come into labour too early because of fibroids.

Types of fibroids and their locations

Fibroids can be described according to their location in relation to the uterus; or according to their type.

Location

Intra-uterine

These fibroids are found within the uterine cavity. They are sometimes called 'sub-mucus' because they are situated below or within the endometrial lining. These fibroids can sometimes be removed via a hysteroscope if they are less than 5–6 cm in diameter. They are frequently associated with heavy menstruation, even if rather small, and can extend through the cervix if they are pedunculated. Problems with fertility may occur because the endometrium around the fibroid does not undergo normal hormonal change. Implantation can be affected and the miscarriage rate is often higher.

Myometrial

These are fibroids found within the muscle wall of the uterus (the myometrium). They are sometimes referred to as intramural fibroids. They can occur at any location within the uterine muscle and vary considerably in size. Symptoms are usually excessive bleeding at menstruation, and if large enough, pressure may be exerted on adjacent organs. Rarely, pressure on a ureter (the tube between the kidney and bladder) may cause a back-flow of urine causing structural abnormalities of the kidney and ureter and abnormal renal function.

Extra-uterine

As their name suggests, these fibroids are attached to the outside of the uterus. They are sometimes called 'sub-serous' because of their positioning under the serous outer lining of the uterus. They can also cause pressure symptoms or be associated with excessive bleeding. Some are found around or on the Fallopian tubes and may interfere with fertility.

Type

Fibroids are of two main types. They can be discrete, fibrous and encapsulated tumours, which are usually roughly spherical in shape; or they might be pedunculated tumours attached to the uterine cavity or the outside of the uterus by a stem or pedicle.

The latter variety can cause problems because of the (fairly rare) tendency to twist on the pedicle (called torsion). If this occurs the blood supply to the fibroid can be cut off, and death of the fibroid tissue will occur. This is associated with extreme pain and increased pressure symptoms as the fibroid swells in its capsule and presses on adjacent organs. Immediate surgery may be needed.

What makes a fibroid grow?

It is not known why muscular fibres start to arrange themselves in the spherical form that is typical of fibroids. What is known, however, is that their growth is dependent upon the presence of oestrogen: they rarely develop before menarche and will almost always shrink after menopause. Women with other conditions which are associated with oestrogen over-activity, such as endometrial hyperplasia and endometriosis, have a greater risk of fibroids, adding weight to the theory that they are somehow reliant on, or caused by, oestrogen levels.[19]

Downgrading oestrogen 'excess' is one of the requirements of a successful treatment. Natural therapists treat fibroids as conditions associated with 'relative oestrogen excess'; and doctors use drugs which will temporarily cause a menopausal state, or suggest surgical removal.

Fibroids have also been found to contain larger amounts of DDT than other uterine tissue.[20] The significance of this is not clear, but DDT has oestrogen-like effects and may in some way initiate the tissue changes.

Factors which affect the incidence of fibroids

Pregnancy

Pregnancy seems to reduce the risk of fibroids developing. With each successive pregnancy, the rate at which fibroids develop reduces and women who have had five full-term pregnancies have only one-quarter the risk of women who have had none.[21]

Coffee

Coffee may increase the likelihood of developing uterine fibroids. Researchers from the company Nestlé gave mice the equivalent of two to three cups of instant coffee per day.[22] They had a slightly higher incidence of fibroids than control mice, but the significance of this for women is not clear.

Obesity

Obesity is associated with an increased risk of fibroids, possibly due to the relative oestrogen excess created by production of non-ovarian oestrogen in fatty tissue.

Use of oral contraceptives

Studies which have investigated the Pill and fibroid incidence have been inconclusive with some studies showing a reduced incidence;[23] one study showing a slightly increased rate (not statistically significant);[24] and two others finding no change.[25]

Smoking

Smokers tend to develop fibroids *less* often.[26] In one study, current smokers were shown to have a 40 per cent lower incidence of fibroids than non-smokers.[27]

Diagnosis

A fibroid could be suspected if the following signs and symptoms are present.

- Heavy bleeding at the time of menstruation.
- Dragging, congestive pain in the lower abdomen at the time of menstruation and premenstrually.
- An enlarged and bulky uterus discovered during a pelvic examination by the doctor.
- A lower abdominal mass discovered by the woman or her doctor.

An ultrasound scan is used to diagnose uterine fibroids. They will show up as masses in or attached to the uterus: their number, size and position can often be precisely determined. An ultrasound is also frequently used to monitor the size and growth-rate of fibroids. Some doctors will also want to perform a laparoscopy to absolutely establish that the pelvic mass visible with the ultrasound is a fibroid. This is particularly the case if the ovaries cannot be clearly seen as ovarian cysts or cancer can sometimes be mistaken for uterine fibroids.

■ ■
■ ■ The medical approach

There are three main options for the management of fibroids.

- Observe, but do not treat.
- Surgical removal involving a hysterectomy or a myomectomy, see Chapter 20 'Drugs and surgery'.
- Drugs to reduce the size of fibroids prior to surgery. These drugs have two different effects, but the overall aim is to reduce the level of oestrogen. The drugs used are Danazol, to produce a predominance of androgens and suppression of oestrogens; and GnRH agonists, which induce a medical menopause.

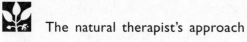 The natural therapist's approach

The treatment of fibroids aims to:

- regulate excess bleeding
- reduce 'relative oestrogen excess'
- contain or reduce the size of the fibroid.

Abnormal bleeding

It is often surprisingly easy to reduce the excessive bleeding associated with fibroids and this may be all that is required. Women who have passed their child-bearing years, those with small fibroids, or those women for whom surgery is not an option may find that this simple approach to managing the fibroid is satisfactory.

All of the herbs mentioned in the treatment of functional menorrhagia, *Trillium erectum*, *Equisetum arvense*, *Achillea millefolium*, *Panax notoginseng*, *Capsella bursa-pastoris*, and *Hydrastis canadensis* are appropriate. Astringents are usually combined with one or more of the uterine tonic herbs to improve the uterine tone and try to normalise uterine function.

Of the nutrients, the bioflavonoids are the most useful for bleeding associated with fibroids. Iron is recommended for anaemia or low serum ferritin, and may also improve bleeding.

Relative oestrogen excess

It is possible to contain or reduce the growth-promoting effects of oestrogen. The main way this is achieved herbally is via competitive inhibition. Other methods, many without scientific trials to verify their efficacy, are also used. Considering the number of women who develop fibroids, the research on treatment and prevention is disappointingly sparse.

In one of the few trials using medicinal herbs to treat fibroids, the herbs *Paeonia lactiflora* and *suffruticosa*, *Poria cocos*, *Cinnamomum cassia*, and *Prunus persica* were given to 110 pre-menopausal women with uterine fibroids. Ninety per cent of the women experienced an improvement of their symptoms and in 60 per cent of the cases, the fibroids were reduced in size.[28] The same formula known as Cinnamon and Hoelen Combination also reduced adenomyosis,[29] another oestrogen-dependent condition, in mice.

It is important to regulate relative oestrogen excess because women who have the tendency to grow fibroids can do so again after the fibroid has been removed or adequately treated, or they may continue to produce multiple fibroids if the hormonal imbalance is not corrected.

All conditions related to relative oestrogen excess seem to respond to the same sorts of treatment and the principles for improving oestrogen clearance are discussed in Chapter 5 'Maintaining hormonal balance'.

Other fibroid treatments

Herbs used to treat fibroids and reduce their size are *Calendula officinalis*, *Thuja occidentalis*, *Ruta graveolens*, and *Turnera diffusa*. Vitamin E is believed to reduce fibroid size, but the reasons for this are unclear.

 Self care

Uterine fibroids are related to relative oestrogen excess. The self-care strategies to reduce this imbalance are discussed in Chapter 15 'Endometriosis and adenomyosis'.

Preventing anaemia is also important and information on iron can be found below.

THE IMPORTANCE OF IRON

Iron and iron deficiency anaemia

Iron requirements for women are around 80 per cent higher than for men because of menstruation and child-bearing. It is estimated that iron deficiency is the commonest nutritional disease worldwide and that more than half of all women consume less than the recommended amount of 10–15 mg daily.

Those at most risk for developing iron deficiency are:

- pregnant women
- women with heavy menstrual loss
- children
- vegetarians
- frequent dieters
- those who are on strict exclusion diets
- those with low gastric acid levels such as occurs after stomach surgery and with ageing
- those who do not have access to good quality food e.g. due to poverty and famine

Iron deficiency vs anaemia

Iron is stored in the body in places other than in the red blood cells. These include the liver, bone marrow, spleen, muscles and in the serum. A test for anaemia will determine whether there is a depletion

---

of iron stored in the red blood cells (the haemoglobin level), but not whether iron stores elsewhere in the body are at sufficient levels.

It is now known that the symptoms of iron deficiency can exist before the red blood cells become depleted of iron and that a considerable number of people are iron deficient even though their haemoglobin is normal. For this reason, many doctors now order a blood test to check both iron stores (in the serum) and haemoglobin levels since haemoglobin alone is an unreliable indicator of the true status of iron in the body.

Symptoms of anaemia and iron deficiency

Many of the symptoms of *anaemia* are related to the inability of the red blood cells to carry oxygen around the body because they lack iron. These include:

- poor stamina
- shortness of breath on exertion
- unreasonable limb fatigue
- dizziness

Other symptoms seem to be related to the lack of iron in the serum, called *iron deficiency*. These might include:

- a red sore tongue and cracks in the corners of the mouth
- concave fingernails
- reduced resistance to infection, particularly in children
- also in children, a failure to thrive, slow learning and poor appetite
- poor digestion caused by low gastric acid levels. Iron deficiency can be both a cause of decreased production of gastric acid and can be itself caused by low gastric acid.

Improving iron absorption

Apart from increasing the amount of available iron in the diet, there are a number of other ways to increase iron levels.

- Eat Vitamin C rich foods, particularly when consuming foods high in iron.
- Add acidic dressings, such as lemon juice and vinegar, to iron rich foods. This is a common Southern Mediterranean practice, where there is a high incidence of inherited anaemia and the traditional diet contains little red meat.
- Eat bitter vegetables or fruit before or during the meal to increase the flow of gastric acid which will in turn improve the absorption of minerals. Alcoholic aperitifs, grapefruit, Swedish bitters and bitter green vegetables can all be used. Bitter vegetables are best

because they usually contain iron as well as stimulate its absorption.

- When low gastric acid levels are accompanied by iron deficiency, taking iron may improve both.
- Avoid tea (especially black tea) or coffee until the iron deficiency improves. The tannin in tea binds with iron making it difficult to absorb. Coffee also reduces absorption, especially if taken with or after a meal, but not when taken more than one hour before eating. Don't take iron tablets with a cup of tea or coffee.

Detecting low iron stores

Iron deficiency causes the symptoms described above and should respond to a low-dose iron supplement. Iron should not be taken unnecessarily as it will accumulate in the body and may become toxic. If symptoms do not respond, seek advice and ask for a blood test which evaluates serum iron levels.

Table 11.1 Sources of iron (mg per 100 g)

RDA 10–15 mg/day

Meat, fish and eggs

eggs	2.0	light chicken meat	0.6
beef, lean	3.4	cod	0.4
lamb, lean	2.7	sardines	2.4
pork, lean	1.3	mussels	7.7
dark chicken meat	1.9	oysters	6.0

Grains

wheat germ	10.0	whole wheat bread	2.5
wheat bran	12.9	All Bran™	12.0
whole wheat flour	4.0	Special K™	20.0
raw oatmeal	4.1	Weetbix™	7.6
soya flour	9.1	rye biscuits	3.7
white bread	1.7		

Legumes and vegetables

haricot beans	2.5	spring onions	1.2
broccoli tops	1.0	parsley, raw	8.0
leeks	2.0	peas	1.2
lentils	2.4	potatoes, jacket	0.6
lettuce	0.9	spinach	3.4
mushrooms, raw	1.0	silver beet	3.0

Fruits

apricots, fresh	0.4	peaches, dried	6.8
apricots, dried	4.1	prunes	2.9
avocado	1.5	prunes, stewed	1.4
currants	1.8	raisins	1.6
figs, dried	4.2	raspberries	1.2
dates	1.6	sultanas	1.8

Other

almonds	4.2	walnuts	2.4
brazil nuts	2.8	curry powder	75.0
hazel nuts	1.1	yeast	20.0
peanuts	2.0		

12

Erratic bleeding

Key words

adaptogen
adenomyosis
anovulatory
biopsy
diagnostic D&C
follicle-stimulating
  hormone (FSH)
haemostasis
hyperplasia
hypothalamic–pituitary–
  ovarian axis

hysteroscopy
luteal phase
luteinising hormone
  (LH)
menorrhagia
mittelschmerz
nervine
peri-menopause
prostaglandins
spiral arterioles
steroidal saponins

Bleeding between periods is often not a problem—caused by hormonal changes at ovulation or by benign lesions on the cervix—but it *could* be caused by cancer, and until that possibility has been investigated and eliminated as the cause, no treatment should be undertaken.

Women sometimes dismiss slight bleeding as trivial; as a mild inconvenience which will 'probably just go away'. But paradoxically, it is the slight bleeding that can be most suggestive of cancer or other serious pathologies: any bleeding between periods, therefore, should be given the same diagnostic priority as a breast lump.

COMMON CAUSES OF BLEEDING BETWEEN PERIODS

1. Dysfunctional uterine bleeding (DUB)

Dysfunctional uterine bleeding is associated with disturbance in the body's hormonal control and feed-back centre in the hypothalamic–

---

pituitary unit. Bleeding is erratic and unpredictable and often associated with failure to ovulate. The dysfunction may be chronic and persistent, or a transient event which lasts for one cycle.

2. Endometrial hyperplasia

This is a condition where the endometrial cells are excessively stimulated by prolonged exposure to oestrogen without sufficient counter-balancing from progesterone. Failure to ovulate is the usual cause. Endometrial hyperplasia can only be diagnosed if a sample of tissue is taken and examined under a microscope. This is usually performed with a hysteroscope or a D&C, both of which usually require a general anaesthetic. The condition can be pre-cancerous in older women. Common symptoms are irregular bleeding, spotting, and/or heavy, persistent flow.

3. Uterine cancer

Cancer of the endometrium is most frequent in women over 40. It is characterised by abnormal or recurrent bleeding between periods, after sex or after the menopause. In this age group, these symptoms should always be investigated irrespective of how scant and transient.

4. Polyps

A polyp is an overgrowth of tissue, which is attached by a stem or pedicle. Gynaecological polyps might originate from the cervix or endometrium. The cells of the polyp are often normal, but can bleed easily or cause pain due to their position. Contact bleeding i.e. bleeding after sexual activity or examination by a doctor, is a common symptom. Women over 40 with cervical polyps may also have endometrial polyps.

5. Abnormalities of the cervix

Abnormalities of the cervix can cause bleeding and/or pain.

i) *Cervical eversion/ectropion*
If the cells which normally line the cervical canal grow down and onto the outer areas of the cervix the abnormally situated tissue is called a cervical ectropion or eversion. These cells are more friable than the usual cells of the cervix and usually bleed more easily, especially on contact.

ii) *Cervical dysplasia and cancer*
Both cervical cancer and dysplasia are detected with a Pap smear. Cervical dysplasia is a pre-cancerous condition which indicates that

the cells are changing and may eventually become cancerous if left untreated. Dysplasia is a common disease of women between the ages of 30 and 40; cervical cancer is more common amongst women in their fifties. Both conditions cause few symptoms, and by the time bleeding has developed, the course of the condition can be quite advanced.

iii) Cervicitis

This is inflammation of the cells of the cervix, usually from chronic infection. Discharge is a common symptom which may be accompanied by pain or contain brownish blood and have an offensive odour.

6. Conditions affecting the ovaries

Conditions affecting the ovaries present less frequently as abnormal bleeding. Usually pain is the initial symptom.

i) Ovarian cysts

Ovarian cysts are sacs of fluid in the ovary. They may be 'physiological' (a consequence of the normal ovarian cycle), they may be benign, or occasionally cancerous. Some cysts can be associated with abnormal bleeding patterns.

ii) Ovulation

Some women experience spotting with or without pain (mittelschmerz) with normal ovulation. The bleeding is presumed to be caused by the oestrogen changes at mid-cycle. If this is a new symptom it should be investigated.

7. Contraceptive causes

i) Hormonal contraceptives

The combined (oestrogen and progesterone) Pill; the sequential Pill (pills containing oestrogen and progesterone which are varied throughout the cycle); the Mini Pill (progesterone only) and Depo-Provera (an injection of slowly absorbed progestogen) can all be associated with abnormal bleeding patterns.

8. Metabolic causes

i) Malnutrition or excess weight loss

This may be due to chronic illness, unavailable food, inadequate food, dietary extremes (anorexia or bulimia nervosa) or excessive exercise. Usually menstruation stops, although infrequent and heavier periods may be the consequence.

9. Pregnancy and bleeding

i) Placental malfunction
Bleeding can occur as a result of placental malfunction, and is of three main types.

- Bleeding associated with abnormal development of the placenta and often foetus.
- Bleeding associated with a normally developing placenta, which is situated in the wrong place. This is referred to as a 'placenta praevia'.
- Bleeding associated with a normal placenta which dislodges from the uterine wall prematurely. This is called an 'accidental haemorrhage' and is associated with considerable pain.

ii) Hydatidiform mole
This results from products of conception which lack an intact foetus. The tissue secretes large amounts of human chorionic gonadotrophin (HCG) hormone which usually causes severe 'morning sickness'. Often heavy bleeding starts about 10–12 weeks into the pregnancy, but will generally continue until all the hydatidiform mole is expelled. As this tissue can become cancerous, most women have a D&C to ensure that all the tissue is removed, and have hormonal (HCG) monitoring for another year.

iii) Ectopic pregnancy
An ectopic pregnancy refers to a pregnancy which has started to develop outside the uterus. If the pregnancy develops in the tube, the increasing size may cause tubal rupture. This can be very serious and requires immediate surgery.

iv) Implantation bleeds
Some women experience bleeding at the time the fertilised ovum implants into the endometrium. As this often occurs at or around the time of the expected period, it can be confused with a light period.

DYSFUNCTIONAL UTERINE BLEEDING (DUB)

DUB, like functional menorrhagia, is a disorder of function, but in this case there is an additional problem with the hormone balance. The reproductive tract remains essentially normal, although the endometrium may not show secretory (progesterone-related) changes. The disorder usually originates from a disorder of the hypothalamic–pituitary unit.

Causes of DUB

In many cases of DUB, ovulation does not occur normally, or fails entirely. This leads to an imbalance in the hormones—oestrogen is still produced, but progesterone production is either far too low or entirely absent. This results in unopposed oestrogenic stimulation of the endometrium ('unopposed' refers to the lack of normal amounts of progesterone) and leads to the characteristic bleeding patterns—an erratic cycle, no obvious signs of ovulation, and irregular or prolonged episodes of bleeding.

In the normal course of events, oestrogen is accompanied (opposed) by progesterone, and it is primarily the progesterone production and withdrawal that maintains the regularity of the endometrial shedding (and therefore the period). When ovulation does not occur, oestrogen continues to stimulate the endometrial cells which grow and thicken. However, the absence of progesterone means that the endometrium does not develop the usual structural features of the secretory phase, including the spiral arterioles. Their function is to nourish the endometrium and to control blood loss once menstruation commences.

Without the development of these blood vessels, circulation throughout the thickened endometrium is incomplete and eventually fails; and the tissue becomes fragile and starts to break down. This does not occur uniformly throughout the endometrium—some sections are shed while others remain intact, resulting in the spotting and erratic blood loss characteristic of the condition.

In a normal cycle, the usual mechanisms for slowing the blood loss are shared by prostaglandins and spasm of the spiral arterioles. With these structures being absent, haemostasis is impaired and excessive flooding can occur. This type of DUB is most common when regular ovulation is at its most fragile: amongst teenage women who have just started to menstruate and around the menopause. It can also be a feature of any condition where ovulation does not occur such as after stress, but can occur in relation to other less common conditions, such as thyroid disease and androgen excess.

Diagnosis

As with functional menorrhagia, the diagnosis of DUB is a diagnosis of exclusion and examinations are performed to eliminate other conditions as the cause of bleeding.

Signs and symptoms highly suggestive of DUB are:

- The age of the woman
  Women who are establishing their normal cyclical pattern at the

menarche, and women whose cycles are slowing down around menopause are more likely to develop anovulatory DUB.

- Normal uterine size and normal cervix
Because spotting is a feature of cervical conditions, a healthy cervix is unlikely to be causing inter-menstrual or premenstrual bleeding. Uterine size and shape will change if the woman has fibroids or adenomyosis which are common causes of heavy menstruation.
- A recent history of persistent or severe stress
Ovulatory failure or disrupted progesterone production can occur after stress because of the effect on the hypothalamic-pituitary function.
- A negative pregnancy test
Pregnancy-related bleeding is the most common cause of abnormal menstrual patterns amongst women who are sexually active.
- No pain during either a vaginal examination or abdominal palpation
Pelvic inflammatory disease and endometriosis are two conditions which can cause symptoms similar to DUB, however they are both usually accompanied by pain during an examination.

■ ■
■ ■ The medical approach

The treatment for DUB is similar to that described for functional menorrhagia. A synthetic progesterone (e.g. Provera or Primolut) is used to try to interrupt the abnormal hormonal pattern and regulate the cycle. Usually a D&C or hysteroscopy is performed for older women to determine whether the bleeding is caused by endometrial hyperplasia or cancer.

 The natural therapist's approach

The treatment of DUB is based on a multi-faceted approach which aims to:

- re-establish ovulation
- support the luteal phase of the cycle
- treat stress where appropriate
- utilise all or any of the treatments for functional menorrhagia as necessary

At the menarche, the occurrence of erratic cycles is so common that it is usually thought of as being physiological—in other words, a normal feature of the physiology of this age group. For this reason, young women with dysfunctional bleeding patterns *do not* normally require any treatment unless the bleeding is particularly severe and causing other problems. Herbal remedies which are appropriate for bleeding experienced around the menarche are *Achillea millefolium, Equisetum arvense, Rubus idaeus* and *Alchemilla vulgaris*.

Ovulation

In order to re-establish ovulation, it is first necessary to identify the reason it stopped. This may be related to the stage of the menstrual cycle, that is, around menopause or the menarche; or ovulation may temporarily stop because of stress, over-exercising, low body weight or a poor quality diet. Sometimes the exact cause is unknown (idiopathic).

(Ovulatory failure can be related to other more complex hormonal irregularities which involve other endocrine glands such as the thyroid or the adrenal gland; or to a major disruption in ovarian function, as is seen in polycystic ovaries; or to abnormal activity of the hypothalamic-pituitary unit, such as hyperprolactinaemia. These conditions are treated by rectifying the abnormal function of the endocrine gland/s involved.)

There is a long herbal history of the use of 'female tonics' to re-establish normal bleeding patterns. These are assumed to have regulatory effects on the hormonal axis and ovulation, but as yet, the mechanisms by which this occurs are largely unknown. Many of these herbs contain steroidal saponins which may interact with the hypothalamus or the pituitary to re-establish ovulation. The important tonic herbs are *Chamaelirium luteum, Angelica sinensis, Cimicifuga racemosa* and *Aletris farinosa*.

A combination of *Chamaelirium luteum* and *Vitex agnus castus* is commonly used to treat DUB. *Vitex agnus castus* has been shown to stimulate ovulation,[1] and is specific to problems of the luteal phase of the cycle and hypothalamic-pituitary function. *Chamaelirium luteum* is the herb of choice for the first half of the cycle and for regulating ovarian function. Since DUB is primarily a relative progesterone deficiency due to an irregularity of ovulation, this is usually an effective combination.

Vitex agnus castus can be used for menstrual irregularity associated with menopause, but in this case is it more favourably combined with *Cimicifuga racemosa*. It is unwise for women to self-medicate with *Vitex agnus castus* because it can *cause* menstrual irregularity if incorrectly administered.

Aletris farinosa and *Angelica sinensis* are both Warming adaptogens for the reproductive organs and have similar effects on ovarian function to *Chamaelirium luteum*. *Cimicifuga racemosa*, slightly Cooler than the other two, is sedative, oestrogenic, adaptogenic and is the herb of choice for peri-menopausal complaints.

The luteal phase

Vitex agnus castus is the primary herb for problems associated with the luteal phase. Trials have verified its use in DUB, endometrial hyperplasia, anovulatory cycles and polymenorrhoea.[2] It should be started as close as possible to day one and continued throughout the whole menstrual cycle including the period. A three-month course is usually necessary and some women may need longer courses to regulate ovulatory patterns. *Vitex* is usually given as a single morning dose of 2 mL of fluid extract.

Although Vitamin B_6 is useful to control symptoms associated with premenstrual hormone irregularities, there is no evidence that it will rectify the causes of DUB. Even so, vitamin B_6 is a useful medication when troubling PMS-type symptoms are associated with the abnormal bleeding pattern, and can be used either alone or in combination with B Complex.

The usual dose of B_6 is 50–100 mg twice daily for 7–10 days before the period, although some authors suggest that doses between 150–200 mg daily are more beneficial.[3] Vitamin B_6 is relatively safe, but there may be side effects at higher doses and the lowest dose that gives the best therapeutic response is recommended.

The nervous system

Nervines are important in the treatment of DUB because of the effect of stress on the hormonal axis. Any of the herbs in these categories will have a beneficial effect, however the nervines which have additional hormone-regulating effects are clinically superior. These include *Hypericum perforatum*, *Leonurus cardiaca* and *Verbena officinalis*.

Nervine herbs can be either Cooling, Warming or neutral. In general, Warming nervines are useful for lack of vitality and debility (*Matricaria chamomilla*, *Verbena officinalis*, *Leonurus cardiaca*, and Cooling nervines have a more sedating effect (*Hypericum perforatum*, *Humulus lupulus*, *Bupleurum falcatum*).

Uterine tone

Trillium erectum contains saponins (plant hormone-like substance) which seem to be capable of regulating both the blood flow and the hormone balance. This herb is considered to be 'specific' to the treatment of DUB which is caused by failure to ovulate, and can regulate both cycle length and menstrual loss within 1–3 cycles. It is often prescribed with *Vitex agnus castus*.

 Self care

The dietary advice outlined for functional menorrhagia is important. It is also necessary to minimise stress because, apart from anything else, erratic and heavy bleeding is stressful in itself and the worry associated with the implications of the symptoms may feed into the stress cycle and worsen the symptoms. Stress management, including 'long slow distance' exercise is discussed in Chapter 10 'The usual suspects'.

ENDOMETRIAL HYPERPLASIA

'Endometrial hyperplasia' refers to overgrown tissue in the uterus and the term is made up of the Greek *endon* meaning within; *metra*—uterus; *hyper*—more than normal; and the Latin *plasia* meaning a tendency to build up tissue.

Endometrial hyperplasia occurs for much the same reasons as dysfunctional uterine bleeding—there is prolonged or excessive stimulation of the endometrial cells by oestrogen—but in this case, the hormonal imbalance causes the cells to change and become overgrown. It can cause erratic bleeding in pre- or post-menopausal women. Other mechanisms may include an abnormal oestrogen metabolism, or obesity.

The *hyperplastic* cells can progress through a range of changes from mildly overgrown and easily treated through to endometrial cancer. A diagnosis is made by taking a biopsy during a hysteroscopy under a general or local anaesthetic. The endometrial cells are examined and graded according to the degree of change from normal to abnormal, usually with a three-stage grading of mild, moderate and serious (often called simple, complex and atypical). Cystic hyperplasia is another term used for the least advanced (simple) form of endometrial hyperplasia.

Once the change in the endometrium has been graded, a treatment is decided upon which will take in to account the severity of the endometrial change, the age of the woman, and whether she expects to become pregnant or not.

It is important to identify the underlying causes of endometrial hyperplasia. These include ovulatory failure secondary to conditions like polycystic ovarian disease, thyroid disease, and ovarian and adrenal tumours. Relative oestrogen excess can occur as a result of obesity and diabetes. Other risk factors for developing endometrial hyperplasia include an early menarche, late menopause, never being pregnant and taking oestrogens without progestogens.

■ ■

■ ■ The medical approach

The aim of treatment is to remove the abnormal tissue and then establish cyclic shedding of the endometrium—initially with drugs. The affected endometrium is removed with a D&C when the hysteroscopy is performed. This will not 'cure' the condition unless the hormonal causes of the endometrial hyperplasia are also dealt with.

To rectify the abnormal hormonal pattern, gynaecologists usually recommend synthetic hormones to simulate a hormonal pattern similar to the normal menstrual cycle. Usually, a progestogen is given by tablet for between ten and twenty days so that the endometrium develops the cells and structures similar to those of the luteal phase, and afterwards, the drug is stopped to allow 'menstruation' to occur. Ovulation often starts spontaneously after a few cycles on progestogens. The reasons for this are not known.

Progestogens are not suitable for women who are actively trying to become pregnant at the time of treatment. When pregnancy is desired, ovulation is often stimulated by short courses of drugs like Clomid. Women taking this drug must be monitored closely because of the risk of hyper-stimulation of the ovary and ovarian cysts.

Endometrial hyperplasia does not always become endometrial cancer, but the risk increases if the degree of cellular change is advanced. Between 1–4 per cent of women with the mildest form—simple or cystic hyperplasia—can develop endometrial cancer; but more than 20 per cent of women progress to cancer if they have the most advanced form.[4]

About ten per cent of all cases of post-menopausal bleeding are caused by endometrial hyperplasia (up to 20 per cent are caused by cancer). This figure increases when women are obese or are given oestrogen without progesterone. When oestrogen is given alone, cell changes occur because the endometrium is continually stimulated by oestrogen without the counterbalancing effect of progesterone.

 The natural therapist's approach

Endometrial hyperplasia is always diagnosed by a medical practitioner. Usually, the same doctor will administer medical treatment, but occasionally a woman will seek the advice of a natural therapist either because she is inclined towards natural treatments whenever possible, or because she fears the side effects of the drugs her doctor has suggested. Endometrial hyperplasia presents specific difficulties in treatment because a pre-cancerous condition has already developed along with the failure to ovulate and shed the endometrium regularly. This condition should always be managed by herbalists and natural therapists with experience in the treatment of the complaint.

A natural therapist's treatment will be similar to that for DUB, but with one major difference: regular cyclic menstruation must be re-established, and with some speed. Even in the mildest forms (cystic hyperplasia), ovulation should be established within the first two cycles; sooner is always better than later.

This can be difficult. Most natural remedies are not capable of stimulating ovulation irrespective of the underlying cause. Some medicinal herbs can regulate the cycle by re-establishing ovulation, but will often fail unless the original cause for ovulatory failure has also been treated. For example, if a woman has developed endometrial hyperplasia because of an underactive thyroid, the treatment will need to be directed toward thyroid gland regulation. Often, ovulation will be delayed for too long (and hence menstruation), and the woman will be at risk in the interim.

A decision to treat with natural remedies should only be made after careful evaluation of all of the risks and benefits for that particular woman. Being over 40, obesity, or having one of the more severe forms of endometrial hyperplasia, should all be considered reasons for *not* using natural therapies. In many cases, the most practical suggestion is for the woman to follow her doctor's advice.

When a decision has been made to treat endometrial hyperplasia, the regime is similar to that outlined for DUB with additional emphasis on:

- re-establishing ovulation *and* menstruation
- protecting the endometrium with phyto-oestrogens which counter the effects of unopposed oestrogens, and anti-oxidants which minimise the risk of the hyperplastic changes becoming cancerous.

Ovulation

When endometrial hyperplasia is mild, the adaptogens, remedies that are capable of returning physiological functioning to normal—in this case ovulation—can be used. This is particularly so if the ovulatory failure is due to stress, a temporarily inadequate diet, or if the woman is approaching menopause. In these instances, it is desirable that return to a normal cycle be achieved within two cycles.

More complex conditions, such as thyroid or adrenal gland disease, or polycystic ovarian disease may take much longer to regulate than is safe for the woman concerned. In these cases, the risks associated with a prolonged anovulatory state are more serious than the proposed medical treatment. A more suitable role for natural remedies may be after medical treatment and could involve the maintenance of normal menstrual patterns, reducing the effects of unopposed oestrogens, and reducing risk factors for cancerous change.

If herbs are to be used to re-establish ovulation, *Chamaelirium luteum*, *Angelica sinensis*, *Cimicifuga racemosa*, *Aletris farinosa* and *Vitex agnus castus* are the important remedies to consider.

Linseeds, which contain phyto-oestrogenic lignans, are also important for women with endometrial hyperplasia. Linseed supplements improved menstrual regularity and ovulation rates amongst women given 10 gms ground linseed daily.[5] The researchers also found that the oestrogen:progesterone ratio improved in favour of progesterone, probably as a result of the improved oestrogen clearance and reduced bio-availability of oestrogens seen when high levels of fibre and phyto-oestrogenic foods are consumed regularly. Linseeds can be suggested after medical treatment for the prevention of endometrial hyperplasia because of their dual effects on lowering oestrogen and improving ovulation.

Menstruation

Sometimes, when regulating ovulatory patterns is not possible, or not possible quickly, herbs can be used which will cause menstruation to occur. These are chosen from the group of herbs called the emmena-gogues.

All emmenagogues are abortifacients, and so due care is needed with their use. They are quite powerful and can cause some unpleasant effects in the wrong hands. They must be prescribed within a definite dose range, and it is necessary to make sure that pregnancy has not occurred prior to their administration. This group of herbs should only be prescribed by an experienced practitioner.

As is the experience of many traditional herbalists, Dr Weiss, a German herbalist and doctor, remarks on the use of the emmenagogues for restoring menstruation:

> . . . medicinal plants get very good results in secondary amenorrhoea and in oligomenorrhoea (no periods or infrequent periods). Hormone therapy is much to the fore in this field, but there are considerable problems; hormone therapy calls for sophisticated techniques and in many cases fails to get results. Medicinal herbs therefore continue to have their place . . . Emmenagogues were very popular before hormone therapy. There remains the fact, based on experience, that emmena-gogues will often restore normal menstrual flow and give very considerable subjective relief.[6]

The popular and reliable emmenagogues are *Ruta graveolens* and *Artemesia vulgaris*. They will usually need to be prescribed for several months until regular menstruation is established. Hormone-regulating herbs can be used at the same time.

Protecting the endometrium

The plant oestrogens occur naturally in foods and herbs and when consumed as part of a normal diet have the potential to protect the tissues from over-stimulation by oestrogens. Medicinal herbs containing steroidal saponins can also be used. Trained herbalists follow traditional guidelines to treat this type of abnormal bleeding. They use specific herbs for the optimum period of time, and prescribe only those medic-inal plants which have historically been used for menstrual disorders of this type. The most important of these is *Trillium erectum*.

Other herbs used include the astringent herbs, *Achillea millefolium* and *Capsella bursa-pastoris* (which contains the same cancer-preventative agents as the cabbage family vegetables).

Numerous studies have been undertaken worldwide to evaluate the effectiveness of the anti-oxidants as protective agents against cancer, or as therapeutic substances in the treatment of cancer. Although there is no definitive evidence, a number of these studies have demonstrated a protective role for some of the anti-oxidants. The effects on the endometrium may prevent endometrial hyperplasia from becoming a cancerous condition. Those shown to have a protective effect are the Vitamins A, E, K and C, beta-carotene and the mineral selenium.

Selenium and Vitamin E seem to work best when adequate levels of both are present in the body. When comparing the blood levels of these two nutrients, one study showed that women with endometrial tumours had 40 per cent less selenium and 23 per cent less Vitamin E than their female relatives who lived in the same household.[7] Selenium-containing foods are garlic, whole grains, meat, eggs, brewer's yeast and fish.

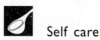 Self care

Improving the regularity of ovulation may be necessary and the type of intervention will depend on the reason why ovulation has stopped. Stress and diet are often important factors. Excessive exercise; BMI below the recommended levels; many drugs (both prescribed or social); alcohol consumption, cocaine and other recreational drugs; and excessive amounts of coffee can all affect ovulation. These factors are discussed in Chapter 10 'The usual suspects'.

Protective foods can be included in the diet as a means of reducing the risk of developing cancer. Healthy colonies of gut bacteria are needed to convert dietary phyto-oestrogens into the active forms needed for the competitive inhibition of oestrogen-binding sites. Yoghurt encourages healthy levels of gut bacteria and may improve conversion of inert lignans into the active forms.

ABNORMALITIES OF THE CERVIX AND SPOTTING

Bleeding from the cervix is often slight, erratic and painless. Sometimes the discharge doesn't resemble blood at all, but is brownish or like stained fluid. It can occur at any time during the cycle, and is more common after sexual activity or examination by a doctor. Many of the common causes of cervical bleeding are not related to cancer and are easily treated. Bleeding caused by cancer of the cervix is less common when women have regular Pap smears.

Cervical eversion

The tissue which lines the inner cervical canal (columnar epithelium) is very delicate in comparison to the tissue lining the vagina and the outer surface of the cervix (squamous epithelium). The junction of the columnar and squamous epithelium is called the transitory zone and is usually situated just at, or just inside the cervical canal.

Cervical eversion occurs when the transitory zone is located on the outer surface of the cervix, leaving much more of the friable columnar epithelium on view and prone to bleed on contact.

Columnar epithelium is normally visible at the cervical opening during adolescence and pregnancy. Women who take the Pill also commonly develop cervical eversion. DES daughters (DES = diethylstilboestrol—a synthetic oestrogen) are sometimes born with a 'congenital' eversion, and can develop a cervical eversion that extends into the vagina. Some doctors also blame irritation from the string attached to an IUD, but this is disputed.

Cervical eversion usually causes few problems and is often discovered at a routine Pap smear. Sometimes the eversion causes an increase in vaginal secretions and the area becomes infected, but sometimes the eversion is *caused* by an infection. When there is an infection in the cervical canal, the swollen membranes are inclined to protrude from the cervical opening. In severe cases and when infection is present, the tissue becomes angry, red and looks unhealthy. Contact bleeding (especially bleeding after sex) is common and an offensive and/or blood-stained discharge may be present.

The bleeding associated with cervical eversion will alter depending on the associated complaints and the amount of blood lost. Slight bleeding may be brownish and thin or sticky. After sexual contact, the bleeding may be heavier and brighter. Cervicitis will often cause the bleeding to be yellowish or brown and offensive.

■ ■

■ ■ The medical approach

Regular monitoring of the cervical eversion is desirable, and some women may have to stop the Pill. Occasionally, the area is treated with diathermy or laser treatment, especially if inflammation or infection are a problem.

 The natural therapist's approach

Local astringent remedies which improve the tone and strength of the mucus membranes, treat secondary infection and stop bleeding are used for cervical eversion. Cervical eversion is considered to be associated with Heat and Moistness, and the remedies chosen are Cooling and Drying.

- *Hydrastis canadensis* is the herb of choice, either in the form of a cream, pessary, or wash. Treatment needs to be continued until all inflammation has reduced. (A repeat speculum examination is warranted.)
- *Calendula officinalis* also in the form of a wash, cream or pessary is also useful. *Phytolacca decandra*, as a combination pessary with *Calendula officinalis* is popular in Europe.
- Agents such as tea tree oil are far too harsh, and should never be used for this condition in dilutions stronger than 1:20 (5 per cent), irrespective of the severity of the secondary infection. A cream containing 5 per cent tea tree oil, 10 per cent hydrastis and 10 per cent calendula in an aqueous or Vitamin E base is useful when applied to the cervix.

Women who are taking the Pill, and who would like to continue to do so, may find that their symptoms are helped with folic acid and B complex vitamins. The reasons for this are not clear, but may be related to improvement of the underlying hormonal triggers.

Cervicitis

Cervicitis is an inflammation or infection that affects the cervix. It is usually caused by bacteria, although the type is not always identified. Often the woman is run-down or her vaginal environment is altered sufficiently for opportunistic infections to develop. The diagnosis is usually on the basis of an offensive or blood-stained vaginal discharge and pain on moving the cervix, either during sex or when the cervix is examined.

■ ■

■ ■ The medical approach

Cervicitis is often treated with antibiotic creams, and in some cases, oral antibiotics as well. Creams and pessaries are inserted at night to keep the medication near the cervix.

  The natural therapist's approach

Astringent and antiseptic creams, pessaries or douches are used for cervicitis. Creams and pessaries which are inserted at night are favoured because they stay in contact with the cervix for longer. The herbs *Hydrastis canadensis*, *Calendula officinalis* and tea-tree oil are effective in the treatment of cervicitis.

Echinacea angustifolia or *E. purperea* can be taken for long-term and recurrent infections, and to support a weakened immune system when the woman is run-down and unable to fight off trivial infections.

ABNORMAL TISSUE TONE

Healthy tissue in the human body forms a barrier between the inner structures of the body and the outside world. When the tissue becomes unhealthy, either through abrasions, poor diet or age, it forms a less efficient barrier, allowing noxious (often infectious) material to pass into the body and the normal body fluids to pass out.

This is an important concept in natural medicine since the integrity, strength and tone of all tissues throughout the body are believed to have marked effects on an individual's ability to maintain health. As examples, a breach in tissue tone of the mucus membranes of the respiratory tract may contribute to hayfever; and poor tissue tone of the cervix can cause infections and discharges such as cervicitis.

Poor tissue tone is treated with herbal astringents—agents which are applied directly to the tissues to 'tighten' and improve the integrity of the barrier between the tissues and the outside world. Creams, pessaries or washes of herbs such as *Calendula officinalis* and *Hydrastis canadensis*, are astringent, anti-microbial, anti-inflammatory and healing to the mucus membranes.

Abnormal tissue tone may also be a feature (but not the cause) of a wide variety of serious cervical pathologies including cervical cancers and *identification of the condition must first be obtained before any treatment is instituted*.

13

Amenorrhoea and oligomenorrhoea

Key words

androgen
androgenic alopecia
dihydrotestosterone
dopamine
galactorrhoea
hyperthecosis
hirsutism
hyperprolactinaemia
imperforate hymen
latent
  hyperprolactinaemia

pilo-sebaceous unit
pituitary
  microadenoma
polycystic ovarian
  disease
primary amenhorrhoea
prolactin
secondary amenorrhoea
vaginal septum
virilisation

The absence of menstruation in a woman during the usual menstruating years for more than six months is called amenorrhoea. This is not a diagnosis, but a symptom of another condition. It can be caused by a wide range of other hormonal, physical and metabolic conditions and the most complex aspect of treating amenorrhoea is to establish the exact cause for the absent period.

Needless to say, treatment should only proceed after identifying the underlying problem. Otherwise a serious condition might remain unidentified—conditions like polycystic ovarian disease or elevated prolactin levels, which commonly cause amenorrhoea, are often not accompanied by any other obvious signs. Alternatively, a pregnancy might be deliberately or accidentally missed and herbs used to 'bring on the period' could result in a dangerous situation for the woman and a difficult problem for the practitioner.

Amenorrhoea is usually divided into two types for the purposes of diagnosis and treatment.

Primary amenorrhoea

- Where menstruation has not commenced by age seventeen.
- When physical maturation, such as breast development, has not commenced by fourteen.

OR

- When the period has not started within two years of physical maturation commencing.

Table 13.1 Medical evaluation of primary amenorrhoea when breast development is normal

Take pelvic ultrasound:
- Uterus absent—chromosomal abnormalities
- Uterus present—examine for obstruction of vagina or imperforate hymen
- Uterus, vagina and hymen normal—take blood tests to evaluate FSH, LH, prolactin:
  - Normal tests = delayed puberty or hypothalamic causes such as low body weight, over-exercising, stress
  - High LH = PCOD
  - High prolactin = prolactinoma
  - High FSH and LH = resistant ovary syndrome

Secondary amenorrhoea

- Cessation of the period for six months or more during any of the years between the onset of menstruation (menarche) and menopause.

OR

- Cessation of the period for more than three menstrual cycles when the cycle is longer than usual, for example, when a woman has a period only every two months.

THE COMMON CAUSES OF SECONDARY AMENORRHOEA

1. Uterine causes

Conditions which affect the uterus or cervix either prevent menstrual blood loss due to obstruction, or are associated with destruction of the endometrial tissue.

i) Asherman's syndrome

Persistent amenorrhoea and infertility which results from intra-uterine adhesions, usually following a curette or from an uterine infection.

ii) Cervical stenosis

Obstruction of the menstrual flow can be caused by extreme narrowing or closure of the cervical canal. Chronic infection, cone biopsy, cauterisation (the destruction of tissue with a hot instrument, or the burning of tissue with a caustic substance), cryosurgery (the destruction of tissue with extreme cold), laser surgery, or irradiation of the cervix can cause this type of obstruction.

---

2. Hypothalamic dysfunction

The hypothalamus usually secretes GnRH in pulses, but a number of conditions can interfere with this secretion. Of these, stress, weight loss and rigorous and prolonged exercise are the commonest causes.

i) *Stress*

Stress can sometimes lead to amenorrhoea (travelling, leaving home, relationship difficulties, for example). The oestrogen levels are in the lower range and often ovulation does not occur.

ii) *Weight loss*

Amenorrhoea occurs if the body fat content drops below 25 per cent. Common causes are anorexia nervosa and serious illness.

iii) *Rigorous exercise*

GnRH is negatively affected by prolonged and rigorous exercise causing amenorrhoea.

iv) *Severe chronic illness*

Chronic renal or liver failure, and other severe or prolonged illnesses can interfere with menstruation because of their effect on the hypo-thalamus.

v) *Drugs*

The phenothiazides (e.g. Largactil, Stemetil, Stelazine) can increase prolactin levels and lead to amenorrhoea or menstrual irregularities. Some anti-hypertensive (blood pressure lowering) drugs can also cause amenorrhoea, especially Aldactone and Aldomet.

vi) *Post-Pill amenorrhoea*

About 80 per cent of women start to menstruate within three months of stopping the Pill, but about 1 per cent will experience long-term post-Pill amenorrhoea. Some of these women have pre-existing conditions such as polycystic ovarian disease which have not been apparent while the Pill caused regular 'menstruation'.

vii) *Pseudocyesis ('phantom pregnancy')*

A phantom pregnancy is usually accompanied by higher than normal levels of prolactin and luteinising hormone which cause amenorrhoea.

viii) *Hypothalamic lesions*

Lesions of the hypothalamus causing amenorrhoea are associated with levels of FSH and LH which are too low to stimulate follicle devel-opment and oestrogen production.

3. Pituitary causes

The destruction of pituitary gland tissue can give rise to amenorrhoea.

i) *Pituitary lesions*

Malignant or non-malignant tumours of the pituitary gland can cause amenorrhoea. The most common of these are associated with increased secretion of prolactin (prolactinomas) which leads to hyperprolactinaemia.

ii) *Pituitary insufficiency*

Rarely the pituitary tissue can be damaged by lack of oxygen, blood clots or severe haemorrhage (haemorrhage after childbirth causing destruction of the pituitary gland is called Sheehan's syndrome). The FSH, LH and oestrogen levels are all low.

iii) *Empty sella syndrome*

In this rare syndrome the membrane that separates the pituitary and hypothalamus is either absent or incomplete. This might be congenital, caused by surgery, irradiation, or be associated with a tumour. The pressure of the cerebrospinal fluid flattens the pituitary gland, which appears on X-ray to be absent. Amenorrhoea can be the result.

4. Failure to ovulate

A number of conditions can lead to prolonged ovarian dysfunction and amenorrhoea.

i) *Polycystic ovarian disease*

This is the most common condition associated with failure to ovulate and is characterised by multiple ovarian cysts, an abnormal hormone profile and amenorrhoea.

ii) *Breast-feeding*

Breast-feeding is initially associated with high prolactin levels which cause ovulation and menstruation to cease.

iii) *Thyroid conditions*

An underactive thyroid causes lower levels of SHBG which leads to an eventual increase in the availability of oestrogen. An overactive thyroid leads to a greater conversion of androgens to oestrogens. Both situations can lead to amenorrhoea due to ovulatory failure, but once the thyroid condition has been treated, menstruation recommences.

iv) *Cushing's syndrome*

A syndrome associated with excess corticosteroids and a wide range of symptoms including obesity, thinning of the skin, abnormal fat distribution around the neck and upper back, high blood pressure, diabetes, hirsutism and amenorrhoea. It can be caused by adrenal or pituitary tumours, or cortisone medication.

v) *Congenital adrenal hyperplasia*

This is a rare congenital condition where the adrenal gland produces too much androgen. An adult-onset form is also seen and is associated with abnormal cortisol production and elevated androgen levels.

vi) *Androgen-secreting adrenal and ovarian tumours*

These very rare, often malignant tumours secrete androgens and can cause amenorrhoea. In the ovary, mucinous cystadenomas, cystadenocarcinomas and Brenner tumours; as well as a number of other malignant ovarian tumours are associated with increased androgen production.

vii) *Premature ovarian failure*

Cessation of ovarian function before 40 is defined as premature ovarian failure. The causes are unknown, but for some women, may arise from an auto-immune response or because of a failure of the ovarian tissue to respond to FSH and LH.

viii) *Destruction of ovarian tissue*

Ovarian tissue can be damaged by impaired blood supply and irradiation. This leads to a failure of ovulation and amenorrhoea.

Primary amenorrhoea

Primary amenorrhoea, or failing to commence menstruation, can be caused by a number of congenital and hormonal factors. In rare cases, patients are found not to have a uterus. Doctors describe four categories which are based on the presence or absence of a uterus and on whether breast development occurs.

No breast development, but a uterus can be seen

In this group, four main conditions are identified.

- The hypothalamus does not secrete GnRH because of a functional disorder.
- The pituitary gland does not secrete FSH and LH.
- Congenital abnormalities of the ovaries lead to absent ovulation and menstruation. This includes the rare condition known as resistant ovary syndrome in which the ovary cannot respond to FSH, and the chromosomal abnormalities like Turner's syndrome.
- Lesions or tumours affect the function of the hypothalamus or pituitary glands.

Breast development, but no uterus

Two very rare conditions are associated with breast development and a congenitally absent uterus. In the first, the uterus is absent, but the ovaries function and ovulation occurs. The other is an extremely rare condition known as androgen-insensitivity syndrome where the foetus has an inherited 'lack of response' to the androgen dihydrotestosterone. This leads to the development of female genitalia, but no uterus. This is almost always undetected until a reason is sought for primary amenorrhoea.

No breast development, uterus absent

These very rare congenital conditions are associated with genetic abnormalities.

Breast development, uterus present

This category is associated with an abnormality of the hypothalamic–pituitary–ovarian axis; or the causes of secondary amenorrhoea listed in Table 13.1 may also be responsible. Rarely, blockages in the vagina, such as a transverse vaginal septum or an imperforate hymen may need correcting so that the outflow of menstrual blood can occur.

Diagnosis

The medical diagnosis of the causes of primary amenorrhoea follows a fairly routine pattern. In many cases, there is no major physical problem, and the onset of puberty has simply been delayed. In these cases, menstruation will commence in due course. Delayed onset of puberty, however, is a diagnosis of exclusion, and most doctors will want to make absolutely sure that this diagnosis is correct.

Breast development indicates that either ovarian oestrogen is being produced or that oestrogens are being produced by conversion of androgens in the fat. Because full breast development will only occur in the presence of ovarian oestrogens, examination of the breasts gives important information about the causes of the primary amenorrhoea.

Attaining a normal height for age is also important because some of the more common chromosomal abnormalities, such as Turner's syndrome, are associated with a short stature.

The next step is an abdominal ultrasound to determine whether a uterus is present. This allows any uterus, tubes, ovaries and vagina to be seen.

When breast development is normal and the uterus is present and looks normal, the next step is to take blood tests to try to determine if a hormonal abnormality is associated with the problem (see Table 13.2). Usually the levels of FSH, LH, and prolactin are checked. Normal levels of all three are seen in delayed puberty; a high LH with a low FSH is seen in polycystic ovarian disease (and the ovarian cysts will usually be apparent on ultrasound as well); a high prolactin level usually indicates a pituitary tumour called a prolactinoma; and a high FSH and LH indicates a possible resistant ovary syndrome.

HYPERPROLACTINAEMIA

Hyperprolactinaemia is characterised by prolactin levels in the higher than normal range which often leads to breast milk production (galactorrhoea) in non-pregnant women, and menstrual irregularities. In fact, the most common symptom of hyperprolactinaemia is the production of breast milk—light or irregular periods or amenorrhoea only occur some of the time. Because high prolactin is one of the more common causes of amenorrhoea, women with absent periods usually have their prolactin levels evaluated in the first round of tests.

It is worth noting, however, that although galactorrhoea commonly accompanies hyperprolactinaemia, many women who are not breast feeding, and who have normal prolactin levels, can express breast milk. This ability commonly persists after breast feeding has stopped, but many women who have never breast fed can also express milk. This is entirely normal and affects an unknown number of adult women. In many cases it requires no treatment, however all women with galactorrhoea should have blood tests to determine prolactin levels and thyroid function.

Causes of elevated prolactin levels

Prolactin levels can rise in response to a number of factors. Elevations above normal might be prolonged, or occur because of an isolated incident, such as breast stimulation, and cause only a transient increase in prolactin.

Factors causing prolonged hyperprolactinaemia
- Pituitary tumours, called microadenomas or prolactinomas, which secrete prolactin, are the most common causes and are believed to be the cause of hyperprolactinaemia where the other abnormalities listed below have been ruled out. (Often the tumours are very small and cannot be seen with a 'Cat scan'.)
- Hypothyroidism (underactive thyroid gland).
- Surgery or chest wall trauma caused by burns, irritation or herpes zoster (shingles).
- Epileptic seizures.
- Spinal cord tumours.

Transient hyperprolactinaemia
- Excessive and prolonged stress.
- Prolonged breast stimulation in non-lactating women increases prolactin levels. This may be the mechanism whereby Deer Massage (a meditative yoga pose which includes prolonged massage around the nipples) inhibits regular menstruation.
- Excessive and prolonged exercise, such as athletic training.

Drugs causing excess prolactin
Some drugs can cause elevated prolactin levels, amenorrhoea or unwanted breast milk production.
- Major tranquilliser therapy such as the phenothiazines (Largactil, Stemetil, Stelazine and Melleril), and haloperidol (Serenace) deplete the hypothalamus of dopamine.

- Anti-ulcer drugs such as Pepcidine, Tagamet, Tazac and Zantac.
- The anti-hypertensive drugs Aldactone and Aldomet.
- High-dose oestrogen oral contraceptive pills.
- Opiates, cocaine and alcohol, especially beer.

Latent hyperprolactinaemia

This syndrome is associated with PMS symptoms and is believed to be related to an oestrogen excess relative to progesterone. This leads to either an increased sensitivity to prolactin in the luteal phase, or a marginally elevated prolactin level. In this regard it is quite different to hyperprolactinaemia where a biochemically detectable increase in prolactin levels is seen.

Signs and symptoms

When prolactin levels are elevated, galactorrhoea is the most common symptom, but low levels of both GnRH and LH can also cause menstruation and ovulation to cease. Oestradiol and most androgen levels are reduced, but the adrenal androgens are elevated.[1] The elevated androgen levels are readily identified with blood tests, but usually do not cause increased hirsutism because of reduced levels of the enzyme (5 alpha reductase) which converts the adrenal androgens into the more potent forms. SHBG levels are also reduced.[2]

Women with hyperprolactinaemia may develop low bone density even when oestrogen levels are normal.[3]

■ ■

■ ■ The medical approach

When a high prolactin level has been identified, a CT scan of the pituitary gland is recommended to evaluate the size of the pituitary tumour. Rarely, very large pituitary tumours might need removal because they can interfere with vision or cause blindness if they damage the optic nerve.

In most cases, however, the course of action is to re-instate a normal cycle by reducing prolactin with bromocriptine (Parlodel) which is the most frequently prescribed drug to reduce elevated prolactin and stop lactation. Ovulation, cyclic regularity and fertility return to normal with the use of this drug. Other conditions which are responsible for the elevated prolactin levels, such as hypothyroidism, will also require treatment.

When women are lactating, but have normal menstrual cycles, treatment is rarely needed and a wait-and-see approach is usually adopted. If the cycle is erratic and long, progestogens are given at regular intervals and then withdrawn to initiate endometrial shedding.

Yearly measurements of blood prolactin levels are often suggested to monitor prolactin-secreting tumours (prolactinomas or microadenomas). These tumours usually do not increase in size and so repeated X-ray imaging is generally unnecessary, and the level of prolactin can decrease over time, even when the tumour size remains constant. Measurements of the optic field to determine whether the tumour is encroaching on the optic nerve may also be necessary.

Normal prolactin levels in non-pregnant women are between 1–25 nanograms per millilitre (ng/mL). These levels normally increase during sleep, especially between 3 a.m. and 5 a.m.; after lunch; after a high fat, high protein meal; during periods of stress; following breast stimulation; and after exercise.

Prolactin levels are also effected by oestrogen levels. When oestrogens are highest in the menstrual cycle during the luteal phase, prolactin levels also increase. During pregnancy, especially in the third trimester, when oestrogen levels are many times the levels in non-pregnant women, prolactin is correspondingly high at around 200 ng/mL. After delivery, the decrease in oestrogen and progesterone levels allows lactation to commence.

Because of these normal variations, the best time to take blood tests to evaluate prolactin levels is during the follicular phase of the cycle and late in the morning. Breast stimulation, heavy meals and exercise should also be avoided before the test. Some endocrinologists take three tests at half-hour intervals to rule out false positive readings.

 The natural therapist's approach

Many women experience side effects from bromocriptine such as dizziness and seek herbal alternatives; others are inclined to try a more natural approach for their complaints before using medication. Herbal, vitamin and mineral treatments for hyperprolactinaemia, however, are quite complex and certainly not as straightforward as taking a drug. There is also a tendency for herbal preparations to regulate menstruation successfully for the first few months, then only with some difficulty after that.

For these reasons, it is necessary to decide in advance on the desired outcome of the treatment. Herbal remedies make quite useful short-term medications where pregnancy is the aim, but may not be appropriate in the longer term to regulate menstruation and prevent osteoporosis, for example.

Nutrients
Nutrients which can normalise prolactin levels are thought to do so because of their effect on dopamine levels:

Zinc and vitamin B_6
Zinc is necessary for the normal synthesis of dopamine. It is not clear whether giving zinc will lower elevated prolactin levels, but zinc should

be considered as a supplement for women who have signs of zinc deficiency. Vitamin B_6 acts as a co-factor with zinc in the synthesis of dopamine. Symptoms associated with a relative progesterone deficiency and latent hyperprolactinaemia respond to these nutrients, and elevated prolactin which occurs secondary to depleted dopamine may also benefit. It is questionable, however, whether hyperprolactinaemia of other causes will respond to these nutrients.

Herbs

A number of herbal formulas, commonly used in traditional Chinese medicine have been trialled for their effectiveness in the treatment of hyperprolactinaemia. These include Rehmannia Eight Combination (Ba Wei Di Huang Tang) and Peony and Liquorice Combination (Shao Yao Gan Cao Tang).

Rehmannia Eight Combination given over three months resulted in lower prolactin levels and pregnancies amongst 11 of the 27 infertile women treated.[4] Peony and Liquorice Combination is thought to act directly on the pituitary gland to counteract hyperprolactinaemia. It stimulates the dopamine receptors, and also directly stimulates the ovarian production of oestrogen by stimulating aromatase (enzyme) activity.[5]

Vitex agnus castus has also been investigated for its effect on prolactin secretion. It has been shown to mimic the action of dopamine, the naturally occurring antagonist of prolactin secretion. The researchers suggested that Vitex agnus castus be considered as a safe and efficient alternative to drugs for luteal phase defects, associated with latent hyperprolactinaemia. In some cases, it will also lower prolactin levels when women have a prolactinoma.[6]

 Self care

Stress affects prolactin levels. Relaxation techniques, stress management, meditation, and increasing exercise of the long slow variety are all useful. Beer also increases prolactin and should be avoided.

ANDROGEN EXCESS

Women usually have much lower levels of androgens that men, but some conditions can give rise to higher than normal levels of androgens in women and lead to erratic menstruation or amenorrhoea. The effects of androgens, where and how they are produced, are discussed in Chapter 4 'Hormones'.

Causes

A number of gynaecological and other conditions can lead to excess androgen production.

- Ovarian causes
  Polycystic ovarian disease, androgen-producing tumours of the ovary, hyperthecosis.
- Adrenal gland disorders
  Congenital or adult-onset adrenal hyperplasia, androgen-producing tumours of the adrenal gland.
- Drugs
  Some drugs can cause androgenising effects and can also interfere with menstrual flow and the regularity of the cycle: Phentoin sodium (Dilantin), and some of the progestogens such as dydrogesterone (Duphaston) and danazol (Danocrine); the corticosteroids and corticotrophins; and the anabolic steroids, such as Deca-Durabolin.
- Metabolic and hormonal states
  Post-menopause, obesity, Cushing's syndrome.

Signs and symptoms

The most common effect from elevated androgens is excess hair growth, also known as hirsutism; or excessive scalp hair loss which is referred to as androgenic alopecia. Acne can also become worse or can be caused by elevated androgens, and in pre-menopausal women, menstrual irregularity or amenorrhoea can also occur.

Hirsutism, also referred to as male-pattern hair growth, is when coarse hair grows on the chin, upper lip, cheeks, around the nipples and between the breasts, the buttocks, lower back, and the lower abdomen. Not all hirsutism is caused by high androgen levels, however, and the amount and distribution of hair is an inherited trait. As a rule, dark-haired and dark-eyed women naturally have more body hair than fairer women or Asian women.

Signs which indicate androgen excess can include acne and/or increased male-pattern hair growth at puberty, accompanied by delayed menarche; or when women are past menarche, *changes* in the amount and coarseness of body or facial hair, especially when this is also accompanied by menstrual irregularity.

Androgenic alopecia is another sign of androgen excess which can occur in pre- or post-menopausal women. It is also known as male-pattern baldness. The hair loss might occur as a generalised thinning all over the scalp or might be localised to the crown. The rate of hair loss is variable and the hair usually becomes thinner and finer. Complete baldness does not occur. Menopausal women can develop androgenic alopecia, facial acne and hair growth even when their androgen levels are not markedly elevated above normal. This is thought to be brought about by the decline in oestrogen levels, which leads to lower SHBG, along with an increase in, or an increased sensitivity to adrenal androgens.

Signs of severe androgen excess, also known as virilisation, such as enlargement of the clitoris and reduced breast size are rare. Usually, androgen-producing tumours of the ovary or adrenal gland are responsible for the extremely high androgen levels. Some drugs such as danazol can also cause virilisation.

Diagnosis

The first step is to test for an elevated serum testosterone level and the levels of the carrier protein, SHBG. Serum testosterone is the best indicator of ovarian androgen production and SHBG gives an indication of how much testosterone is unbound and therefore able to exert androgenising effects. Ovarian androgen production is elevated in polycystic ovarian disease and androgen-producing ovarian tumours.

DHEA sulphate is the most reliable test for evaluating abnormal adrenal androgen levels when adult-onset adrenal hyperplasia or androgen-producing adrenal tumours are suspected. Women with adult-onset adrenal hyperplasia often have a short stature, elevated blood pressure, menstrual irregularities and hirsutism.

In many cases of hirsutism, acne or male-pattern baldness, androgen levels are normal, and the problem seems to arise because of an inherited sensitivity to androgens in the pilo-sebaceous unit. The treatment for elevated androgens or for an increased sensitivity to normal androgen levels is the same.

■ ■
■ ■ The medical approach

The treatment of androgen excess is dependent on the causes. Obesity requires weight loss; post-menopausal women are often prescribed HRT; drugs can be withdrawn or changed; congenital adrenal hyperplasia and adult-onset adrenal hyperplasia are treated with low doses of dexamethasone (a type of corticosteroid). Adrenal or ovarian tumours will usually require removal. Oestrogen is often prescribed to increase levels of SHBG.

The common medications used for hirsutism are either Aldactone (spironalactone), Androcur (cyproterone acetate) or the Pill called Diane which contains a small amount of cyproterone acetate. Aldactone, Androcur and Diane block the effects of androgens by competitive inhibition—these drugs prevent the androgens from being able to interact with tissues which are normally responsive to androgens (such as the hair follicle and the skin) by blocking the receptor sites on the cells.

Some of the new 'third generation' Pills—which contain the progestogens norgestimate, desogesterol and gestodene (Femoden, Marvelon, Minulet, Triminulet and Trioden) have low androgen potency. The use of these types of Pill, however, can increase the risk of blood clot formation[7] and they may not be suitable for all women.

Often, when these drugs are stopped, the hair will grow again, and they may need to be continued for long periods of time to successfully control the problem.

The progestogen levonorgestrel, which has androgenising effects, is contained in many oral contraceptives, and in many cases is unsuitable for women with androgen excess. A gynaecologist should be consulted about the suitability of these Pills when contraception is needed and androgen excess is a concern. The amount of progestogen in the Pill used, however, will influence its androgenic potential. For instance, Triphasil and Triquilar, which have low levels of levonorgestrel, usually do not exacerbate symptoms of androgen excess.

Other progestogens with androgenising effects such as Duphaston, Primolut and danazol are discussed in Chapter 20 'Drugs and surgery'.

 ## The natural therapist's approach

Again, the treatment depends on the cause. Women with polycystic ovarian disease (PCOD) will need advice to help to regulate hormonal balance and re-establish regular menstruation. Post-menopausal women can use vegetarian diets[8] and phyto-oestrogens[9] to increase SHBG (which falls in conjunction with the fall in oestrogen levels) to reduce the masculinising effects of androgens. Women who are taking androgenising drugs should be referred to their GP to discuss a change of medication if possible.

Excess male pattern hair growth or the hair loss associated with androgen excess can be difficult to control. The Smilax species (sarsaparilla) and *Turnera aphrodisiaca* seem to block the effects of androgens by preventing them from interacting with receptor sites on cells. This is known as competitive inhibition. They are not as reliable, nor do they work as quickly as drugs. When excess hair growth or loss is a serious problem, drugs first, followed by herbal remedies to maintain the status quo, can be the most effective combination.

Another method is to increase the rate at which androgens are converted (aromatised) to oestrogens. *Glycyrrhiza glabra* and particularly a component of *Paeonia lactiflora* called paeoniflorin, increase the aromatisation process and reduce testosterone levels. Peony and Liquorice Combination, a formula used in traditional Chinese medicine, is suitable for excess production of ovarian androgens, but its effects are often short-lived.[10]

Reducing weight or maintaining an ideal weight will help to control androgen levels when women are obese or have PCOD. Regular meals, a low-fat intake and 30–40g of fibre daily, will help. Morning exercise, such as brisk walking or multiple repetitions of weights that increase the heart rate also increase the rate of weight loss. Losing weight, and a high fibre and phyto-oestrogen-containing diet increases the levels of SHBG which binds to androgens, making them relatively unavailable.

When excess hair growth or androgenic alopecia is the primary concern, treatment must be continued for many months, and in some cases indefinitely. It is important that the chosen remedies are considered safe for long-term administration. This is not a condition for self-treatment. The advice of a practitioner with knowledge in this area is essential.

BLOOD QUALITY

Over the centuries, traditional medicine developed an understanding of the actions of blood by observing people during and after blood loss. Those who looked as though they had lost blood and were pale, weak, tired and vague were said to have 'weak' blood; those who were red-faced, overstimulated, irritable and energetic, were said to have an excess of blood.

A large number of women's complaints were attributed to blood because women not only lose blood every month and during childbirth, but also were believed to lose the essence of blood when they breastfed. (Many early cultures thought of breast milk as blood with the redness taken out.)

A relatively modern name for weak blood, dating from around Shakespeare's time until the turn of this century was 'chlorosis'. Chlorosis means 'greenish colour' and was a common diagnosis of young menstruating women. The symptoms were fatigue; a yellowish face with dark rings around the eyes and menstrual symptoms such as amenorrhoea or menorrhagia.[11]

The opposite condition, 'plethora', indicated an excess of blood. It was characterised by over-indulgence generally and of alcohol in particular, irritability, headaches and a red face. It was a condition common to the older generation, usually men, and was believed to be the precursor to strokes.

A diagnosis of either chlorosis or plethora was cast aside when it became possible to test for anaemia. Technically, anaemia means a lack of iron in the red blood cells or insufficient numbers of red blood cells. The common causes are lack of dietary iron or excessive blood loss. The term is often used (incorrectly) in common language to describe a number of symptoms including tiredness, inability to concentrate, paleness, dizziness, or a lacklustre attitude to life.

A natural therapist's diagnosis of poor blood quality (also known as 'blood deficiency' in traditional Chinese medicine, and 'anaemic' or 'nutritionally depleted' by naturopaths) is *not* the same as anaemia. It is a rather more complex syndrome characterised by:

- frequent exhaustion and poor stamina
- unusually debility around the time of menstruation, and especially afterwards
- an increased tendency to infection around the period, especially thrush and recurrent viral infections such as herpes
- frequent headaches often with or after the period
- dizziness
- pale face and tongue
- dry skin and unhealthy lank hair
- menstrual irregularities, especially amenorrhoea or infrequent periods, occasionally menorrhagia

The aim of the treatment is to improve the overall quality and activity of the blood. Iron, though important, is not the end of the story.

- The quality of blood is corrected with appropriate dietary changes, nutritive herbs and supplements as required.
- The general energy levels are improved with the female tonic herbs.
- Where infrequent periods or amenorrhoea occurs, hormonal regulatory herbs are used.
- Assimilation of nutrients is assisted with the Warming digestive herbs and foods.
- Circulation is enhanced with circulatory stimulants and Warming herbs.

Many of the common herbs used to treat abnormal bleeding are also nutritive herbs and are high in the blood-building and anti-haemorrhagic nutrients iron, Vitamins A, K and C, and folic acid. Some important examples are *Rubus idaeus* and *Petroselinum crispum*.

Chamaelirium luteum, *Aletris farinosa*, and *Angelica sinensis* as well as *Rubus idaeus* are general female tonics and assist with regulation of all aspects of the menstrual cycle.

Anaemia is related to blood quality and is a common complaint affecting menstruating women. The iron-containing foods, and information on iron and anaemia can be found on page 189.

14

Period pain

Key words

adenomyosis
anodyne
antispasmodic
bioflavonoid
congestive
   dysmenorrhoea
emmenagogue
endometriosis
hysterectomy
irritable bowel
   syndrome

laparoscopy
nervine
PID
proanthocyanidins
prostaglandins
pycnogenol
spasmodic
   dysmenorrhoea
spasmolytic
uterine tone

Pain is the most common symptom to accompany disease, and it is the symptom that brings people to their health-care practitioners quicker than any other. And not only because it is uncomfortable and unpleasant—we all know that pain means that something is wrong, and that it needs remedying.

That is, unless the pain is period pain. Many women, and their doctors, think that a 'bit of period pain is normal'. 'Grin and bear it', 'you'll just have to get on with it', 'it will be better once you have a baby' are the sorts of comments they hear regularly. A bit of period pain is *usual*, but being common doesn't make it normal.

The two questions to ask about period pain are: 'Does it bother you enough to want/need to do something about it?' and if so 'Are you happy with the treatments you are using?'. After all, on average, a woman will have twelve or thirteen periods annually and if she has pain on two or three days of these, she will experience about a month of pain every year.

Period pain is frequently called dysmenorrhoea. Dysmenorrhoea means painful periods and the term is made up of the Greek *dys* meaning difficulty with, and *menorrhoea* indicating that the difficulty is associated with menstruation. Dysmenorrhoea is a symptom, not a disease—and the first aspect of any successful treatment of dysmenorrhoea is to determine exactly what is causing the pain. Period pain can be associated with two major categories of complaint.

- Functional disorders where the uterine muscle is behaving abnormally, but is otherwise healthy. This is called *primary dysmenorrhoea*. (Primary dysmenorrhoea is sometimes also called functional dysmenorrhoea.)
- Organ disease where the pain is caused largely by the underlying complaint. This is called *secondary dysmenorrhoea*. Common causes of secondary dysmenorrhoea are endometriosis and pelvic inflammatory disease (PID).

Severe pain cannot be assumed to have a secondary origin. Sometimes the most severe pain of all is caused by primary dysmenorrhoea, and sometimes conditions which seem like they should cause pain, like endometriosis, are pain free.

PRIMARY DYSMENORRHOEA

Primary dysmenorrhoea is caused by uterine contractions which are too strong and occur too frequently. Between the contractions, the uterine muscle does not relax properly, and there is an abnormally high 'resting tone'. (For a description of uterine tone, see pages 236–7.) The overall effect is a reduction in the amount of blood flowing through the uterine muscle (ischaemia) which causes the pain known as primary dysmenorrhoea.

The most usual cause of primary dysmenorrhoea is an imbalance in the prostaglandins levels. Prostaglandins are complex hormone-like substances which are found in most body tissues. There are many different types of prostaglandins which control bodily functions by working together as an integrated team. When the different types of prostaglandins are present in normal ratios, menstruation proceeds normally. An imbalance in the ratios in favour of the type of prostaglandins which increase muscle spasm will cause period pain. Their role in menstruation is complex and is discussed in Chapter 6 'Prostaglandins'.

The symptoms

The quality and severity of period pain can vary dramatically from woman to woman, and even from period to period. The most usual description of period pain is a continual, dull, 'background' ache or sense of heaviness (congestive dysmenorrhoea), over which is superimposed episodic, cramping pain (spasmodic dysmenorrhoea). The pain is usually central and located in the lower abdomen. Sometimes a heavy aching pain extends to the groin, the back, and down the thighs.

The pain may start before the menstrual flow has become established. It may be of either type, but is more frequently congestive and aching. Sometimes this sort of dysmenorrhoea is accompanied by a heavy dull sense of dragging in the vagina or a sense of fullness in the bowel. It is often described as feeling as though 'everything will fall out'.

Most commonly, the pain starts with the beginning of the period and intensifies as the flow becomes heavier, or when clots are passed. Some women describe this pain as being 'like labour'. Usually the spasmodic, crampy-type pain is the shortest-lived, but it is generally the most debilitating. Sometimes cramps can be accompanied by vomiting or diarrhoea, possibly caused by a reflex irritation of the gastrointestinal tract.

Bowel complaints often aggravate dysmenorrhoea. The bowel tends to be affected by hormone changes as well as by the muscular activity of the uterus. Many women become constipated premenstrually and a full bowel can exacerbate the sense of fullness and heaviness felt with congestive dysmenorrhoea. Irritable bowel syndrome both aggravates period pain and is in turn aggravated by it. The bowel and uterus share a similar nerve supply and when either organ is in spasm, the other will spasm in sympathy. (This knowledge was used in the past to bring women into labour by giving them castor oil and enemas to irritate the bowel and start uterine contractions.)

Diagnosis

Primary dysmenorrhoea is a diagnosis of exclusion—the exclusion of other complaints as the origin of the pain. An appraisal of the individual features of a woman's medical, menstrual and obstetric history; age; and sexual activity are the first steps in locating the cause. For example, a sexually active woman has a higher risk of PID, and an older woman is more likely to have adenomyosis than a younger woman.

The history of the pain gives other important clues. Where it is, how long it lasts, which other symptoms accompany the pain, whether it radiates and whether it occurs predominantly before, during or after bleeding, are all important in establishing the causes of the pain.

Pelvic examinations

Once a woman is sexually active, a doctor may suggest an internal examination of the pelvic organs. This usually involves looking at the cervix with a speculum to see whether it looks normal and healthy, and examining the pelvic organs by inserting a gloved hand into the vagina to feel the size, state and position of the organs. These examinations and the reasons they are performed are described in Chapter 3 in 'The Well Woman's Check List'.

Laparoscopic investigations

Sometimes surgery is needed to make a diagnosis, usually in the form of a laparoscopy. This may be used if the history is suggestive of secondary causes of pain, or if the pain fails to respond to the medication used for primary dysmenorrhoea. The laparoscopic procedure is described in Chapter 20 'Drugs and surgery'.

When to see the doctor

- Pain changes in character or is present for the first time.
- Pain is unilateral and/or radiating.
- Pain is associated with pregnancy or has occurred after a missed period where pregnancy is likely.
- Usual pain control measures are no longer useful (in other words, the pain has changed in character).
- New symptoms accompany the pain e.g. vomiting or diarrhoea, faintness.
- Pain worsens towards the end of the period.
- Pain is aggravated by pressure, bowel motions or sexual activity.
- A fever or discharge accompanies the pain.

■ ■ The medical approach

There is a hierarchy of treatments used by medical practitioners to treat dysmenorrhoea. Prostaglandins-inhibiting drugs are the most likely first suggestion, but the Pill and some other forms of pain killers are also commonly used. Sometimes, if the pain is severe and fails to respond to the usual treatments, drugs like Duphaston are used. These drugs are discussed in Chapter 20 'Drugs and surgery'.

A hysterectomy is sometimes suggested for women who are past their child-bearing years or who do not want to have children, when pain does not respond adequately to drugs. Another surgical procedure, rarely used, is to cut the uterosacral nerve to destroy the perception of pain in the uterus.

The natural therapist's approach

Sometimes even severe dysmenorrhoea will improve with dietary changes and exercise, and this is always the best place to start. Limiting animal fats and increasing essential fatty acids in the diet can reduce period pain, perhaps because of the relationship between prostaglandins imbalance and fat intake; or maybe it is related to oestrogen levels and fats. Whatever the reason, many women reduce their period pain just by changing their diet and exercising.

When dysmenorrhoea does not improve with diet and exercise, herbs or supplements are the next option. Herbs are combined so that the formula treats both the symptoms and the cause of the dysmenorrhoea. Supplements may also be appropriate in some cases.

Herbs

The uterine tonics
The uterine tonics, *Chamaelirium luteum*, *Aletris farinosa*, *Caulophyllum thalictroides*, *Angelica sinensis* and *Rubus idaeus*, are used to treat pain because they are believed to regulate the muscular activity of the uterus and help initiate contractions which are regular, rhythmic and more orderly. They are combined with other herbs which are indicated by the symptoms.

The antispasmodics
Antispasmodic herbs are indicated for period pain which is crampy, colicky and comes in intermittent waves of pain. They are also useful for the vomiting and diarrhoea that sometimes accompanies dysmenorrhoea. Antispasmodics are more effective if given to stop the onset of spasm, rather than to treat pain that has already started. They should be started several days before the expected onset of the period. There is no reason to take antispasmodics throughout the whole cycle.

Viburnum opulus and *V. prunifolium*, *Caulophyllum thalictroides*, *Dioscorea villosa*, *Ligusticum wallichii* and *Paeonia lactiflora* are useful antispasmodics. *Paeonia lactiflora* is usually combined with liquorice root to obtain the best effect. *Caulophyllum thalictroides* is used when the spasm seems to be localised in the cervix, resulting in acute crampy pain with very little flow. Women with this pain pattern usually experience relief once the flow becomes established.

Emmenagogues
Emmenogogues are herbs which can increase the strength of uterine contractions. They are used to increase the expulsive activity of the uterus and start the menstrual flow. *Artemesia vulgaris*, in combination with any of the uterine tonics, is particularly indicated for period pain which is dull and congestive and which occurs in conjunction with periods which are slow to start.

Warming herbs

Herbs which are Warming improve the action of the antispasmodic herbs, especially when the period pain is aggravated by cold, relieved by heat, or the woman has a tendency to 'feel the cold' easily. Two herbs are specific for the pelvic region: *Zingiber officinale* and *Cinnamomum zeylanicum*. Both can be added to a herbal mix in the form of a tincture, or taken as a tea, either alone, with other therapeutic herbs or in an ordinary cup of tea.

Warming herbs are best if taken hot. To make ginger tea, grate 2–4 cm green root ginger, place in a stainless steel saucepan with 1–2 cups of water, cover and bring slowly to the boil. Keep covered and simmer for about ten minutes. Strain, add honey to taste and sip while still hot. If possible, also have a bath. Other herbs can be taken at the same time. Ginger also eases nausea and is useful for period pain accompanied by vomiting. Commercial tablets such as Travel Calm™ (Blackmores), are quite useful for mild period pain.

Relaxing herbs

Nervine (relaxing) herbs are useful, especially where anxiety or tension accompany the pain. Some nervine herbs are also antispasmodics, the best being *Valeriana officinalis*, *Paeonia lactiflora*, *Piscidia erythrina*, *Corydalis ambigua*, *Verbena officinalis*, and *Matricaria recutita*. Even when anxiety is not a problem, nervine herbs in the formula potentiate the actions of the antispasmodic and pain killing herbs.

Herbs to reduce pain: the anodynes

Anodyne is the term used in herbal medicine to describe herbs that have analgesic (pain reducing) effects. *Corydalis ambigua* from the Chinese *Materia Medica* is the most potent of these, and can be used for pain anywhere in the body. It also reduces heavy menstrual flow. Other important anodynes for menstrual pain are *Piscidia erythrina*, *Lactuca virosa*, and *Anemone pulsatilla*.

It may seem strange that the anodynes herbs are included so far down the list of herbs used to treat period pain. There are very good reasons for this. Anodynes are much weaker than conventional analgesics and must be prescribed with other herbs for the best effect. Also, a herbalist never tries to treat painful conditions by just stopping the pain. The aim is to rectify the underlying causes so that the problem is cured, rather than the symptom abolished.

Prostaglandins-inhibiting herbs

There is no herbal tradition to use prostaglandins-inhibiting herbs for dysmenorrhoea. (Prostaglandins were only discovered in the 1930s, and by this time herbal medicine had been used for thousands of years.) However, a number of commonly used herbs for period pain have been discovered to have prostaglandins-inhibiting effects similar to those of drugs. *Zingiber officinale*, *Tanacetum parthenium* and *Curcuma longa* are commonly prescribed herbs, and there are probably others, but there is little research in this area. In fact, *Tanacetum parthenium* was suspected of having prostaglandins-inhibiting effects when women taking it for migraines noticed an improvement in their period pain. *Curcuma longa* is used in Chinese and Indian herbal medicine and has a long tradition of use for period pain. It has proven prostaglandin-inhibiting effects.[1]

Hormone-regulating herbs

Herbs which regulate the hormone levels can improve period pain. Regulating hormone levels is believed to have an indirect effect on the prostaglandins levels and is one of the reasons that the Pill is effective for pain. The most valuable of the herbal hormone regulators is *Vitex agnus castus*, which is very useful for congestive dysmenorrhoea, particularly when the pain is accompanied by premenstrual tension. *Vitex agnus castus* is a very difficult herb to prescribe successfully and should only be taken while under the supervision of an experienced herbalist.

A number of other herbs have subtle effects on hormonal balance and are also effective for the treatment of pain. The exact reasons for their actions is often unknown, but it is likely that they work at a variety of levels. Included in this group are *Paeonia lactiflora* and *P. suffruticosa*, and *Cimicifuga racemosa* which are antispasmodics and may also competitively inhibit the activity of oestrogen; and *Verbena officinalis* which is sedative and has been traditionally used for menstrual disorders which have a hormonal origin.

Treating the liver

Congestive period pain; the heavy, dull, dragging type of pain experienced by many women before their period, is often improved when women are given Liver herbs or bitters. Historically, the Choleric (liverish) woman was described as being inclined to be irritable, hot-headed, constipated, as suffering from headaches and 'congestive complaints', like congestive dysmenorrhoea, with heavy, fiery-red menstrual flow. She was given bitter and Cooling herbs to expel Heat and remove the Yellow Bile humour.

These herbs are still used today for the same kinds of symptoms, even though we don't know exactly why they work. They may have an indirect effect on hormone balance and improve the excretion of oestrogens from the bowel and through the liver and bile. *Berberis vulgaris* seems to be particularly useful, but as it is also an emmenogogue, the positive results may come from multiple effects.

Treating bowel-related symptoms: constipation and irritable bowel syndrome

Spasmodic or congestive dysmenorrhoea accompanied by constipation is difficult to treat successfully unless the constipation is improved as well. The aperient herbs such as *Cassia senna*, *Rhamnus purshiana*, and

Aloe barbadensis can be used but will often aggravate spasm if taken during the period. Bitters are safer and equally reliable, especially *Taraxacum officinalis*, *Silybum marianum* and *Berberis vulgaris*.

By far the best method to treat constipation is to increase the level of fibre and fluids in the diet. About two litres of water should be taken every day when fibre intake is increased.

Irritable bowel syndrome frequently becomes worse around the period and can aggravate period pain—sometimes it is even mistaken for period pain. A diet and regime for treating irritable bowel syndrome follows.

IRRITABLE BOWEL SYNDROME

These dietary recommendations help to reduce spasm, pain and bloating associated with irritable bowel syndrome, and to regulate bowel function.

Seed breakfast
The seed breakfast consists of a combination of seeds, pectin-containing fruit and yoghurt.

Seeds and rice bran
- Linseed meal
- Almond meal
- Ground pumpkin seeds
- Ground sesame seeds
- Sunflower seeds
- Rice bran

The seeds and bran are combined together in quantities equal by weight after being ground to a consistency of coarsely ground coffee. They should be used immediately or kept refrigerated.

Fruit
- Grated raw apple
- Stewed apple, pear or plums

Yoghurt
- Plain (unsweetened) low-fat yoghurt with live cultures. (Jalna, Lesna, Hakea and Hellenic are all good brands.)

In winter, the seed mix can be added to cooked oatmeal (porridge) or rice and eaten with warmed stewed fruit and yoghurt.

Herb tea
Melissa officinalis, *Matricaria recutita* and *Mentha piperita* in equal quantities are prepared as for ordinary tea (2 teaspoons per cup).
    Dose: 1–2 cups between each meal.

Making a herbal formula for dysmenorrhoea

Every woman experiences period pain differently and has combinations of symptoms that are peculiar to her. Herbal formulas which are individually prescribed should attempt to deal with as many of these symptoms as possible. This is one of the reasons that over-the-counter herbal remedies for period pain can be less than successful—they simply can't have the right combination of herbs for every single woman.

It can be quite complicated to design a remedy for period pain, but the formula is made up with the following rules in mind.

- One of the uterine tonics should always be included because these herbs are believed to have a regulatory and normalising effect on uterine muscle.
- Antispasmodics, relaxing, pain-relieving and prostaglandin-inhibiting herbs are included if the symptoms indicate their use.
- Emmenagogues may also be used if the pain is accompanied by late or slow-starting periods.
- Almost always, Warming herbs will also be needed.

These herbs are combined together and given for a few days before, and in frequent doses during the period. It is also usual to prescribe the uterine tonics throughout the whole cycle because their action on uterine muscle is slow and progressive. They are frequently prescribed with hormone regulating or Liver herbs.

This first group of herbs treat the uterus, but generally it is also necessary to treat the whole person to ensure that the underlying causes of the pain are removed. Herbs for hormone regulation and the Liver, and remedies to improve constipation or irritable bowel syndrome, are usually needed throughout the month rather than just around and during the period. It may also be necessary to use herbs for congestion of the pelvic blood vessels. These are discussed later in this chapter in the section on 'Pelvic congestion syndrome'.

Diet and supplements

Prostaglandins cause menstrual pain, but prostaglandin levels can be influenced by hormones and diet. When the diet contains too many saturated fats and not enough of the 'good fats', the levels of prosta-glandins associated with muscle spasm are more likely to increase. Hormone imbalances are also likely to alter prostaglandins ratios, again usually in favour of the prostaglandins which increase muscle spasm and the volume of menstrual flow. (One of the reasons the Pill is effective in the treatment of dysmenorrhoea is because it alters hormone levels.)

Dietary changes which encourage high levels of the essential fatty acids can reduce the levels of the series 2 prostaglandins (see Chapter 6, 'Prostaglandins') which are associated with an increase in muscle spasm. The dietary precursors to these series 2 prostaglandins are animal products, especially meat, organ meats, egg yolk and prawns. If a restriction in animal fats is combined with the dietary precursors to the series 1 prostaglandins, there is often a reduction in menstrual pain.

Essential fatty acids

The oil of evening primrose and fish oils can improve dysmenorrhoea. Usually a dose of 3 g of either in capsule form is necessary to achieve good results. For the first few months, taking the supplements daily is recommended. This dose can be reduced once pain control is achieved. The role of essential fatty acids for dysmenorrhoea is discussed in Chapter 6, 'Prostaglandins'.

Calcium and magnesium

Calcium and magnesium supplements will sometimes relieve menstrual cramps, but whether this is related to a dietary deficiency of these nutrients is not clear.

Calcium can be taken in the form of an orotate, citrate, chelate or phosphate. Follow the recommended dose on the label. Usually, a combination of calcium and magnesium together is best.

Acupuncture

Acupuncture can help with dysmenorrhoea. The treatments are usually given twice weekly and may involve moxibustion as well (the burning of herbs to warm certain acupuncture points). Some women respond well to acupuncture, others not.

Chiropractic and osteopathy

Chiropractors and osteopaths believe that period pain can be aggravated by pressure on the spinal nerves that supply the uterus. They treat this problem by manipulating the lower back. A positive response is usually obvious within one or two treatments.

Self care

Relaxation
Being able to relax doesn't stop pain, but it does improve a person's ability to cope with pain. Some women use relaxation tapes (hypnotherapists and psychologists will sometimes make a personalised relaxation tape) either when they have pain or in the week prior to the period. Guided imagery and meditation can be useful as well.

Massage
Massage just before or during the period can help, either from a qualified practitioner or from a friend. Some people use massage as a way of relaxing, but some specific massage techniques like shiatsu, acupressure, and foot reflexology can be used to relieve pain, pelvic congestion and improve symptoms related to hormone imbalance.

Aromatherapy
Clary sage, lavender, and chamomile oil are all useful for period pain because of their antispasmodic, and relaxing properties. They can be used regularly in the bath, as a component of massage oil or as a warm compress, but should not be taken internally. These oils are not used 'neat', and are always diluted with other oils or water.

To make a massage oil, add between 1–3 mL or 20–60 drops of each essential oil to 100 mL of massage oil (olive, almond or apricot kernel oil are good choices). Massage into the lower abdomen and back when pain is a problem. Some women find it is useful to have a hot bath first, then use the massage oil.

A hot compress is made by adding about 5 drops of each essential oil to a bowl of very hot water, soaking a cloth and then applying it to the painful area after wringing out the excess water. The cloth can be repeatedly dipped in the water each time it cools. Alternatively, a hot-water bottle can be placed over the compress to keep it warm.

Another very useful way to use these oils is in the bath water. Usually only about 5–10 drops are needed in a full bathtub. Valerian oil can be very useful if the period pain prevents sleep, or when it is useful to 'sleep the pain off'. It can make some people quite drowsy, so don't expect to be the life of the party afterwards.

Warmth
Heat of any sort will help to relieve muscle spasm. A hot-water bottle or a hot bath is cheap and easy to arrange. It is also possible to buy small hot packs that can be worn close to the skin—some manufacturers even sell them with specially made underwear which has a little pouch to hold the pack in place. (Warmease is the name of one product.)

A warm ginger pack on the lower abdomen, while messy, can be useful. Place grated root ginger on several layers of cloth and place a hot-water bottle over the top. A little oil on the skin first will prevent burns from the ginger juice. Remove the pack if the skin starts to burn or sting.

While warmth is helpful, getting cold can increase pain. Swimming in cold water can be a problem, but only because of the temperature of the water. The swimming itself can relieve pain.

Food quality

Period pain which becomes worse with exposure to cold, or improves with warm applications, can be aggravated by iced drinks, ice-cream or cold food from the refrigerator. Raw foods, like salads, can also be a problem. Women with this type of period pain can try warm food which is at room temperature or hotter; and adding warming spices to food, like ginger, cardamom, coriander, turmeric and cinnamon.

Sex

Having sex or an orgasm can sometimes help to reduce menstrual pain by reducing muscle spasm and pelvic congestion.

Smoking

Smoking can either increase or decrease pain. Smokers tend to have period pain less often than non-smokers, possibly because of an inhibition of the prostaglandins responsible for triggering the pain.[2] But if a cigarette smoker does get dysmenorrhoea, her pain is likely to get worse if she smokes during her period.

PELVIC CONGESTION SYNDROME

Definition

Pelvic congestion syndrome is poorly defined and poorly understood. The most frequent symptoms are a dragging or heavy lower abdominal pain, congestive period pain, low backache and pain during sex. Some women develop a vaginal discharge. The pain can become worse towards the end of the day when the blood pools in the veins, or might occur primarily around and during the period. Often anxiety, fatigue, headache and insomnia, in other words premenstrual syndrome, accompany the pelvic symptoms. Typically, the complaint is most common after the age of 35 and after a woman has had a number of pregnancies.

In many cases, when a pelvic examination or laparoscopy is performed, the pelvic blood vessels are engorged, and the uterus is enlarged and tender. Even so, no consistent relationship has been seen between pelvic blood vessel engorgement and pain—some women have swollen blood vessels without pain, while others have the same sorts of symptoms without any evidence of physical changes.

A number of causes of pelvic congestion syndrome have been suggested. It may be related to tension and stress;[3] and can also occur when women have chronic pelvic inflammatory disease.

The medical approach

Some doctors treat pelvic congestion with progesterone (Provera or Primolut) because they believe that it has a hormonal origin; or sometimes a hysterectomy is suggested. Other doctors think it is a psychosomatic condition.

The natural therapist's approach

In natural medicine, pelvic congestion is believed to be related to constitutional weakness, hormonal imbalance, lack of exercise, constipation, or stress and tension.

Herbs for pelvic venous congestion

Hamamelis virginiana, *Aesculus hippocasticum* and *Ruscus aculeatus* are used to treat any condition associated with venous congestion or blood vessel inflammation. These herbs have additional anti-inflammatory, anti-haemorrhagic, and astringent effects and are useful when pelvic congestion is accompanied by heavy menstruation, or when other blood vessels are affected and the woman complains of aching haemorrhoids or varicose veins.

Older women or women who have had repeated pregnancies often develop symptoms similar to pelvic congestion syndrome which are caused by pelvic floor or uterine prolapses. The specific herb in this case is *Aletris farinosa*. This herb also contains bitters and is a general tonic. It is ideal for women who are tired and who have heavy, dragging pain; prolapses or low back pain. A combination of *Astragalus membranaceus*, *Bupleurum falcatum* and *Angelica sinensis* is frequently used in Chinese medicine.

Diet and supplements

The bioflavonoids are a group of naturally occurring compounds often found in vitamin C-rich foods which improve the integrity of blood vessels. Rutin and hesperidin are often combined with vitamin C supplements and also occur in fruit, especially citrus fruits, capsicum and buckwheat leaf tea.

The proanthocyanidins are a class of bioflavonoids quite recently recognised as having an even more potent effect on blood vessel fragility and permeability. They are found in many berries, fruit, seeds and barks with a red or purplish colour. These compounds are anti-oxidants and have the ability to prevent collagen destruction, including the collagen of tendons, ligaments, cartilage and bone; the collagen in the skin; as well as that found in the blood vessels. Blueberries are a particularly rich source, and the herb *Vaccinium myrtillus*, which is a combination of the fruit and the leaves, can be used as a medicinal agent.

The pycnogenols, which are extracted from grape seed skin, the bark of Lindes' pine, the bracts of the lime tree and the leaves of the hazelnut tree, are available in supplement form and are believed to be the most effective of all of the classes of bioflavonoids. The supplemental dose is between 150–300 mg per day.[4]

The bioflavonoids are unlikely to have a direct affect on the pain, but can be used to improve blood vessel integrity and reduce tissue oedema caused by lymphatic fluid leakage.

A high fibre intake will also help to prevent constipation which will aggravate the symptoms of pelvic congestion.

 Self care

Exercise assists with the return of blood to the heart and helps to prevent blood from pooling in the pelvic blood vessels. When symptoms are severe, it may be necessary for the exercise to be non-weight bearing, such as swimming. Alternatively, exercise such as walking should be taken in the morning before the veins become too engorged.

Sometimes sleeping with the foot of the bed elevated on a brick helps relieve the symptoms of pelvic congestion by assisting venous blood drainage overnight.

UTERINE TONE

Uterine tone is the term used by natural therapists to refer to the muscular activity of the uterus. When uterine tone is normal, muscular contractions are orderly, regular, neither too strong nor too weak, and there is a resting phase between each contraction. This muscular activity continues all the time, even when the uterus is apparently at rest. During menstruation, or the birth of a child, the uterine activity is amplified many times, but when this muscular activity is normal, both the resting phase between the contractions, and their regularity, means that pain is kept within normal limits.

The 'resting phase' or 'resting tone' between contractions is important. Normally, the blood flowing through the uterine muscle carries oxygen and other nutrients. When the muscle fails to relax adequately, the diminished oxygen supply causes pain.

The quality of the pain can be crampy and spasmodic, and some women describe it as being 'labour-like'. Many women also develop

---

diarrhoea, frequent desire to urinate, or vomiting due to the reflex spasm in adjacent organs.

Poor muscle tone, on the other hand, is frequently accompanied by heavy bleeding or 'flooding' at the time of menstruation, There may be a sense of heaviness or pelvic congestion, often described as dull dragging. Lack of tone can be caused by:

- frequent pregnancies
- the recent birth of a child
- conditions which prevent adequate contraction of the uterus such as fibroids, polyps and adenomyosis.

Treatment

There are three classes of herbs which effect uterine muscle: the uterine tonics, the emmenagogues, and the spasmolytics. Each class has a specific action on uterine tone and is discussed in more detail in Chapter 19 'Herbs'. In summary, spasmolytics reduce amplitude of contraction, frequency of contraction and the resting tone. Emmenagogues have the opposite effect. They increase strength and frequency of contraction, and at high doses increase the resting tone. Uterine tonics normalise uterine activity. If tone is too high, they relax the muscle, if it is too weak, they improve it. Uterine tonics also ensure contractions are regular and rhythmic. They are the most important class of uterine herbs used in gynaecology and obstetrics.

Table 14.1 Uterine tone

	Hypertonicity	Normal	Hypotonicity
Tone	Excessive with contraction		Relaxed
Uterine size	Normal	Normal	Bulky
Pain	Spasmodic, cramp-like or colicky		Congestive and dull pain
Flow	Tardy with crampy pain		Excessive with dull pain
Herbal Treatment	Spasmolytics, uterine tonics and prostaglandin-inhibiting herbs		Uterine stimulants or emmenagogues and uterine tonics

15

Endometriosis and adenomyosis

Key Words

adhesions	laparoscopy
adenomyoma	laparotomy
auto-immune disease	leukotriene
dysmenorrhoea	IVF
endometrioma	peritoneal fluid
emmenagogue	peritoneum
endometrium	pouch of Douglas
functional	prostaglandins
hypoglycaemia	spasmolytic
hysterectomy	ultrasound

Normally, the endometrium lines the inside of the uterus and is expelled during each menstrual period, but in endometriosis and adenomyosis, the endometrial tissue starts to grow elsewhere in the body, most commonly in the pelvic region.

Endometriosis occurs when endometrial growths develop on the ovaries, the tubes, the outer wall of the uterus, the uterine or ovarian ligaments, the bowel, the ureters or the bladder. The term is made up of the Greek *endon* meaning within which refers to the endometrium; *metra* for uterus; and *osis* meaning a process, usually a disease process.

Adenomyosis is endometrium growing between the fibres of the muscular wall of the uterus.

Endometriosis is a perplexing complaint. No one knows for sure why it happens; and so prevention is difficult. It causes a multitude of different symptoms; making it hard to diagnose. The course the illness follows is unknown; therefore decisions about treatment are complex and sometimes conflicting. And predictions about future fertility are almost impossible.

Incidence

The number of women with endometriosis is unknown, but most estimates suggest a figure between 1–10 per cent. This may not be representative of true incidence, however, because only women with infertility or pain usually have investigative surgery. For instance, between 16–22 per cent of women having a laparoscopy for tubal ligation were found to have mild endometriosis,[1] and when doctors deliberately look for endometriosis during a laparoscopy, the number of women diagnosed almost doubles.[2]

Almost all menstruating women who have patent (non-blocked) Fallopian tubes have some menstrual fluid in the pelvic cavity, but in the majority of cases, endometriosis does not develop. This has led to speculation that factors other than menstrual fluid in the pelvic cavity (also called refluxed endometrium or retrograde menstruation) are involved.

Some researchers believe there may be different types—and that some of the time, endometriosis may not be severe enough to be classified as disease. Many women seem to have endometrial implants when conditions are favourable (oestrogen and menstruation for long enough), but only some of these women have endometriosis which causes pain or infertility.[3] For largely unproven reasons, probably related to the immune and inflammatory responses, these other (well) women are capable of preventing the endometriosis from progressing further and becoming a serious problem to their health and well-being.

Symptoms are reliable indicators of endometriosis—it is the cause of up to 80 per cent of pelvic pain or infertility. Endometriosis also tends to recur and about half of all women with endometriosis develop the condition again within five years of completing a successful treatment regime.[4]

Possible causes

Almost all women who develop endometriosis, do so during times in their lives when they are producing oestrogen and menstruating regularly. But other factors are clearly involved in the development of endometriosis—otherwise every woman would have it.

Relative oestrogen excess

Women who develop endometriosis might do so because they have a relatively higher level of exposure to oestrogen than other women. Endometriosis is associated with menstruating more times per year, starting to menstruate at a younger age, and delaying pregnancy and breast feeding. Relatively high levels of oestrogens might be capable of stimulating a thicker endometrium and more severe pelvic contamination because of increased menstrual volume. Oestrogen also influences the activity of the immune system.

Retrograde flow

Retrograde flow is probably normal. Almost all women who are examined laparoscopically while menstruating have refluxed endometrium in their pelvic cavity. The difference between women who do and do not develop endometriosis may be related to the volume of the menstrual fluid which is regurgitated up the Fallopian tubes.

The ability of the menstrual blood to pass easily through the cervix and into the vagina is an important factor in limiting the volume of retrograde flow.[5] Women who have an outflow blockage (either partial or complete) from congenital abnormalities, adhesions within the uterus or cervix or an imperforate hymen, may have excessive volumes of refluxed endometrial cells, and seem to have a higher incidence of endometriosis. One woman with endometriosis recovered completely after surgery was performed to correct a congenital abnormality which had been restricting her menstrual flow.[6]

Prostaglandins imbalance may also allow excessively large amounts of endometrium to reflux up the tubes by increasing uterine spasm *and* increasing Fallopian tube diameter. Women with endometriosis have higher levels of prostaglandins in their peritoneal fluid, and have Fallopian tubes with a wider diameter than usual.[7]

The immune system

The immune system appears to be involved in the development of endometriosis. The number of white cells—leucocytes—which are found in the peritoneal fluid, increase in the early stages of endometriosis. These white cells normally engulf and/or otherwise destroy cells which should not be found in the peritoneal fluid. Of these, the macrophages and the T-lymphocytes are the most important.

Macrophages congregate in tissues to clean away the debris caused by infection or inflammation by engulfing bacteria and cells like damaged red blood cells. In early-stage endometriosis (stages 1 and 2), these cells increase in number and activity to remove the endometrium shed into the pelvic cavity and to suppress the growth of the endometrial implants.[8] In the later stages, macrophage activity declines[9] and may be associated with a reduced ability to suppress the growth of the endometriosis.

Macrophages have many effects. In the early stages of endometriosis, macrophages can prevent fertilisation of ovum; reduce sperm motility; or engulf and destroy sperm, ovum, and embryo. This may contribute to the infertility associated with early-stage endometriosis.[10] Macrophages are also believed to increase the rate of adhesion formation associated with endometriosis,[11] and after surgery.[12] Later in the course of the disease, their activity is reduced[13] which may allow the endometriosis to become more invasive.

Macrophages also produce a number of factors which regulate immune activity and inflammation. Important amongst these is prostaglandin E 2 (PGE 2) which increases uterine muscle spasm and increases blood loss by dilating blood vessels. Another substance produced by macrophages is believed to act as growth factor for the implantation and maintenance of endometrium in the pelvic cavity.[14]

The other white cells of interest are the lymphocytes, especially the T-helper lymphocytes and the natural killer cells. The T-helper cells help in the functions of the immune system and serve as regulators of virtually all immune function. To do this they produce a number of proteins called lymphokines which, among other functions, stimulate the growth and proliferation of the natural killer cells, and improve the surveillance and engulfing activities of the macrophages. These important functions of the T-helper lymphocytes are depressed in endometriosis.[15]

The natural killer cells are also affected. Natural killer cells can attach themselves to foreign or malignant cells, bacteria or virally-infected cells and inject the cell with a substance to destroy it. When women have endometriosis, the activity of natural killer cells is reduced.[16] This has been linked to oestrogen levels,[17] and to substances produced by the endometrial tissue itself.[18] High levels of oestrogen diminish natural killer activity, but this improves spontaneously as oestrogen levels fall. Treatments which reduce oestrogen levels are believed to improve the activity of the natural killer cells.

Another theory about endometriosis and the immune system is that endometriosis is an auto-immune condition. Auto-immune literally means that the body has antibodies to its own tissues, but as yet it is unclear whether the auto-immunity develops because of the endometriosis, or whether it preceded the endometriosis and caused it to occur.

Prostaglandins

Prostaglandins may be involved in the pain, the increased menstrual loss and some of the altered immune responses seen when women have endometriosis. These substances are so important to the normal function of the reproductive tract and as causative agents in disease that they have been given a whole chapter. See Chapter 6 'Prostaglandins'.

Cellular change

Some researchers believe that the cells which line the pelvic cavity alter and become identical to endometrial cells.[19] These cells then behave in the same way as the normally placed endometrium. No-one can say exactly why these cells might start to change, but this theory does help to explain the rare cases of endometriosis found in the lungs and other distant sites.

Risk factors for developing endometriosis

A number of dietary, inherited and lifestyle factors seem to contribute to the risk of developing endometriosis. Risk needs to be kept in perspective: not all risk factors carry the same weight; some will need to occur in combination with other risks for a cumulative effect to occur.

Menstrual characteristics

Risk of endometriosis seems to be associated with the frequency, length and regularity of the period. Starting to menstruate at an early age, long (more than seven days) and heavy *periods* are associated with an increased risk of endometriosis. Long and irregular *cycles* are associated with a lowered risk.[20]

Family

An immediate family member, either the mother or sister, of a woman with endometriosis is seven times more likely than other women to also have the condition. Daughters of women with endometriosis are also believed to have an increased risk of endometriosis.[21]

Exercise

The amount and timing of physical activity effects the chances of endometriosis developing. Women who engaged in strenuous physical activity during menstruation had an increased risk of endometriosis, thought to be related to an increased volume of retrograde flow.[22] Conversely, women who do regular exercise may have a reduced risk of endometriosis because exercise is thought to decrease the rate of oestrogen production.[23]

Pregnancy

Full-term pregnancies are associated with a decreased risk of endometriosis, and the reduced risk increases with each successive full-term pregnancy.[24] This does not mean that pregnancy will 'cure' endometriosis and there are cases of endometriosis being found in the pelvic cavity when a Caesarean section is performed. Breastfeeding for as long as possible after delivery is useful to delay the onset of the period and perhaps the incidence of endometriosis.

Type of contraception used

The use of the IUD has been associated with an increased incidence of endometriosis, possibly because the device increases the degree of retrograde flow[25] and may temporarily alter prostaglandins levels.[26]

It is not clear if there is a link between taking the Pill and endometriosis. Some studies have reported an increased risk, others a reduced risk, and still others no change.[27] In one study of more than 17 000 women, the incidence of endometriosis was lower in women currently taking oral contraceptives, but higher in former Pill users when they were compared with women who had never taken the Pill.[28]

The Pill might influence the risk of endometriosis in three ways: the oestrogen component could potentially increase risk (although the amount of oestrogen has steadily reduced over the past 30 years); the progesterone component might decrease risk; as might the reduced amount of menstrual bleeding observed when women take the Pill.

Caffeine

When 1000 women with infertility were asked about their caffeine consumption, researchers reported a significant increase in the risk of infertility due to tubal disease or endometriosis in the group of women who consumed between five and seven grams of caffeine per month.[29] (A strong cup of tea contains 50 mg, and a cup of coffee contains, on average 100 mg. Five to seven grams per month is roughly equivalent to two cups of coffee or four cups of tea a day.)

Alcohol

Two recent studies examined the relationship between alcohol and endometriosis. One found alcohol consumption was higher in women with endometriosis and that they also tended to drink more when they were experiencing gynaecological problems.[30] The other reported a decreased fertility rate with moderate alcohol consumption which was associated with either ovulatory disorders or endometriosis.[31]

Sex while menstruating

One American study asked nearly 500 women about their sexual practices to determine whether there was a relationship between sexual activity and the incidence of endometriosis. They found an increased rate of endometriosis when women had intercourse during their period, and an increased rate of infertility related to abnormalities of the Fallopian tubes.[32]

Tampon use

Tampons probably have no effect on the risk of developing endometriosis,[33] however, a link between long-term (more than fourteen years) tampon use and endometriosis has been found.[34]

Cigarette smoking

Smoking reduces risk by altering the levels of oestrogen, but needless to say is not a recommended practice.[35]

What it looks like

The ovary

About 60 per cent of women with endometriosis develop ovarian cysts which vary in size from microscopic spots to cysts the size of tennis balls. When small, the endometrial growths look a bit like blood blisters and are reddish-blue or brown (if the blood is old). Both ovaries are usually affected.

The ovary usually tries to contain the growth of the endometrial tissue by creating a capsule around it, and a cyst is formed. These cysts are either called endometriomas, 'chocolate cysts' or endometrial cysts, and are filled with the endometrial blood shed at each period. Even when small, these cysts have a tendency to rupture and spill their contents into the pelvic cavity.

If early rupture does not occur, the cyst/s grow within their thickened capsule. The encapsulated endometrial tissue still responds to hormonal change in the same way as normal endometrium and bleeds with each period causing the cyst/s increase in size every month. Over time the blood becomes thick, sticky and dark brown—hence the term 'chocolate cyst'.

Until the cyst ruptures, there will be little scar tissue formed. Instead, there may be increasing pain as the ovarian cyst becomes larger and presses on other organs, blood vessels and nerves. Alternatively, the cyst may grow painlessly, but either way, because the size of the cyst typically increases at each period, the risk of rupture multiplies as the months go by.

When large cysts rupture, they usually cause symptoms of acute abdominal pain and shock which has to be treated by immediate surgery. Occasionally, the cysts shrink spontaneously because the internal pressure becomes so great that the endometrial tissue is deprived of a blood supply and wastes away (atrophies). Atrophied cysts cause ovarian scarring which looks like multiple small whitened areas within the ovarian tissue.

Much more frequently, however, the cysts will rupture before they grow to any great size, shedding small amounts of menstrual blood. Even a very small amount of blood is extremely irritating to the lining of the pelvic cavity and causes inflammation and pain. Rupture often occurs during or just after the period, and may account for a large percentage of the pain felt with endometriosis.

The Fallopian tubes, ligaments and the peritoneum

Endometriosis in other locations can occur in conjunction with endometriosis on the ovary or independently. Common sites are in the pouch of Douglas, on the uterine ligaments (the round, broad, and uterosacral), and the pelvic peritoneum. These 'raspberry-like' lesions of varying number and size can be reddish-blue or brownish-black. As the endometriosis worsens, the lesions tend to merge together and form larger islands of endometrial implants.

The endometrial tissue will usually 'menstruate' for some months, but as the disease advances, scar tissue develops and fibrous, solid lumps form over the tissues and organs that have become invaded by the endometrial implants. These are called adhesions.

During a laparoscopy it is common to find multiple adhesions; endometrial implants at various stages of development and activity; and the drawing together of adjacent organs which have become increasingly immobilised by the bands and sheets of fibrous tissue.

The uterus

Endometrial growth within the muscle fibres of the uterus is termed adenomyosis. When the uterus is palpated, it feels larger and may have an irregular shape. Pain is common because the irritant menstrual blood is shed into a confined space between muscle fibres. This causes a combination of pressure-like symptoms (described as heavy pain) and cramping of the uterus due to muscle spasm. Occasionally, the endometrial implants form a well-defined benign tumour-like mass called an adenomyoma.

The uterus becomes retroverted (tilted backwards) and fixed (difficult to move) if endometrial growths are located on the ligaments which hold it in place.

Other sites

Endometrial implants can develop in the lower bowel and cause progressive scarring. This can become severe enough to cause constriction in the colon and occasionally even an obstruction in the bowel.

Irritation, severe intestinal cramps and bleeding can occur when moving the bowels, especially during the period.

Infrequently, endometrial implants are found in the bladder or the urethra, and can cause painful, frequent passing of urine. Blood may be detectable in the urine during menstruation. In the vagina or on the cervix, endometriosis looks like small raised patches of bluish tissue which is firm to touch, but which frequently breaks down and bleeds with the period. It may be associated with pain, particularly during intercourse. Occasionally these types of lesion may develop on the vulva.

Endometrial implants found in scar tissue or around the navel are called endometriomas. These also look like bluish swellings under the surface of the skin or within the scar tissue, and may break through the surface and bleed during the period. These are sometimes a long way from the pelvic region, for example in the arms and legs, or in the lungs. Endometriomas vary in size and can become quite tender to the touch when they swell as menstruation approaches.

Adhesions

One of the ways the body protects healthy tissues from irritant body fluids or infective material is to 'wall off' the problem area with a protective barrier. Adhesions (scar tissue) are the result. Blood is the irritant when a woman has endometriosis and the normal response (triggered by the macrophages) is to attempt to confine it to as small an area as possible.

Adhesions typically solidify over time and become thickened and fibrous. If the endometriosis progresses unchecked, more and more adhesions are formed. Eventually, the tissue and organs near the endometriosis are totally covered and plastered down by scar tissue and the pelvic organs become one large immoveable mass. Any movement of these constricted organs, for example during sexual activity or an examination by a doctor, can cause pain or discomfort.

Endometriosis and the menstrual cycle

Endometrial tissue, irrespective of its location, is continually influenced by the cyclic variation of hormones. During the follicular phase, oestrogen has the major effect on endometrial tissue. This is particularly so for the most stimulatory form of oestrogen, oestradiol. Increasing levels of this hormone during the first weeks of the cycle are responsible for the normal thickening of the endometrium, as well as for the growth of endometriosis and adenomyosis.

Endometrial tissue starts to produce microscopic glandular structures under the influence of progesterone during the luteal phase. This causes an increase in the volume of endometrial tissue and the increase in tissue mass can cause bloating and pelvic discomfort or pain before the period.

When menstruation begins and the (normally placed) endometrium is shed vaginally, the misplaced endometrium also starts to break down and is shed into the pelvic cavity (endometriosis) or between the muscle fibres of the uterus (adenomyosis).

What it feels like—the symptoms

Adenomyosis and (especially) endometriosis are both extremely variable diseases with diverse symptoms ranging from debilitating and recurrent pain, pelvic discomfort, painful sex, abnormal bleeding, premenstrual tension, and infertility to none at all.

Pain

The quality, timing and severity of pelvic pain is extremely variable; and there is no relationship between severity of endometriosis and the severity of the pain. About one-third of women with endometriosis have no pain.

The quality of pain is often described as a congestive, heavy, or a dull, dragging sensation in the pelvis. During the period, the pain can become sharper, more crampy and labour-like—sometimes pain is severe enough to cause fainting, vomiting and diarrhoea. The timing of pain varies from woman to woman. It can occur randomly throughout the month; at ovulation; before, during or after the period; or all the time. Many women report pain during intercourse or during bowel movements.

Hormonal imbalance

Most women with endometriosis have symptoms of PMS including anxiety, mood swings, bloating, breast soreness, constipation, food cravings, and headaches. These symptoms are believed to be related to an imbalance between oestrogen and progesterone. Symptoms may occur from a few days premenstrually or start just after or at ovulation and last for up to two weeks.

Cycle length and menstrual flow

Some women with endometriosis have long cycles, but a short cycle with a heavier period is common. The flow is characteristically slow to start and may be thick, black and tarry at first. Irregular cycles, spotting, and/or mid-cycle bleeding can be common.

Making a diagnosis

The 'suggestive' signs and symptoms

Some symptoms occur so commonly that they indicate the need for a pelvic examination and possibly, further (surgical) investigations. The *suggestive* symptoms, in decreasing order of significance, are:

- severe dysmenorrhoea
- infertility
- pain associated with sexual activity
- pain increasing in severity toward the end of the period
- pain before period and at ovulation
- one-sided pelvic pain
- a mother or sister with endometriosis

Pelvic examination
A fixed and retroverted uterus, as well as nodules or swellings along the uterine ligaments, increases the likelihood of endometriosis. A large, bulky or irregularly shaped uterus can indicate adenomyosis. Referral to a specialist gynaecologist is likely when the combined symptoms and physical findings strongly indicate endometriosis or adenomyosis.

Ultrasound
An ultrasound can be used to aid diagnosis. This is a type of imaging using high frequency soundwaves to show the contents of the pelvic cavity. (An ultrasound for endometriosis or adenomyosis is performed with the same instrument that is used during pregnancy.) The ultrasound image might be taken abdominally or vaginally. Ultrasound imaging will not reveal endometriosis in the pelvic cavity, but it can be used to diagnose adenomyosis or ovarian cysts. Endometriomas (the particular type of ovarian cyst associated with endometriosis) are blood filled and appear as denser lesions than other fluid-filled cysts.

The definitive diagnosis

Laparoscopy
A laparoscopy is the only way that a diagnosis of endometriosis can be absolutely confirmed. The procedure is described in Chapter 20 'Drugs and surgery'.

Treatment

■ ■

■ ■ The medical approach

Surgery

Laparoscopic removal of endometrial lesions or small cysts is the commonest way to manage endometriosis surgically. Occasionally, some women will need microsurgery to remove adhesions from the pelvic cavity or the tubes; and serious endometriosis or intractable pain may require a hysterectomy.

Laser laparoscopic surgery for the treatment of pain associated with endometriosis is very successful. In one study of pain relief following laparoscopic laser, 62.5 per cent of women said that their pain was reduced or resolved. There were no complications related to either the operation or the laser.[36]

However, surgical treatment of endometriosis will not necessarily increase fertility. Similar pregnancy rates were shown with laparoscopy for observation, and laparoscopy for diathermy or laser. In fact, a number of studies suggest that neither the medical nor surgical treatment of mild endometriosis improves the fertility rate more than no treatment at all. In severe endometriosis, laser treatment seems to be superior to laparotomy or diathermy in improving fertility rates.[37] The common surgical procedures used to treat endometriosis are described in Chapter 20, 'Drugs and surgery'.

Drugs

The aim of drug treatments for endometriosis is to either reduce the volume of menstrual flow (the Pill), to create a pseudo-pregnancy state (the progestogens Provera and danazol, or the Pill when given continuously) or to cause a temporary menopausal state (the GnRH agonists). The decision to use one type of medication over another depends on the woman's history, the severity of the condition and her desire to become pregnant. These drugs, and the prostaglandins inhibitors used for the treatment of menstrual pain are discussed in Chapter 20 'Drugs and surgery'.

 The natural therapist's approach

The aims of treatment are to improve relative oestrogen excess and immune system irregularities; to regulate prostaglandin synthesis; to ensure normal uterine function and menstrual flow; and when appropriate, to improve fertility. Appropriate dietary and lifestyle changes are usually ongoing to minimise chances of a recurrence.

The amount of pain and the desire for pregnancy are the characteristics of a woman's history that determine the type of treatment she is to be given. For instance, some categories of herbs, such as the emmenagogues, cannot be given when pregnancy is desired; and when pain is severe, it will be given priority of treatment.

Many of the complaints associated with endometriosis are covered in detail elsewhere in this book. For instance a whole section is devoted to the management of period pain, another to the treatment of excessive bleeding, and another to PMS. In this chapter, only the essentials will be given if the treatment is covered in another section, and the reader will be directed to that section for further information.

Reducing the growth-promoting effects of oestrogen

Endometriosis is believed to be related to a relative oestrogen to progesterone ratio imbalance which causes the PMS-type symptoms as well as the abnormal production of endometrium. Oestrogen levels are influenced by 'competitive inhibition' with plant oestrogens; and dietary changes and exercise to improve oestrogen clearance. This is discussed in the section on relative oestrogen excess in Chapter 5 'Maintaining hormonal balance'. The aim is to keep oestrogen within normal limits, rather than reduce the levels below normal as with medical treatments.

In essence the regime involves increasing dietary fibre intake; eating bitter foods such as chicory and radicchio; cabbages; yoghurt; reducing fat intake; and exercising regularly.

Some women will not respond adequately to dietary or herbal manipulation of oestrogen. For them an oestrogen-deprived or oestrogen-free environment produced with drugs is the best place to start. In the meantime, all of the other aspects of treatment can be started (apart from hormone regulation which cannot be undertaken while women are on drugs) in preparation for the time when they are taken off medication.

Uterine tone

Uterine tone is primarily effected by the prostaglandins balance and is responsible for the ease of menstruation and the amount and type of menstrual pain. Herbal and other remedies are selected from those which:

- initiate orderly uterine contractions, the uterine tonics
- encourage an expulsive uterine action, the emmenagogues
- reduce excessive and abnormal uterine spasm, the spasmolytics
- rectify prostaglandins imbalance.

Uterine tonics
Uterine tonics initiate regular and orderly uterine contractions and regulate uterine tone. *Angelica sinensis* is the principal herb used for

endometriosis; *Caulophyllum thalictroides*, *Chamaelirium luteum*, and *Rubus idaeus* are also indicated.

Emmenagogues

Sluggish menstrual flow, which is thick, tarry and dark is a common symptom of endometriosis and indicates a need for emmenagogues (uterine stimulants). Emmenagogues have an expulsive effect on the uterus, and can hasten the menstrual flow. They are indicated for congestive symptoms which include heavy dragging pain, especially when menstruation is late. They are always prescribed with the uterine tonics. *Artemesia vulgaris* and *Ruta graveolens* are amongst the most useful.

Spasmolytics

Spasmolytics reduce uterine muscle spasm, relieve pain and ensure orderly uterine evacuation. The most important for endometriosis include the Viburnums, *Paeonia lactiflora* and *Corydalis ambigua*.

Prostaglandins regulation

The omega-3 essential fatty acids found in oily fish have the greatest impact on menstrual pain and retrograde flow caused by prostaglandins or leukotriene imbalance. Between three and five 200 g serves of fish per week, or 2–3 capsules of fish oils daily containing around 200 mg of EPA and 100 mg of DHA are beneficial.

The herbs *Tanacetum parthenium* and *Zingiber officinale* also have prostaglandins-inhibiting effects and can improve menstrual pain. *Tanacetum parthenium* is a Cold herb, *Zingiber officinale* is Hot, and as most menstrual pain is worsened by cold, *Tanacetum* is often combined with *Zingiber*.

PMS

PMS is common when women have endometriosis or adenomyosis. Natural therapists use these symptoms to determine the degree of hormonal imbalance and as an indication of the success of treatments. PMS is often associated with relative oestrogen excess and progesterone deficiency. The treatment of this type of hormonal imbalance is outlined in the 'PMS' section in Chapter 8.

Mood swings

Episodes of depression and irritability often accompany endometriosis. Common symptoms are feeling overwhelmed, tearful and irritable; feeling inadequate and as though everything is too much; inappropriate tiredness; irritability and 'on a short fuse' all the time. These may become worse premenstrually when other physical symptoms are at their peak, and are often confused with PMS, but unlike PMS, these symptoms last all month.

There are a number of reasons why women have these sorts of feelings, not the least of which is continual pain or the anticipation of the arrival of the period. Infertility, the constant recurrence of the condition and the inevitability of PMS are also common triggers. Many women feel worn down by their repeated experiences with surgery and the frustration of a condition which seems so totally out of their control.

These types of feelings are called 'reactive' to indicate that they have occurred as a reaction to an event, in this case to some aspect of endometriosis.

Although counselling is one way of dealing with reactive depression—probably the best way for most people—it is not always acceptable. *Hypericum perforatum*, the B complex vitamins, and the common nervines such as *Avena sativa*, *Scutellaria lateriflora* and *Passiflora incarnata* are useful. Exercising often helps, especially exercise first thing in the morning and of the 'long slow distance' variety. Functional hypoglycaemia often aggravates mood swings or depression. A hypoglycaemic diet is included on pages 129–30.

Infertility

Many women consult natural therapists for infertility associated with endometriosis. Often they have been treated by gynaecologists and have tried in-vitro fertilisation (IVF) without success and try natural medicine as the last resort. All of the problems associated with endometriosis-related infertility—prostaglandins imbalance, luteinised unruptured follicle syndrome, failed ovarian follicle development, infrequent ovulation, immune dysfunction and adhesions need to be treated to provide the most stable environment for conception to take place.[38]

Immune system irregularities

The traditional treatment for conditions such as endometriosis were based on symptoms rather than any knowledge of the underlying causes. The common and recurring symptom of lower pelvic discomfort, heaviness and dragging pain was referred to as pelvic congestion and was said to be, in part, related to lymphatic congestion. It has since been discovered that the herbs used for lymphatic congestion, the 'lymphatic drainage herbs', all have an effect on the immune response.

Calendula officinalis is the favoured lymphatic drainage herb. It reduces muscle spasm, lessens menstrual bleeding, and reduces inflammation. It also has well-known effects as a wound healer and antiseptic when applied to the skin, and has an immune-stimulating effect when taken internally. It is useful when there is dull, congestive pain with heavy bleeding; and in any case of menstrual disorder with altered immune function. All of these factors are common to endometriosis.

Fish oils, star flower oil and evening primrose oil alter prostaglandins and leukotriene levels and may be capable of improving fertility. Evening primrose, from between 2000–3000 mg daily, and/or fish oils also between 2000–3000 mg daily, can be taken as supplements. A high essential fatty acid diet is also recommended.

Grape seed extract
A number of practitioners have reported improvement in the severity of endometriosis with the use of grape seed extract. The exact mode of action is unknown, but may be related to an inhibition of the release of prostaglandins, leukotrienes and other compounds that promote inflammation. The standard dose of grape seed extract is between 150 to 300 mg per day of the oligomeric procyanidins (pycnogenol).

Problems with ovulation
A number of problems are associated with ovulation when women have endometriosis. In the follicular phase, ovulation can either be delayed or the follicle might not develop normally. Luteinised unruptured follicle syndrome—where the follicle develops but the egg is not expelled—is thought to be one of the causes of infertility which effects the luteal phase.[39] The other, lower than normal progesterone levels, is often referred to as a luteal phase defect and is commonly seen in association with luteinised unruptured follicle syndrome. These conditions are associated with ovulatory infertility or early miscarriage.

Chamaelirium luteum is known in herbal circles as a herb to regulate ovarian function during the follicular phase. It is used for ovarian cysts and for infertility (years ago, its use was forbidden if a woman was unmarried). *Vitex agnus castus*, is also useful for infertility associated with failure to ovulate, and for problems of the luteal phase. It should never be self-prescribed as it can over-stimulate ovarian follicles.[40]

Other herbs known to non-specifically enhance fertility include *Aletris farinosa* and *Angelica sinensis*. Vitamin E also seems to improve fertility, possibly by reducing adhesion formation.

Adhesions
Adhesions increase when women have endometriosis. Vitamin E has been shown to reduce adhesion formation.[41] It is likely that the reduction in adhesion formation is related to the inhibition of the series 2 prostaglandins production (which increase inflammation)[42], and better removal of debris in the pelvic fluid by white cells.[43]

Doses of 500–1000 IU of vitamin E can be used to prevent adhesion formation, although doses at this level should be supervised. Large doses of vitamin E (exceeding 500 IU) should not be given in the immediate pre- or post-operative period as there is a slight chance that bleeding may occur due to reduced platelet adhesiveness.

Irritable bowel syndrome and constipation

Irritable bowel syndrome commonly accompanies endometriosis, and can aggravate the severity of period pain. Because some of the symptoms of endometriosis are so similar to irritable bowel syndrome, many women do not realise that they have bowel spasm, and treat their pain and bloating inappropriately.

When irritable bowel syndrome is suspected, the diet outlined on pages 230–1, and especially the seed breakfast, is useful. The seed breakfast also has the advantages of being rich in trace minerals, calcium and essential fatty acids.

Constipation is also a common problem for many women when they are expecting a period. Apart from a sense of pelvic discomfort, constipation usually aggravates dysmenorrhoea and reduces the capacity for oestrogen clearance via the bowel. Bitter green vegetables and dietary fibre are the best remedies for constipation.

Analgesics containing codeine are very useful for pain control, but are inclined to aggravate constipation. A chemist or doctor can give advice on the most suitable codeine-free preparation.

CASE STUDY

Deborah is 28 and has had endometriosis since her early twenties. She has had one endometrioma removed and has had a variety of drugs including Provera and the Pill. She has recently decided to come off all medication, but has had bad period pain. Recently she fainted while doing aerobics during her period because of the severity of the pain. Her other symptoms are premenstrual acne, PMS and a tendency to constipation.

For the last four years she has been studying, but now has her first job which she finds very stressful. She and her partner would like to start a family in about two years (this is the reason for coming off medication), and are using condoms for contraception. She had one termination nine years ago.

Her treatment
Diet: Low-fat, high-fibre diet with no coffee, chocolate or alcohol. Bitter greens every day as a salad or cooked vegetables. Chinese or other cabbage at least three times a week. Review of diet after three months.
Exercise: 30 minutes of rapid walking every second day, no exercise during the period, and one class of aerobics weekly.
Herbs: Vitex agnus castus, Chamaelirium luteum, Angelica sinensis, Berberis vulgaris and *Cinnamomum zeylanicum,* one dose morning and night. Period pain mix consisting of *Viburnum opulus, Corydalis ambigua, Zingiber officinale, Anemone pulsatilla, Paeonia lactiflora* and *Glycyrrhiza glabra,* taken 2–3 hourly for period pain as needed.
Supplements: Vitamin B complex, one tablet daily and increased to two daily (divided dose) for ten days prior to the period. Vitamin E 500 IU for adhesions.

Self care

The possibilities for relief of some of the symptoms associated with endometriosis by adopting simple dietary and lifestyle changes are very good. Many women also seem to be able to reduce their recurrence rate by continuing to adhere to these changes.

- Reducing risk factors, where possible, taking regular exercise, reducing caffeine and alcohol intake.
- Adhering to a low fat, high fibre and high essential fatty acid diet.
- Having a regular intake of the cabbage family vegetables, phyto-oestrogens and lignans for competitive inhibition of oestrogens.
- Adopting a lifestyle which balances work and relaxation, and allows for some time to have fun, relax and a good laugh.
- Finally, make sure of good reliable professional back-up. This is too complicated to be taken on alone.

THE LIVER

In antiquity, the liver was considered to be the 'seat of the mind' and a liver imbalance could give rise to grave emotional states. The humoral theory described two personality types (temperaments) related to bile (and directly or indirectly to the liver)—the Choleric and the Melancholic.

The Choleric person was hot-tempered and irascible. So common has this concept remained that we still describe people who are bad tempered as being 'liverish'. Melancholic was the temperament associated with the Black Bile. An excess of Black Bile might cause introversion, depression, or even insanity.

The humoral theory also described a wide range of physical complaints, including problems associated with menstruation. A Hot womb caused by an excess of Yellow Bile, caused fiery and red menstrual loss; a Cold womb led to too little menstrual loss and a feeling of coldness and heaviness in the pelvic area.[44]

The symptoms associated with the Liver are not peculiar to Western thought and the humoral theory. The symptoms of Liver disharmony described by traditional Chinese medicine include irritability, depression, frustration, anger, and digestive upsets; and common gynaecological complaints such as PMS, irregular menstruation, light periods or amenorrhoea, infertility and dysmenorrhoea.[45]

Many of the broader concepts of the humoral theory and Liver dysfunction are incorporated into the herbalist's diagnosis and treatment today. Herbs and foods which improve liver function are used to treat conditions accompanied by emotional symptoms, such as

---

PMS; and conditions caused by hormonal imbalance such as fibrocystic breast disease, endometriosis, fibroids, and some types of excessive bleeding. Liver function is adversely affected by poor diet, over-eating, excessive intake of fats, sugars, alcohol, and coffee; and the burden of environmental poisons.

As the major organ of detoxification in the body, the liver must be ready to process the (approximately) 3000 chemicals which can be added to foods during processing, and around another 12 000 chemicals which can be used in food packing materials; the pesticides, fungicides and antibiotics which commonly contaminate food and the environment; and the prescribed, recreational and social drugs. Since early this century, an estimated four million new chemicals have been introduced into the environment. For about 80 per cent of these, the long-term effects on the body are unknown.[46]

Functions of the liver

- Detoxification of drugs, chemicals and poisons.
- Bile production.
- Storage of vitamins (especially the fat-soluble vitamins A, E, D, and K) and minerals.
- Storage of sugar in the form of glycogen.
- Storage of blood which can be quickly released if needed.
- Heat and energy production from the breakdown of fats, proteins and carbohydrates.
- Production of the plasma proteins.
- Break down, excrete and/or recycle hormones.

Optimising liver function

Protection of liver cells
- *Silybum marianum* seeds contain the most potent liver cell protective compounds known to exist.
- Anti-oxidants, such as vitamins A, E and C, betacarotene and selenium.
- Phosphatidyl choline, or lecithin, is a major component of healthy cell membranes. It protects liver cell membranes from damage from the continual attack of toxins and free radicals.

Improved bile flow
- Bitter foods and herbs (see Table 15.1) increase the flow of bile which is the vehicle for removing the substances broken down by liver cells.

Improved detoxification
- Specific herbs can improve liver enzyme activity such as *Silybum marianum* and *Schizandra chinensis*.
- Sulphur compounds found in cabbage family vegetables, garlic,

and dandelion, can induce enzymes reactions in the liver which assist with detoxification. Brussels sprouts and cabbage, for example, can improve the breakdown and removal of some drugs.

- An adequate protein intake is necessary to bind (conjugate) some toxic materials.
- Carbohydrates assist with detoxification pathways. Low kilojoule diets may not provide enough carbohydrate for the liver to function as an organ of detoxification.
- Minerals such as magnesium, calcium, zinc, copper and iron are essential components of many of the enzymes needed in detoxification pathways and are also involved in biochemical reactions which help to prevent free radical damage in liver cells.
- Ingestion of the foods which inactivate oestrogens through methylation—a chemical reaction which occurs in the liver, especially methionine in beans, eggs, onions and garlic.

Table 15.1 Bitter foods and herbs

Foods	Herbs
Endive	St Mary's thistle (*Silybum marianum*)
Chicory	Gentian (*Gentiana lutea*)
Silverbeet	Barberry (*Berberis vulgaris*)
Radicchio	Centaury (*Centaurium erythraea*)
Cos (outer leaves)	Hops (*Humulus lupulus*)
Mustard greens	Artichoke leaves (outer) (*Cynara scolymus*)
Dandelion leaf	
Dandelion root (coffee)	
Grapefruit	

16

Ovarian cysts

Key words

aromatisation
cystadenoma
fibroma
follicular cyst
FSH
hyperprolactinaemia
insulin resistance
LH
luteal cyst
oestradiol

oestrone
pedicle
pedunculated cyst
peripheral conversion
polycystic ovarian
  disease (PCOD)
SHBG
teratoma
torsion

The ovary consists of many complex tissues which perform a variety of cyclic functions such as ovum (egg) production and hormone secretion. Sometimes ovarian tissue begins to develop abnormally and cysts or tumours form. Ovarian cysts range from cancerous to completely harmless, requiring no treatment.

Ovarian cysts can be structurally different from each other and often have unique behaviour patterns. For example, if the cells that produce ovum develop abnormally, they may become a dermoid cyst which contains teeth and hair, a rather bizarre, but common ovarian cyst. If the cells which produce hormones for the natural cycle develop abnormally, the resulting cyst may produce large amounts of unnecessary hormones. Some cysts are associated with painful conditions like endometriosis; others may develop and resolve spontaneously without the woman ever knowing.

Many ovarian cysts are symptom-free. Often women only discover they have an ovarian cyst because of a routine examination, or when an examination is being performed for another reason. Sometimes pain during intercourse can be a warning sign, and very large cysts can cause pressure symptoms, abdominal enlargement and discomfort.

An ultrasound will detect most ovarian cysts and a doctor can sometimes make an 'educated guess' about the type because some types of cysts are characteristically solid, semi-solid or fluid-filled. However, many of the different types of cysts have forms which can be benign, malignant or 'borderline', and it is usually not possible to differentiate between these different forms without surgery.

The most reliable method of telling whether a cyst is malignant, benign or somewhere in between, is to examine it under a microscope. This will require a general anaesthetic and either a laparoscopy or laparotomy so that the cyst can be removed. Because of the many different cyst types, and the possibility that some of these may be cancerous, it is essential that women with ovarian cysts know which type of cyst they and their practitioners are dealing with.

THE DIFFERENT TYPES OF OVARIAN CYSTS

Benign

There are many different types of benign ovarian cyst. The most common ones are the physiological cysts and those associated with polycystic ovarian disease (PCOD) both of which develop as a result of a disturbance in the normal processes associated with ovulation. They are discussed later in this chapter. Other less common varieties include the cystadenomas, fibromas, dermoid cysts and Brenner cysts. Many are symptom-free unless they rupture or twist on their stem or pedicle.

Serous and mucinous cystadenomas

These types of ovarian cyst frequently grow to very large sizes and are sometimes attached to the ovary by a stem or pedicle which carries the blood supply to the cyst. Pain or rupture of the cyst can occur if the cyst twists on its pedicle.

Torsion can be complete or occur intermittently as the cyst twists and then untwists again. Complete torsion is usually accompanied by extreme pain and often vomiting. There is a high risk of rupture because the cyst tends to swell. Incomplete or intermittent torsion usually causes episodic pain.

The serous cysts are filled with a thinnish liquid, while the mucinous ones contain a much stickier mucus-like substance. Rupture of both types is associated with pain, but the mucinous cyst causes more irritation of the pelvic lining and adhesions are more common. They do not affect ovulation, but rarely reabsorb by themselves and surgery is advisable.

These ovarian cysts have a malignant form called serous or mucinous cystadenocarcinoma. These should be removed as soon as possible.

Fibromas

Fibromas are fibrous, often solid and sometimes produce oestrogen. Absolute confirmation of their type can only be made after they are examined under a microscope, and as they rarely go away of their own accord, doctors usually recommend that they be removed.

Dermoid cysts (teratomas)

Dermoid cysts form as a result of abnormal multiplication of the cells which produce the ovum. These ovum-producing cells have the capacity to give rise to any of the many different types of tissue normally found in the body. Erratic growth of these cells, as occurs in dermoid cysts, can produce structures including hair, teeth, bones and skin fragments. Dermoid cysts can be pedunculated, sometimes become malignant, and will not resolve spontaneously. They rarely rupture, but when they do their contents are extremely irritating and they cause severe pain. They are best removed surgically.

Brenner tumours

These are usually small and benign, but can sometimes become malignant. They can occur at any age, but are more common when women are post-menopausal. They are sometimes associated with abnormal periods and surgical removal is usually recommended.

Malignant (ovarian cancer)

Ovarian cancer is quite rare, but carries serious implications because it is usually symptom-free until it is relatively advanced. The earlier ovarian cancer is diagnosed, the greater the chances of survival—the early removal and treatment of a cancerous cyst can result in a complete cure in some cases. Ovarian cysts can be 'borderline'—neither benign or malignant, but somewhere between the two, and some benign ovarian cysts may become malignant. Some tumours might metastasise to the ovary, but have their origin elsewhere.

To reduce the risk of undiagnosed ovarian cancer, women over 40 should have an annual internal examination and all women should have an internal examination when they have a Pap smear. Routine pelvic ultrasound screening was also suggested as a way of reducing the risk of ovarian cancer, but was not found to be cost-effective.

Hormone-producing

Hormone-producing cysts, also known as functioning cysts, have the ability to produce oestrogens or androgens and therefore interfere with the cycle or fertility. They are usually diagnosed because of their effects on the period or, in the case of those cysts which produce androgens (male hormones), because they have masculinising effects including male-pattern hair growth, deepening of the voice, decreased breast size and the development of a male-type body shape. These androgen-producing cysts are rare. Removal of the cyst should rectify all of these problems, although the voice changes may persist.

The ovarian cysts which produce oestrogen are the more common of the two. They can cause irregular and heavy bleeding and abnormal cell changes in the endometrium which can progress to endometrial cancer. All of these symptoms are related to the prolonged and elevated exposure to oestrogen. These cysts vary in size, but are often quite small. Ovulation can still occur despite the excess oestrogen levels, albeit erratically.

Treatment

The treatment of ovarian cysts needs to be adapted to prevent the complications associated with each type. Complications can include the spread of cancer; rupture; twisting of the cyst on its pedicle, commonly known as torsion; interference with the regularity of the cycle; destruction of ovarian tissue; and infertility. The three strategies often adopted are surgical removal, hormonal treatments, or 'wait and see'.

Many cysts require no treatment. If the cyst is small, and there is a very good chance that it is benign and will reabsorb of its own accord, it is safe to observe and not treat. This is especially so for young women who develop benign physiological cysts, which usually reabsorb within two cycles. However, when any cyst is present for more than two cycles, surgery is often recommended because benign and trouble-free cysts are less likely to persist for this long. The Pill may be recommended when recurrent cysts are a problem or for some cases of PCOD because it prevents ovulation which is the source of these cysts. Long-term use of the Pill is also associated with a lower risk of developing ovarian cancer.

Surgical removal of a cyst is advised if it has characteristics which indicate possible complications or serious illness. Cysts which continue to grow, fail to reabsorb or which might be malignant fall into this category. Some women seek natural treatments to 'dissolve' or 'shrink' the cyst as an alternative to surgery. This is not a good policy—treating ovarian cysts without specific knowledge of their type is asking for trouble.

Torsion of ovarian cysts is associated with severe pain and will require surgery. Torsion is when the ovary containing the cyst twists and cuts off its own blood supply, causing death of the ovarian tissue.

Large cysts, especially those larger than 5 cm, can rupture at any time causing pain and adhesions. Blood-filled cysts associated with endometriosis (endometriomas) tend to grow with each period and are prone to rupture, even when quite small. Growing or large ovarian cysts are removed because they can destroy normal ovarian tissue, sometimes so severely that the entire ovary atrophies and becomes incapable of ovulation or hormone production. If malignancy is suspected, surgical removal is also recommended.

Ovarian cancer is a concern for all women. Although the incidence is very much less for younger women, one in every three ovarian cysts which occur from 45 onwards are cancerous. In this age group, when a small benign-looking cyst is discovered the doctor may wait for one cycle, but if it persists or if there is any doubt about the type of cyst, the doctor will suggest immediate removal.

Ovarian cysts when women are post-menopausal women are suspicious (because ovulation has stopped, ovarian cysts should not form) and there is a high likelihood of malignancy. They should be removed as soon as possible. Hormone 'markers' are often produced by ovarian cancers and these can be used as diagnostic aids and, after surgical removal, as a way of telling whether the malignancy has been completely eradicated.

PHYSIOLOGICAL CYSTS

Physiological cysts are also known as simple cysts or functional cysts (and should not be confused with 'functioning cysts', which produce hormones). Functional cysts represent a deviation in the normal functioning of the ovary rather than an expression of abnormal cell growth. There are two sorts of physiological cysts, follicular and luteal, which are named after the time they appear in the menstrual cycle.

Follicular cysts

Follicular cysts are formed due to a deviation of the normal ovulation and occur quite frequently. They develop as a consequence of a developing follicle (egg sac) and may occur either because the most mature follicle fails to release its ovum and continues to grow, forming a cyst; or one/some of the other developing follicles fail to disintegrate and form a cyst instead.

In most cases they are small, cause few symptoms, and may only be discovered because of a routine examination. They generally require no treatment and are usually re-absorbed without causing any problems. Occasionally these cysts may rupture, but since they are small and don't often contain blood, they usually require no further treatment.

Luteal cysts

Luteal cysts develop in the second phase of the cycle after the corpus luteum has formed. If large enough they can cause dull pain on one side, but most of the time they are only discovered because of a routine examination. They require no treatment and will usually be re-absorbed uneventfully.

Very occasionally luteal cysts rupture. When the cyst is small, the pain is generally mild, requires no treatment, and ceases once the period starts (due to the degeneration of the corpus luteum which is the source of the minor blood loss). However large blood-filled cysts can be associated with quite a degree of pain and may be confused with ruptured ectopic pregnancy or other causes of abdominal pain.

Luteal cysts may interfere with progesterone production and can cause irregularities in the cycle. The progesterone stimulates the uterine lining and can delay the onset of menstruation; or can cause an alteration in blood loss during the period. Luteal cysts usually disappear after one cycle, and the menstrual cycle will return to normal without any treatment.

■ ■

■ ■   The medical approach

Physiological cysts are diagnosed with ultrasound imaging. They rarely require treatment, however, some women develop these cysts very regularly and sometimes suppression of ovulation with the Pill is suggested as a treatment.

 The natural therapist's approach

Physiological cysts require no treatment unless they occur frequently and interfere with the cycle or cause pain. The herbs used most often for physiological cysts are *Chamaelirium luteum* and *Paeonia lactiflora*. *Chamaelirium luteum* is believed to normalise ovarian function including the processes of ovulation (it is also used for infertility associated with erratic ovulation) and is specific for the treatment of ovarian cysts. The way that it works is not fully understood because, unlike the Pill, it does not stop ovulation, but it will usually prevent the formation of recurrent cysts.

Paeonia lactiflora has been shown to normalise follicular development because of its effect on aromatase enzyme and may prevent cyst formation. These herbs are discussed in Chapter 19 'Herbs'.

POLYCYSTIC OVARIAN DISEASE (PCOD)

Polycystic ovaries literally means a condition associated with many (poly) cysts in the ovary or ovaries. PCOD, however, is a more complex condition—in fact a series of conditions or syndromes—each of which has the common finding of multiple ovarian cysts. Unfortunately, there is a degree of confusion surrounding these terms and the conditions they describe because many writers, doctors and natural therapists do not differentiate between polycystic ovaries and polycystic ovarian disease.

With the use of ultrasound, it has been possible to identify that up to 20 per cent of all women have multiple ovarian cysts. Some of these women have both normal cycles and periods and experience no problems; others may have a range of symptoms including irregular menstruation or amenorrhoea. All of these women have polycystic ovaries, *but only those with additional hormonal irregularities have polycystic ovarian disease*. To reduce confusion, the condition which presents as multiple simple cysts on the ovaries is referred to as polycystic ovaries. The more complicated syndrome or disease which includes a variety of additional hormonal abnormalities *and* ovarian cysts is called polycystic ovarian disease (PCOD). This section deals only with PCOD.

PCOD is accompanied by a *tendency* to produce too much androgen (male hormones) and to ovulate erratically. Other symptoms of PCOD can be failure to menstruate, failure to ovulate, hirsutism and obesity; and women with PCOD might have none, any or all of these complaints.

Making a diagnosis of PCOD is complicated because the combination of symptoms commonly encountered—the ovulatory failure, hirsutism, obesity etc.—is not unique to PCOD. Women who have other endocrine disorders may develop similar symptoms. These conditions include Cushing's syndrome; inherited adrenal disorders such as congenital adrenal hyperplasia; hormone-producing cysts or tumours of the ovary and adrenal gland; hyperprolactinaemia (excess prolactin production); and disturbed function of the thyroid gland.

Diagnosis

PCOD is usually suspected because of the symptoms of menstrual irregularity or amenorrhoea in conjunction with male-pattern hair growth (for example, facial hair, hair around the nipples and navel, and more pubic hair than usual), obesity and infertility. An ultrasound of the ovaries will detect multiple ovarian cysts and blood tests usually reveal an elevated LH with relatively constant or low FSH levels. Before a firm diagnosis of PCOD can be made, all of the other possible types of endocrine abnormalities need to be excluded as causes. This usually involves a physical examination, blood tests and X-rays in addition to the ultrasound.

Causes

Although it is now generally agreed that PCOD originates in the ovary, a number of other factors seem to make important contributions. For instance, excess weight gain seems to be able to initiate hormonal changes that can transform a symptom-free condition into a full-blown case of PCOD. The hypothalamic-pituitary unit and the adrenal glands are also involved in PCOD, but their relative importance may vary in each case. It has been suggested that other endocrine glands like the thyroid might be associated with PCOD some of the time, or that a number of different triggers may interact in susceptible women.[1] PCOD may also be related to blood sugar abnormalities or be inherited. Around 40 per cent of the women in families with PCOD will have the condition, but not all of these women develop symptoms.

Abnormal ovarian function

Women with PCOD produce low levels of ovarian oestrogen (oestradiol) and excessive levels of ovarian androgens. This seems to support the view that the condition originates as an abnormality of the ovary. The androgens produced within the follicle seem to prevent ovulation and normal follicular development (see Figure 16.1). The end result is the formation of small cystic follicles instead of mature follicles with the capacity to ovulate. Some woman with PCOD have one ovary that is normal and one that is polycystic. This also suggests a primary ovarian problem because a hormonal imbalance which originated in other endocrine glands would affect both ovaries.

Excess weight gain

The fatty tissue, muscle and the brain have the capacity to convert androgens into oestrone, by a process known as aromatisation. Importantly, when women are overweight, the conversion of androgen to

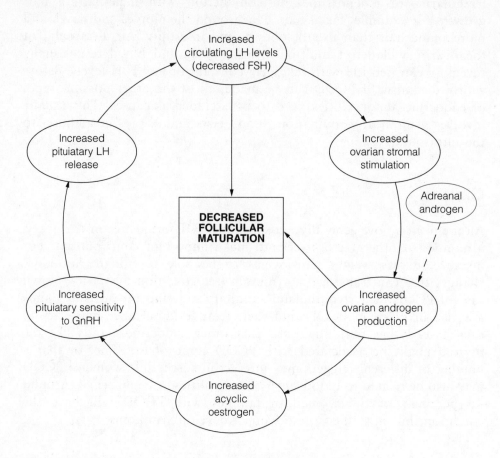

Figure 16.1 The causes of ovulatory failure in PCOD

oestrone is enhanced and much more oestrone is produced. This leads to the chronically high and non-variable levels of oestrogen.

This increased conversion of androgens in fatty tissue may affect PCOD,[2] and some women control the severity of the condition and the regularity of their menstrual cycle by reducing weight. It is likely that this tendency is inherited.

Women with PCOD tolerate being thin better than other women. They maintain their bone density even when their body mass index (BMI) is low, and continue to ovulate (or start to) when they are thin. For these reasons, some researchers speculate that women with PCOD will reproduce better in famines, and pass on this tendency to their daughters who will also have the reproductive edge when times are grim. Women without PCOD and 'normal ovaries' function best when there is an abundance of food. They do not have the hormonal profile to tolerate thinness easily; they stop menstruating or ovulating if they lose weight or are too thin;

and are most fertile and have better bone density when the food supply is regular and their body weight is within the normal range.

Many women with PCOD and obesity also have problems associated with insulin, known as insulin resistance. Insulin resistance develops because of an insensitivity of cellular insulin receptors to insulin. Insulin levels are normal or even elevated, but the insulin is incapable of transporting glucose into the cell. This leads to elevated *blood* glucose levels (but low *cellular* glucose levels), which further down—regulates the receptivity of cells to insulin. Insulin resistance is often seen in combination with obesity with a high abdominal distribution of fat (apple-shaped).

The adrenal gland

Another theory is that PCOD can be triggered by excessive *adrenal* production of androgens. These androgens are converted to oestrone in the fatty tissue, causing the blood levels of oestrone to rise. The elevated oestrone levels, which do not have the usual cyclic variations, stimulate the production of excessive amounts of luteinising hormone and insufficient follicle-stimulating hormone. The luteinising hormone triggers *ovarian* androgen production, and so the cycle is perpetuated.

The hypothalamic and pituitary hormones

Elevated levels of LH are generally accepted as being caused by androgen excess. Some researchers, however, have suggested that there may be a primary problem in the hypothalamus or the pituitary gland. Inappropriate hypothalamic secretion of GnRH can cause an increase in the pituitary's production of luteinising hormone which then causes an increase in the production of androgens. Excess androgens increase the secretion of luteinising hormone, and so the cycle becomes self-perpetuating.

The other pituitary hormone, FSH, is chronically low when women have PCOD. Low FSH is usually thought to be a casualty of the chronically elevated and unvarying oestrogens. Low FSH reduces the capacity of the cells in the follicle to convert androgen to oestrogen, and creates another self-perpetuating source of imbalance in the hormone levels.

Associated hormone changes

Elevated acyclic oestrogen

In PCOD, oestrogen levels are elevated and non-variable—unlike the fluctuating levels that are secreted from the ovary during a normal cycle. These oestrogens arise from the peripheral conversion of androgens to oestrogen, predominantly androstenedione to oestrone. Ovarian oestrogen production is chronically low due to the abnormal follicular development.

Androgen excess

Androgens can exert masculinising effects, but usually circulate in small amounts in the blood of all women without causing any problems. If a woman has PCOD, however, the levels of androgens are elevated, and though still well below the normal male levels, they contribute significantly to the hormonal imbalance and the symptoms of PCOD. These androgens arise from the ovary and the adrenal gland.

Sex hormone-binding globulin

SHBG is the carrier protein for both oestrogen and testosterone, but is reduced by high levels of androgen and obesity. Normally, most of the circulating testosterone would be bound to SHBG, making it less capable of exerting masculinising effects on skin and hair. When the level of SHBG is depressed, unbound testosterone circulates in the serum and causes acne and male-pattern hair growth.

Early patterns of PCOD

Many women with PCOD have similar early menstrual patterns. The age of menarche (when menstruation starts) is similar to other young women who do not develop PCOD, but:

- the menstrual cycle does not become regular several years after menarche occurs and continues to be erratic
- increased growth of hair in the male pattern (referred to as hirsutism) is seen around or before the onset of menstruation
- excess body weight is evident at or before the time of the menarche

When these early signs are not evident, excessive adult weight gain has been shown to be one of the common triggers for PCOD to become symptomatic. A body mass index (BMI) at 21 kg/m² can often maintain normal cycles.[3] (See page 165 for BMI calculations)

Signs and symptoms

A number of common signs and symptoms characterise PCOD.

- PCOD is the most common cause of ovulatory failure, and about 75 per cent of women with PCOD develop infertility.
- 60 per cent of those with PCOD have excess body hair.
- About half will not menstruate.
- Around 40 per cent are overweight.
- Nearly one-third have abnormal bleeding patterns.
- About 20 per cent develop signs associated with male hormones such as a deeper voice and changes in body shape.
- Only about 15 per cent have the temperature changes which indicate ovulation if they take and chart their temperature every morning (basal body temperature).
- Only about 10 per cent have regular cyclic periods.

■ ■
■ ■ The medical approach

There are three main aspects to the medical treatment of PCOD:

- Reduce the likelihood of cancerous change occurring in the lining of the uterus (the endometrium)
    The risk of endometrial cancer is minimised by the administration of cyclic hormones such as the Pill; or by small doses of progesterone for 7–10 days of each month. The progesterone, either taken alone or in the Pill, initiates changes in the endometrium which are similar to those in the normal cycle. When progesterone is stopped, menstruation occurs.
- Induce ovulation with drugs if the woman wants to become pregnant
    The most common prescription is Clomiphene Citrate or Clomid.
- Reduce masculinising effects of androgens
    Androgen excess can accompany a number of other gynaecological complaints. Recommendations for treatment are outlined in Chapter 13 'Amenorrhoea'.

 The natural therapist's approach

The natural therapist's treatment of PCOD is also directed at reducing the masculinising effects of the excess androgens, stimulating ovulation, and protecting the endometrium. About three-quarters of women with PCOD have blood lipid and blood sugar abnormalities which require treatment, and some women also have thyroid gland abnormalities or hyperprolactinaemia as well.

    The tendency to develop PCOD cannot be 'cured' or eliminated—the best that can be hoped for is the regulation of hormone levels so that symptoms are minimised. When the condition is severe, natural remedies may not be sufficient to improve the hormonal imbalance. A more suitable treatment may be to combine natural remedies and drugs, especially when there is serious risk of endometrial change or severe masculinising effects from androgens.

The emphasis of natural treatments depends on the combination of the symptoms and the desired outcome. Women who want to become pregnant will be given treatments to stimulate ovulation; when amenorrhoea is a problem, initiating menstruation is necessary to protect the endometrium; and when excess hair growth is a concern, the treatment should focus on the androgen levels.

Protecting the endometrium

For the endometrium to be adequately protected against cellular change caused by the elevated and unvarying levels of oestrogens, menstruation should occur at regular intervals. These intervals vary depending on the weight and age of the woman.

Women who are within the normal range for weight, and who are 35 or less, should have at least three periods every year; women who are older, and particularly when they are overweight should menstruate about twice as often. Obese women, who are likely to have more problems with PCOD, should menstruate as close to monthly as possible. For this reason, the Pill may be their best treatment option when women are obese and at increased risk of endometrial hyperplasia or cancer.

Natural remedies which may be useful to protect the endometrium are outlined in Chapter 12 'Erratic Bleeding' in the section on endometrial hyperplasia.

Normalising ovulation

The herbs which have been historically used for ovulatory disorders are the 'female tonic herbs'. Principal amongst these are *Chamaelirium luteum* and *Paeonia lactiflora*, both of which may have additional benefits in normalising follicular development and reducing the incidence of ovarian cysts. Female tonics usually contain phyto-oestrogens or steroidal saponins. They exert a much weaker effect than oestrogen and may normalise ovulation by improving the function of the hypothalamic–pituitary unit. Included in this group are the dioscin-containing herbs and *Angelica sinensis*. Their hormonal effects are discussed in Chapter 18 'Phyto-oestrogens'.

Androgen excess

The herbal and dietary treatment of androgen excess is outlined in Chapter 13 'Amenorrhoea'. *Vitex agnus castus* is often prescribed for menstrual irregularities and for conditions assumed to be associated with androgen excess, such as acne.[4] Its role in the treatment of PCOD, however, is unclear. *Vitex* stimulates ovulation, but has always been thought to increase LH levels, although this has recently been disputed by researchers who found that prolactin is the only pituitary hormone altered by administration of this herb.[5] Caution is warranted because some women with PCOD seem to improve initially (more regular cycles), but may regress after some months of *Vitex agnus castus* administration. At this stage it is not possible to make firm recommendations either way as more research is needed.

Normalising other aspects of hormonal profile

Luteinising hormone (LH)
Elevated LH occurs in association with excess androgen production and will decline once androgen production slows down. Three herbs, *Cimicifuga racemosa*, *Humulus lupulus*, and *Lycopus virginiana* have a direct impact on LH.

Of these, *Humulus lupulus* and *Cimicifuga racemosa* are most useful. *Humulus* is useful when stress and nervous tension accompany PCOD. *Lycopus virginiana* is usually given to treat hyperthyroidism, but will also reduce the levels of luteinising hormone as well as follicle-stimulating hormone. It is unsuitable for long-term administration and should not be given to re-establish ovulatory cycles.

Blood sugar abnormalities
Women with PCOD are prone to blood sugar abnormalities which develop as a result of obesity and insulin resistance. It is not entirely clear why the abnormal insulin response occurs but the treatment is weight reduction and to also assist the insulin to pass into the cells. The nutrients which help in this regard are magnesium, zinc, manganese and chromium. Herbs are *Gymnema sylvestre*, *Galega officinalis*, *Trigonella foenum-graecum* and the bitters.

Increasing fibre intake also stabilises blood sugar levels. Thirty to forty mg daily as part of whole foods is usually adequate, especially when spread over the entire day. Fibre has the additional advantage of increasing SHBG which reduces the levels of biologically active androgens; and lowers blood lipids.

Regulating the blood lipid levels
The general principles of blood lipid regulation are discussed in the dietary section. In addition, the bitter herbs, *Trigonella foenum-graecum*, high fibre foods, and the legumes (soya products, lentils) all contribute to a blood fat lowering effect.

MAGNESIUM

Magnesium is vital for the maintenance of bone density, the prevention of heart attacks and the functioning of all muscles.

- Bone health
  Magnesium is almost as important for bone health as calcium. It can suppress the activity of hormones which normally encourage the removal of calcium from bone. It also improves the absorption of calcium from food and increases its retention in the body.
  A high intake of calcium inhibits the absorption of magnesium. Foods traditionally thought of as being useful for bone density, such as dairy products, are also relatively low in magnesium (100 mLs of whole milk contains 115 mg of calcium, but only 10–15 mg of magnesium) which raises doubts about the suitability of large intakes of dairy products for bone health. Magnesium, either alone or with calcium, offsets the usual overnight bone mineral loss.

- Heart disease
  Magnesium protects the heart muscle from excess excitability which can cause irregularities in the heartbeat.

- PMS
  Magnesium can reduce the symptoms associated with premenstrual tension.

Deficiency signs and symptoms

- Weakness and/or tiredness, poor muscle coordination, apathy.
- Insomnia, hyperactivity.
- Susceptibility to toxic effects of digoxin, abnormalities of the heart's rhythm, abnormal heart tracing (ECG).
- Premenstrual tension.
- Muscle cramps, grimaces, tremors of the tongue, 'flickering' eyelids.
- Loss of appetite, nausea, constipation.
- Confusion, disorientation and memory impairment, learning disabilities.
- Vertigo.
- Difficulty swallowing or throat constriction (globus hystericus).

These symptoms can have serious causes, but when no obvious cause can be found, magnesium supplements or improved dietary magnesium intake may help.

Table 16.1 Sources of magnesium (mg per 100 gm)

The RDA for magnesium is 400–800 mg daily

Grains		Vegetables	
wheat bran*	520	beet tops	106
wheat germ	300	silver beet	65
whole wheat flour	140	spinach	59
oatmeal	110	raw parsley	52
muesli	100	beans	35
rye flour	92	green peas	33
white flour	36	broccoli	24
Seafood		beetroot	23
shrimps	110		
		Fruit	
Beans and nuts		dried figs	92
brazil nuts	410	dried apricots	65
soya flour	290	avocado	30
almonds	260	banana	20
peanuts	180	grapefruit juice	18
walnuts	130		

* Foods such as bran, which are rich in magnesium, may not provide the best source of minerals. Magnesium can become bound to the phytates in bran which reduce absorption. Whole foods from a wide variety of sources is the best way to attain a good intake of easily assimilable magnesium.

Section F

Setting it right

17

Food for health

Key words

alpha-linolenic acid

anti-oxidant

atherosclerosis

caffeine

carcinogen

cardiovascular disease

cellulose

eicosanoid

essential fatty acid

gamma-linolenic acid

HDL cholesterol

lactose intolerance

LDL cholesterol

lignans

linoleic acid

monounsaturated fat

omega-3 fatty acid

omega-6 fatty acid

phyto-oestrogen

polyunsaturated fat

saturated fat

theophylline

therapeutic diet

trans-fatty acid

triglyceride

xanthines

The idea that food can be used as a therapeutic tool is a foreign one to medicine, but natural therapists often incorporate dietary suggestions into the treatment plans of their patients. Eating a sensible, regular and highly nutritious diet will not fix all ills, but can contribute to good stamina and minimise the risk of illness.

The following dietary recommendations are amongst the most common dietary changes suggested by natural therapists. The daily diet is based on the now widespread knowledge that diets high in complex carbohydrates, fruits and vegetables, and low in saturated fats, are associated with the lowest rate of developing degenerative diseases.

TWENTY IMPORTANT DIETARY RECOMMENDATIONS FOR WOMEN

1. Eat a varied and interesting diet

A good diet does not have to be boring or taste like chaff—and there's certainly no need to eat foods that are unpalatable just because 'they're good for you'. Some of the healthiest and longest-living people in the world eat the most interesting and tasty diets. Southern Europeans, for instance, have low levels of cardiovascular disease; and Japanese women have much lower levels of breast cancer than Western women—and neither of their diets are boring.

2. Drink plenty of fluids every day

Water is vital. About two litres of water every day is the minimum amount of fluid a person should drink, and this should increase in hot weather and when exercising—as a general rule, a dry mouth means that dehydration has already started.

Fluids, like food, should be varied and should not come from coffee, tea and alcohol alone. Two or three glasses of plain water, preferably filtered, throughout the day are essential. Fruit juices (some of which have as much sugar as soft drinks) should be diluted. 'Fruit juice' drinks usually contain added sugar.

3. Eat fresh and organically grown foods where possible

The average volume of food consumed has reduced dramatically in comparison to past generations, making quality all important. Fresh is best—there are less preservatives, the food is less likely to be rancid, nutrient levels are higher and it tastes better. It is easier to see if fresh food has been spoiled or is old and past its 'use by' date. Where possible, buy organic foods to minimise exposure to chemicals.

4. Stay on 'therapeutic diets' only until the desired outcome is achieved

A therapeutic diet is prescribed with a particular outcome in mind, lowering cholesterol or improving anaemia, for example. Therapeutic diets need not be lifelong (fortunately, because some are very strict) and should only be maintained until the desired results have been obtained. Occasionally, some of the basic principles will need to be maintained— lower saturated fat intake is sensible for everyone, especially those with a high cholesterol—but it should not be necessary to stay on a rigid regime indefinitely.

Sometimes therapeutic diets do not work and it may be necessary to take additional medication or try an entirely different approach. If there are undesirable side effects such as excessive weight loss, weight gain, bloating or diarrhoea, the diet should be stopped. Therapeutic diets are not appropriate for all conditions and a failure to respond is often the fault of that diet and not the person on it.

5. Have at least five to seven different types of vegetables and three pieces of fruit daily

Vegetables and fruit contain a good range of vitamins, minerals, trace elements, essential fatty acids, anti-oxidants and fibre. They are also good sources of a variety of components which impart specific health-giving properties: cabbages and tomatoes reduce cancer risk; legumes contain phyto-oestrogens; bitter components flush the gall bladder; fruit pectin lowers cholesterol; and celery lowers blood pressure and reduces acid build-up in joints.

Vegetable consumption should be varied. Preparation by steaming, stir-fry or baking reduces nutrient loss. Two to three orange, red or yellow vegetables, a minimum of two green vegetables, and at least one of the cabbage family such as broccoli or cabbage—and some garlic or onion should be included daily because of their cancer-preventing and blood lipid-lowering properties.

Fruit should not be eaten instead of a vegetable-filled meal (fruits are generally lower in minerals and higher in sugars than vegetables). Fruit is best consumed whole and not juiced, to retain the fibre and slow the absorption rate of sugars.

6. The main energy foods should be complex carbohydrates

Carbohydrates are energy foods which can be consumed either as whole foods (this means that the food is unrefined—brown flour instead of white flour, for example), or as refined carbohydrate. Complex carbohydrate from whole grains and legumes, dried beans and peas, nuts and seeds, soya products and some of the root vegetables, should constitute the major part of any diet. Commonly eaten energy foods include breakfast cereals and muesli, bread, rice, beans, tofu, pasta and potato.

These complex carbohydrates are high in fibre and many also contain phyto-oestrogens. They can lower blood cholesterol, stabilise blood sugar, regulate bowel movements, reduce the appetite and ensure a good supply of regular energy. The slow energy release leads to greater stamina and fewer energy slumps after eating. This is important for anyone troubled by blood sugar symptoms, especially women who have premenstrual sugar cravings.

The milling of grains removes the husk and the germ as well as most of the nutrients, leaving the highly palatable, but nutritionally depleted refined carbohydrate (as in white flour, for example). Refined carbohydrates are the biggest source of 'empty' foods in the diet (an empty food contains very few nutrients but plenty of kilojoules) and tend to contribute to weight gain. They are a rapid source of energy for a 'quick-fix', but the blood sugar increases quickly and then drops rapidly causing fatigue, vagueness and irritability.

Complex carbohydrates contain some of the amino acids which make up proteins and can be combined in a meal so that they become a substitute for animal protein. Carbohydrate combining should be used by vegetarians to make sure that adequate amounts of protein are available on a daily basis. Here are the common combinations:

- Grains with beans: tofu and rice (Asia), lentils and rice (India), tortilla and beans (Mexican).
- Grains and nuts: peanuts and rice (Southern Asia), nut butters and bread (bread-eating countries); rice and cashews (Asia).
- Beans and seeds: sesame seed paste and beans (Middle East).

This doesn't have to be as complicated as it first appears. Many people instinctively cook like this or follow traditional recipes which incorporate these food combinations. Combining carbohydrates gives the energy benefits of protein, as well as the positive benefits of complex carbohydrates without a high animal fat intake.

7. Ensure that the diet contains adequate fibre

Fibre is no longer considered to be the indigestible and unprofitable part of food. Its health benefits include a reduced incidence of constipation and other bowel complaints, and a reduction in the incidence or severity of diabetes, gall stones and cardiovascular disease. A high fibre diet lowers the risk rate of breast and colon cancer.

All plant foods contain different types of fibre intermingled with proteins, fats and carbohydrates. The type and concentration of fibre varies in different parts of the plant and as the plants age. The main types of fibre are celluloses, hemicelluloses, pectin, gums, mucilages, and lignins.

Cellulose is probably the best known fibre and is a component of all plants. It attracts water which results in an increase in stool size and a decrease in transit time. Cellulose is broken down in the gut to form important substances called short chain fatty acids, which seem to protect the bowel wall and lower the incidence of colon cancer. Wheat bran is an important source of cellulose, as are all 'fibrous' vegetables like celery and carrot.

Most of the other types of fibre are referred to as soluble fibre. They disperse in water and are found in relatively high concentrations in dried beans, oat and barley products. They have provoked a lot of interest because of their role in reducing cholesterol by binding to bile acids (bile acids are required for the digestion and absorption of fats—less bile acids means less fat uptake and lower cholesterol levels).

Lignins are also important forms of fibre. They are found in a large variety of fibrous foods including wheat and rye fibre and linseed meal and are converted in the body into mammalian lignans. They can also be converted into the weak oestrogens, enterolactone and enterodiol, by bacteria in the gut, and their consumption is associated with a reduced incidence of oestrogen-dependent cancers and menopausal hot flushes.

Dietary fibre increases the numbers of healthy intestinal bacteria (*lactobacillus*, for instance). Bacteria comprise a significant proportion of the stool weight and their presence tends to reduce the tendency to constipation. Wheat bran, for instance, increases stool weight and volume by supplying bulk as well as by stimulating an increase in the numbers of intestinal bacteria.

The best source of dietary fibre is from whole foods, but occasionally it may be necessary to use processed fibre products (wheat bran, oat or rice bran, for example), to effectively treat some diseases.

8. The 'bad fat', 'good fat' dilemma

The low-fat diet is the answer to all our health problems—or so we are led to believe. If we eat fat we will become obese and unloved, develop cholesterol problems and ultimately, heart disease. So far has this craze gone that a synthetic oil has been developed that provides no kilojoules and is not absorbed. (Probably just as well!) But reducing fat intake without an understanding of the differences between fats is likely to cause more problems than it solves.

In reality, we all need a reasonable level of fats in our diet in order to thrive. The question then becomes: which are the 'bad fats' and which are the 'good fats'?

Saturated fats
Saturated fats are abundant in animal products (pork, beef, lamb, chicken, and dairy foods) and in the tropical oils (coconut and palm oils). They build cell membranes and are an energy source to be used, or stored as fatty tissue. Saturated fats are not essential and can be made from other fats, sugars and starches. They are often solid at room temperature, or become solid when they are refrigerated. Excessive saturated fat intake is associated with elevated cholesterol levels, heart disease, obesity and an increased risk of some cancers.

Reduce saturated fats in the diet by selecting low-fat dairy products, using lean cuts of meat trimmed of all visible fat, removing chicken skin, reducing or avoiding saturated fat spreads such as butter, and checking for fat content of commercially produced foods.

Unsaturated fats
The unsaturated fats are chemically different from saturated fats because they contain one or more double bonds. This means they have a structure which makes them less inclined to aggregate or stick together, and more inclined to disperse and remain liquid at room temperature. The fluidity of the unsaturated fats confers beneficial properties.

Unsaturated fats are found in cooking oils and margarine, seeds, nuts, fish and some vegetables. They are more unstable than saturated fats and susceptible to oxidative damage (rancidity) or structural changes when they are exposed to heat, light or oxygen.

There are two main types of unsaturated fats—the monounsaturates containing one double bond; and the polyunsaturates which have more than one double bond.

Monounsaturated fats

Monounsaturated fats are the best vegetable oils to cook with. They are the most stable of the unsaturated fats when exposed to heat, light or oxygen. Pour them into a pre-heated pan to reduce heating time and store them in the refrigerator in opaque or dark glass bottles. Never re-use oils. Olive oil is the best known monounsaturated oil and when used as a substitute for saturated fats, helps to lower cholesterol and reduce the risk of heart disease. Canola, peanut and avocado are other monounsaturates.

Polyunsaturated fats

The polyunsaturated fats are extremely important. There are two types—the omega-6 group and the omega-3 polyunsaturated fatty acids. See Figure 6.1.

Two of the individual polyunsaturated fats are known as 'essential fatty acids' because they cannot be manufactured by the body and must be eaten in foods. They are linoleic acid which is the first fatty acid in the omega-6 pathway; and alpha-linolenic acid, at the beginning of the omega-3 pathway.

Essential fatty acids are necessary for the normal function and development of most tissues including the kidney, liver, blood vessels, heart and brain. Deficiencies lead to excessive scaliness of the skin, reduced growth rates and infertility in both males and females; and can also cause a greater susceptibility to infection and fragile red blood cells.

The omega-3 and omega-6 fatty acids are the precursors to the production of all eicosanoids (prostaglandins, leukotrienes and thromboxanes) and many of their actions are associated with these end-products. The omega-6 fatty acids, which are usually consumed in large quantities in the diet, tend to produce eicosanoids which are relatively more pro-inflammatory than those eicosanoids derived from the omega-3 fatty acids. For this reason, the dietary ratio of omega-3 to omega-6 fatty acids should be 1:5 (which is approximately the ratio of fatty acids in breast milk) rather than the current dietary ratio of about 1:14. Inreasing oily fish, reducing cooking oils which contain high levels of omega-6 (sunflower, safflower and corn oil) and replacing them with oils containing omega-3 (canola oil) or low levels of omega-6 (olive oil) will improve this ratio.

The omega-3 fatty acids

There are three important omega-3 fatty acids. The first is called alpha-linolenic acid (ALA) and is found in linseed, hemp, canola, soy bean, walnut and mustard seed oils, as well as dark-green leafy vegetables. The other two important fatty acids in the omega-3 series are usually known only by their initials—EPA (eicosapentaenoic acid) and DHA (docosahexaenoic acid). They are found in the oils of cold water fish and marine animals. All omega-3 fatty acids can be made in the body from alpha-linolenic acid, the only *essential* omega-3 fatty acid.

The omega-3 fatty acids are used as supplements to treat conditions which have an inflammatory or allergic component including rheumatoid arthritis, asthma, psoriasis, and other skin complaints. They are also used to prevent and treat cardiovascular disorders, and are especially indicated when an individual has a tendency to blood clot formation.

- Linseeds or linseed (flax seed) oil
  These are very rich sources of the plant-derived omega-3 essential fatty acids (ALA). As a supplement to the diet, flax seed oil can be taken at between 1–2 tablespoons daily. Linseeds can be ground and included in the diet. They must be refrigerated immediately after grinding.

Alpha-linolenic acid content of some oils and seeds

Linseed (flax seed) oil	60 per cent
Pumpkin seeds	15 per cent
Canola oil	10 per cent
Mustard seed oil	10 per cent
Soya bean oil	7–9 per cent

- Oily fish
  Include oily fish in at least four meals a week.

Fish containing high levels of EPA and DHA

Atlantic salmon	Ocean trout
Blue eye	Pilchards
Blue grenadier	Rainbow trout
Blue mackerel	Redfish
Blue warehou	Sardines
Gemfish	Sea mullet
Golden perch	Silver trevally
Herring	Silver warehou
King George whiting	Tuna
Luderick	Yellowtail kingfish

The omega-6 fatty acids

The omega-6 essential fatty acids

The important omega-6 essential acids are called linoleic acid, gamma-linolenic acid and arachidonic acid. Of these, linoleic acid is the only true essential fatty acid because the others can be synthesised from it. However, gamma-linolenic acid (GLA) is often lacking in the modern diet and its synthesis from linoleic acid is very easily disrupted. Supplements are often necessary to rectify this imbalance. Arachidonic acid is found in animal products and is usually present in abundance in the normal diet.

- Seeds and seed oils: Linoleic acid is found in abundance in seed oils such as safflower, soya bean, corn, sunflower, canola and grape seed oils.

  Linoleic acid content of some oils

Safflower oil	75 per cent
Sunflower oil	60–70 per cent
Walnut oil	60 per cent
Corn oil	55 per cent
Soya bean oil	50 per cent
Peanut oil	35 per cent
Canola oil	20 per cent
Olive oil	8 per cent

  Evening primrose, star flower oil and black currant seed oils are all very good sources of linoleic acid and also contain beneficial amounts of GLA. These oils are available in capsule form and serve as precursors to the series 1 prostaglandins.

- Vegetables: Although the levels are low when compared to seeds, most vegetables are sources of linoleic acid.

Cholesterol

Cholesterol is a fat-like substance in the same chemical family as the steroid hormones (oestrogen, progesterone, testosterone). It is found in all animal fats but not vegetable fats. Hidden sources are in manufactured foods such as biscuits, chips, muesli bars and other convenience foods. Cholesterol is utilised in the body to make steroid hormones, myelin nerve sheaths and cell membranes. It is synthesised in the liver from fats in the diet and circulates in the blood in combination with protein and fat (lipoprotein).

Atherosclerotic (vessel-narrowing) plaques contain large amounts of cholesterol, suggesting a relationship between cholesterol intake and heart disease. However, cholesterol metabolism and excretion is very complex. Increased dietary intakes of cholesterol lead to a reduced synthesis of cholesterol in the liver, but higher excretion rates.[2] Reducing cholesterol intake lowers blood cholesterol, but does not affect overall mortality rates,[3] or reduce the incidence of atherosclerosis.[4]

Other dietary factors appear to be more important than restricted cholesterol intakes to both reduce blood cholesterol levels and the incidence of cardiovascular disease. Reduced intakes of saturated fats and *trans*-fatty acids (both discussed in this section), lower blood cholesterol levels more than a restriction of dietary cholesterol. Increasing fibre intake and exercising also reduce cholesterol levels.

The type of cholesterol is also an important factor in the development of heart disease. Cholesterol is transported into the blood vessel walls by a carrier molecule called low-density lipoprotein (LDL). This is one of the initial stages in plaque formation. Fortunately, there is another of these carriers called high-density lipoprotein (HDL) that transports cholesterol back to the liver for storage or conversion.

When LDL levels are high in comparison to HDL, cholesterol is more likely to be deposited in an atherosclerotic plaque. Conversely, high levels of HDL are protective. Women with *lower* HDL levels are at significantly more risk of developing cardiovascular disease than women with *elevated* LDL levels.[5] Low fat diets, or substituting saturated fats with polyunsaturated fats, decreases *both* LDL and HDL cholesterol,[6] and is not good dietary advice to reduce risk of heart disease.

Oxidised LDL cholesterol is also a risk factor for cardiovascular disease because it increases the formation of atherosclerotic plaque in arteries. Anti-oxidants such as vitamin E[7] and compounds found in red wine and grape seed extracts[8] protect against LDL oxidation.

On the other hand, a diet rich in monounsaturated fatty acids significantly reduces total cholesterol and LDL cholesterol but does not alter HDL cholesterol.[9] Certain types of the polyunsaturated fats, such as the omega-3 series, and especially oily fish, also reduce the risk of cardiovascular disease, by reducing blood clotting and artherosclerotic damage to the blood vessels.

Triglycerides

High serum triglycerides are a risk factor for cardiovascular disease. Fats, sugars, alcohol or refined carbohydrates consumed to excess are converted into triglycerides and stored in the fat. High levels of circulating triglycerides can cause blood cells to clump together, and increase the risk of diseases such as cardiovascular disease, kidney failure, hypertension and cancer.[10] Lowering the intake of fats, added sugars, alcohol and refined carbohydrate lowers tri-glyceride level.

Oxidative damage

Oxidation occurs when free radicals cause damage to foods or cells in the body. This process can cause foods to 'go off' or become rancid. In the body, free radical damage is associated with a large number of problems such as ageing, cancer and heart disease.

Anti-oxidants are components found in foods which protect both food and cells from oxidation and free radical damage. The principal anti-oxidants are vitamins E and C, beta-carotene, the flavonoids and the phenolics. Correct storage of foods, particularly oils, also reduces the tendency to oxidation or rancidity by minimising exposure to heat, light and air.

Trans-*fatty acids*

Oils can be processed so that they become solid, for example margarine and vegetable shortening. This process requires high temperatures and hydrogenation to produce the saturates and *trans*-fatty acids which result in a hardened product. Hydrogenated vegetable oils are also common components of manufactured foods.

In their unaltered state, nearly all unsaturated fats are in the *cis*-configuration. When oils are heated, particularly the polyunsaturated oils, their shape changes to the *trans*-configuration. Oils in the *trans*-configuration (a description of their shape) cause platelets to become sticky, blood cholesterol to increase, and an alteration in the ratio of LDL cholesterol to HDL cholesterol. *Trans*-fatty acids can also interfere with the production of the useful group of prostaglandins which may reduce the severity and incidence of PMS, dysmenorrhoea and a host of inflammatory problems.

What to buy and eat

An overall reduction in fats is advisable for most people. Animal fats contain cholesterol as well as saturated fats and should be restricted. The overall levels of polyunsaturated fats as 'vegetable oils' should be reduced as well. Some of the polyunsaturated fats which contain the essential fatty acids (unrefined linseed or flaxseed oil, pumpkin, walnut, soya bean, safflower and sunflower oils, for example) should be included in regular, small amounts, preferably added to cooked or raw foods such as salads. Regular fish consumption reduces the risk of degenerative diseases such as heart disease, arthritis, some cancers and auto-immune diseases.

The best oils to buy are those which have been manufactured without heat and which are stored correctly in dark glass bottles. All oils and oil-containing foods should be refrigerated. Monounsaturated fats such as olive and canola oils are the best oils for cooking and general consumption.

'Best practice' cooking, preparation and storage

- Avoid excessive consumption of heated oils: Heating induces irreversible changes to oils which leads to oxidation or free radical formation.

- Rediscover alternatives to cooking with oils: Many foods can be cooked in just a little water, or even dry fried in a non-stick pan. Fish, eggs and vegetables can be poached in water or a fruit or vegetable puree, and fish and vegetables can be baked rather than roasted in oil.
- Add oils before serving: Food with an adequate oil content can be recognised as satisfying. Rather than cooking in oils, however, add oils to food *after* cooking. Oils with a high essential fatty acid content can be made into dressings or sauces and added to cooked food prior to serving. This will improve the sense of satiety when eating steamed, baked or poached foods.
- Add cold-pressed oils of linseed, safflower and canola to the diet: These can be taken in tablespoon doses once or twice a day or added to the seed breakfast (see page 230), used in salad dressings, poured on cooked food such as steamed vegetables, pasta or potatoes, or mixed with yoghurt in a ratio of about one to two parts oil to ten parts yoghurt. Try following the European tradition. Spread breads with oils such as olive oil, but add a little of the oils rich in essential fatty acids too—canola or linseed oils, for example.
- Make your own spreads: Satisfying alternatives to butter and margarine can be made from avocado, tahini, yoghurt, chickpeas, nut butters or vegetable-based dips.
- Store oils carefully. Omega-3 and omega-6 oils are highly susceptible to damage, so they must be treated with care. For maximum therapeutic benefit, they should be bought in small quantities as oils that are unrefined, mechanically pressed, and in opaque or dark glass bottles. This ensures that the fatty acids are not adversely affected by light, heat or oxygen. They are not for cooking and should be stored in the refrigerator. They can be used as salad dressings or added to food after cooking.

9. Include dairy products in moderation

Many people are confused about dairy products—are they 'good for you' or not? Dietitians often see the enormous potential for improving nutrient intake, especially calcium, and recommend a high intake. Some people, however, are sensitive to dairy products, or at least some aspects of them, and may be wiser not to eat them at all.

It is possible to have difficulty with lactose (milk sugar), or to one of the proteins, usually casein or beta-lactoglobulin (the curds and whey of nursery rhymes). Rarely, an apparent intolerance to all types of dairy products is seen.

Lactose intolerance

Lactose is milk sugar and is found only in animal milks, including human breast milk. Only one-third of the world's population inherit the ability to digest it after weaning. They are usually descendants from Northern European, Middle Eastern or Central African peoples, and maintain high levels of intestinal lactase (the enzyme to digest lactose) as adults. Descendants from most other communities, lose this ability early in childhood.[11]

A transient lactose intolerance can develop after a bout of infectious diarrhoea, particularly if caused by *giardia lamblia* which often affects young children and travellers. Lactose-containing foods should be avoided until symptoms disappear. The incidence of lactose intolerance also seems to increase with age; about 30 per cent of the elderly are affected.

Sufficient quantities of lactose-containing foods need to be eaten before symptoms develop (the 'threshold level'). Dairy foods have differing amounts of lactose. Low levels are found in most cheeses including parmesan, cheddar, edam, gouda, and reduced-fat Swiss. Nimbin™ brand cheese contains no lactose and butter has very little. The highest amounts are in milk (especially low-fat milk) cream and low-fat creamed cottage cheese. Yoghurt also contains large amounts of lactose, but rarely causes intolerance (see following).

Symptoms of lactose intolerance develop because the accumulation of undigested lactose irritates the bowel wall and causes bloating, abdominal discomfort, flatulence, and sometimes diarrhoea. Osteoporosis is more common if a person has lactose intolerance, possibly because they avoid dairy products to prevent the symptoms. Lactose intolerance may also be associated with an increased risk of cataracts.[12]

Proper management of lactose intolerance requires a reduction in the intake of dairy products which have a high lactose content. Complete abstinence is unnecessary. Cultured milks, yoghurt, and cheeses are usually well tolerated and can be eaten in small portions throughout the day to keep the lactose below threshold levels where symptoms develop.

Milk protein intolerance and allergy

Milk products can cause either *acute allergic reactions* or *intolerance* in susceptible individuals. The main culprits seem to be either of the milk proteins beta-lactoglobulin or casein. Beta-lactoglobulin is the main protein in whey. It is present in milk, yoghurt, and in all but the hardest of cheeses. Casein makes up the 'curd' or solid part of milk when cheese is being made. It is present in all milk products apart from those which consist solely of whey such as whey powder.

Acute allergic reactions cause wheezing and difficulty breathing, or in milder cases, acute allergic skin reactions. *Dairy intolerance* is at this stage poorly understood, but can cause a wide range of symptoms which include:

- excessive catarrh, phlegm, wheezing, sneezing, cough, blocked nose or ears
- diarrhoea, stomach cramps, bloating, nausea, or discomfort; colic in infants[13]
- joint pains, muscular aches and pains, or more serious complaints such as rheumatoid arthritis
- eczema, hives
- migraines, mood changes or depressive states.

It is sometimes possible to identify which constituent is causing a problem by selectively withholding and then reintroducing different types of dairy product. This is complicated and a practitioner skilled in food intolerance may need to be consulted—or try yoghurt.

Yoghurt

Yoghurt is an important food. It is easily digestible, provides bacteria which assist with the growth of healthy intestinal bacteria, has more calcium per unit volume than milk, and may help to reduce the risk of breast and other oestrogen-dependent cancers.[14]

It is also well tolerated by those with a dairy or lactose intolerance. Bacteria in the yoghurt starter cultures (usually *Lactobacillus bulgaricus* and *Streptococcus thermophilus)* produce enzymes which convert lactose into the non-irritant lactic acid,[15] and 'digest' the proteins in milk which are related to many of the sensitivity reactions.

When protein molecules are split into smaller amino acid components by the bacteria, they are not recognised by the body as allergy-promoting substances. Lactic acid also acts on casein and breaks it down into smaller components, making the milk protein more digestible as well as less allergenic.[16]

Additional milk solids added to yoghurt during manufacture increase the calcium and protein content of yoghurt, but all dairy products are relatively magnesium-poor and should not be used as the sole source of minerals for bones. (Bone needs magnesium to ensure that calcium is maintained within its structure and not excreted again.) Additional magnesium-rich legumes, vegetables and nuts, are needed in the diet to balance the poor calcium/magnesium ratio of dairy products.

Yoghurt should contain live cultures; many of the snack-type yoghurts, especially the flavoured and 'fruit yoghurts', do not.

10. Include phyto-oestrogenic foods in the diet

Phyto-oestrogens (plant oestrogens) are structurally similar to animal oestrogen and are found in a large and growing number of common foods and medicinal plants. Dietary phyto-oestrogen intake is associated with a reduced incidence of oestrogen-related disease. They are discussed in the next chapter.

11. Ensure an adequate and regular intake of protein foods

When people go on 'healthy' or 'weight loss' diets, they often drastically reduce or stop most of their protein intake. Protein is found in animal products such as meat, eggs, fish, milk and cheese, and also in the vegetable proteins. Neither type is better or worse—both categories have additional qualities and characteristics which determine which type is more or less acceptable.

Vegetarians (lacto-ovo), for example, can obtain protein from eating vegetable proteins, dairy products and eggs; vegans from eating combinations of vegetable proteins. There is a greater difficulty (but not impossibility) for vegetarians to obtain iron, and for vegans to get enough vitamin B_{12} as well. The advantage of being a vegetarian is a lower intake of fat and less likelihood of developing many of the chronic degenerative diseases; the disadvantage is a tendency to anaemia and fatigue.

Meat eaters have an advantage when it comes to iron intake. Iron in meat is easier to absorb and it is present in much greater quantities. Animal protein is also of a better quality and meat-eaters can have a more relaxed attitude to nutrient intake, but still maintain energy levels. On the downside, eating meat increases the intake of saturated fats and the risk of a number of diseases, such as heart disease and cancer. Deep sea fish is beneficial because it contains high levels of essential fatty acids. A suggested diet could contain lean red meat in small quantities, some free-range chicken without the skin, plenty of fish, a few eggs (no more than three a week) and low-fat dairy products. Animal proteins such as these can be consumed at one meal daily. The protein intake at the other meals should come from properly combined vegetable sources.

Deciding how much protein to eat in grams is quite difficult. Young women between the ages of eleven and twenty, should eat about 1 g of protein for every kilogram of their body weight. Women from twenty onwards need about 0.75 g for every kilogram. On average, this means a woman should consume between 45 and 55 g protein each day.[17]

Table 17.1 Approximate levels of protein in common foods

Meat (100 grams)	20–25 grams
Fish and seafood (100 grams)	15–20 grams
Beans/legumes (1 cup)	7.5–15 grams
Whole grains (1 cup)	5–12 grams
One cup of milk or yoghurt	8 grams
An egg	6 grams
Cheese (30 grams)	6–8 grams
Vegetables and fruits (1 cup)	2–4 grams

12. Develop an awareness of the important minerals

Key pages outlining the important minerals are included throughout this book. Calcium is included in Chapter 9 'Menopause'; magnesium is discussed in relation to hormone and blood sugar abnormalities in Chapter 16 'Ovarian cysts'; iron in Chapter 11 'Heavy menstruation'; and zinc in Chapter 7 'Adolescence'.

13. Be aware of the relationship between food and the seasons

Before commercial food preparation, refrigeration and improved transport facilities, most people ate seasonal foods from their area. We can now get most foods most of the time and the idea of eating only seasonal fruits and vegetables probably seems like an unnecessarily restrictive practice.

All fruits and vegetables can be assigned with certain qualities in the same way that medicinal herbs are. Summer foods are generally juicy and light, in the cooler months foods tend to be dense and compact with a high component of carbohydrate and protein. Compare lettuce with cabbage, zucchini with carrot, or peaches with apples, for example. In summer, moist, easily digested raw foods make sense, but in winter they don't provide enough carbohydrate to counterbalance the energy expenditure needed to stay warm.

Winter foods should be mainly beans, legumes and root vegetables; salads can be made from root vegetables and cabbage. These are Warming and comforting foods on a cold winter's day. Summer foods need to be lighter and have a higher moisture content. Most summer fruits and vegetables have Cooling properties—melons are particularly Cooling while bananas which tend to be dense and compact are Warming.

14. Try to vary food flavours

There are five main flavours in the diet: bitter, sweet, sour, salty and spicy or pungent. In Australia we rely heavily on the sweet and salty flavours (just look into the shopping trolleys at the supermarket). Some cultures include all or most of the flavours in their cooking as a matter of course—Thai food for example, is cooked with the addition of salty, sweet, spicy and sour flavours.

Each of the flavours has subtle effects on digestion and health. Bitter foods for example improve digestion and bowel function by stimulating the bile flow. Bitter green vegetables are commonly used in some parts of Europe and radicchio, chicory, dandelion leaves and silverbeet are often included in the diet to aid digestion. (Spinach is not a bitter because it doesn't taste bitter.) Grapefruit is sour and bitter, and the old practice of having half a grapefruit before a fatty breakfast such as bacon and eggs makes a lot of sense. (Not eating a fatty breakfast makes even more sense!) Dandelion coffee is a gentle and effective bitter that is available as a beverage.

Warming spices in the diet improve sluggish digestion and can be used for complaints of the upper gastrointestinal tract such as nausea, dyspepsia (belching) and indigestion. Ginger, cardamom, cumin and coriander are all useful—ginger tea is particularly helpful for nausea. These spices can be brewed in ordinary black tea to assist with digestion. Warming spices are useful for those who feel cold, have difficulties with cold weather, or catch colds easily.

Sour foods are drying and can be used to prevent excessive mucus membrane congestion and moistness. Excessive consumption of sweet foods often causes phlegm or catarrh in susceptible individuals which sour foods can help to counteract. Many sour foods, such as citrus fruit, are useful to protect the mucus membranes from infections. Sour foods also aid digestion.

15. Do not overeat

Overeating is associated with obesity and a shorter life expectancy. The digestive tract is chronically overburdened and the incidence of gall bladder disease increases. The heart has to work harder, and blood lipid profiles are more likely to be abnormal. The risk of high blood pressure also increases.

16. Avoid foods that cause digestive upsets or a sense of ill-health

This should be obvious, but sometimes the desire to 'do the right thing' overcomes commonsense and people try to eat what they think they should rather than what they can. Numerous diets in recent years have been offered as the panacea of all ills—some people benefit from such diets, but others will develop obvious problems such as abdominal upsets, diarrhoea, or become excessively tired. It is simply not possible for one dietary regime to be suitable for all people, or even for any one individual forever.

Raw food diets can be a problem, for example, because raw food is quite difficult to digest. Bloating, flatulence or even diarrhoea can occur, depleting the uptake of nutrients and leading to a deterioration, rather than an improvement in health. Substitutes should be found if foods cause intolerance or are disliked—anaemic women don't have to eat meat if they don't want to, and dairy products might cause problems for someone with osteoporosis. Trading one health problem for another isn't a good idea.

17. Limit intake of sugar and salt in cooking and food choice

Sugar
Sugar is not considered an essential food, and was not a major part of our diet until the mid-nineteenth century. All types of sugar should be minimised, including brown and unrefined sugars; as well as the foods

which are prepared with sugar such as cakes, biscuits, puddings, soft drinks, fruit juices, cordials, jams, ice-cream and lollies.

Many commercially prepared foods contain added sugar which is not apparent on tasting. Canned foods such as peas, bean mix, beetroot; cereals, dry biscuits, and many condiments such as sauces, pickles, mayonnaise are common examples. Sugars are included to increase flavour, or as a preserving agent.

Between 25–50 per cent of Australian women eat more than the recommended amount of refined sugar. The amount of sugar consumed between 1985 and 1990 increased according to nutritional surveys conducted in Victoria. The increase coincided with an advertising campaign by the sugar industry and women between 18–29 years were the most affected.[18]

Excess consumption of sugar has been linked to coronary heart disease, hypertension, and increased serum cholesterol and triglycerides; an increased risk of breast cancer, hyperactivity, dental caries, mineral loss via the urine, obesity, formation of cholesterol gallstones and functional hypoglycaemia.

Salt

Between 40–60 per cent of Victorian women consume more than the recommended daily allowance of salt.[19] Salt intake is associated with high blood pressure and increases the excretion of minerals in the urine. Most sodium enters the diet by way of manufactured foods (cheese, sausage, processed and canned vegetables, biscuits, spreads etc.) and not through adding salt during cooking or at the table. Salt should be limited to around 3–5 g daily.

18. Limit intake of caffeine-containing beverages

Caffeine-containing drinks have an honoured place in our society as a tonic for body, mind and spirit. They contain highly active substances known as xanthines which are alkaloids and are stimulants to the central nervous system. Caffeine is the major active ingredient in coffee; tea contains theophylline and caffeine; and cocoa and chocolate contain theobromine as well as caffeine. Of the xanthines, caffeine is the most pronounced stimulant and theophylline is milder.

Caffeine-containing beverages increase anxiety and aggravate insomnia. The blood lipid profile is altered by their consumption (and with decaffeinated coffee but not filtered coffee[20]) and the blood pressure increases. In the long term, caffeine may effect mineral retention and lead to an increased risk of osteoporosis (due to increased excretion of calcium and magnesium).

Excessive caffeine intake is also associated with a number of common gynaecological conditions including endometriosis, fibroids, PMS and benign breast disease. Caffeine has also been shown to lower fertility,[21] and there has even been a proposed link between caffeine consumption and cancer. Gynaecological problems have been associated with the equivalent of two cups of coffee or four cups of tea every day. 'Plunger' coffee has the least harmful effects. Boiled (Turkish) coffee should be completely avoided if there are problems with high cholesterol levels.

19. Alcohol consumption should be limited

Alcohol-related problems were described by the Australian Senate Standing Committee on Social Welfare (1977) as being of epidemic proportions. Deaths directly related to alcohol make up 26 per cent of all drug-related deaths (71 per cent from tobacco, 2 per cent from others, 1 per cent from opiates). A host of other more subtle health problems are caused or aggravated by alcohol. Some are caused by depletion of minerals such as calcium, magnesium, potassium and zinc, and vitamins A, C and the B complex, especially B_1.

Women are more affected by alcohol and for longer than men. They have a lower body water content (a woman's body contains approximately 49 per cent body water, a man's about 58 per cent) and so a given volume of alcohol is diluted into a smaller volume of body water. They also metabolise alcohol more slowly because they have a smaller liver cell mass than men.

Government authorities acknowledge these differences by issuing different warnings for women and men. Two standard alcoholic drinks will take a woman to the legal blood alcohol limit for driving, but this figure may be influenced by hormonal fluctuations associated with the menstrual cycle (around the period and ovulation, alcohol is thought to be metabolised more slowly), cigarette smoking and dietary habits.

Excess alcohol consumption has been linked to cancers, hypertension, heart disease, foetal abnormalities, and liver disease. The National Health and Medical Research Council have made the following recommendations for women:[22]

- Women should not exceed two standard drinks or fourteen standard drinks a week on a regular basis.
- Two to four drinks a day or 14–28 drinks a week are to be considered hazardous and more than four drinks a day or 28 drinks a week are to be considered harmful.
- Abstinence from alcohol is highly desirable during pregnancy.
- Everyone should have at least two alcohol-free days a week. (A three-day break between drinking to allow the liver time to recover might be even better for a woman.)

20. Be aware of which foods reduce or increase cancer risks

Regular consumption of some commonly eaten foods, especially fruit, vegetables and cereals, is associated with a lower incidence of cancer at many body sites including the uterus, breast, cervix, ovary, lung, skin, stomach and colon.

Although researchers have not identified all of the factors associated with tumour growth, it is known that there are two critical stages, called the 'initiation' and 'activation' stages of cell growth. A carcinogen can make a cell susceptible to change or 'initiate' change, but abnormal cell growth will not occur unless 'activators' stimulate the altered cell. For breast cancer to develop, for instance, the known activators include oxidative cell damage, oestrogen, and some types of prostaglandins.

Some foods may reduce cancer risk because they contain one or more of the numerous anti-carcinogens found in plant foods. In the past decade, over forty foods have been identified as having cancer preventive properties.

Protective foods

Fruit and vegetables

Although it is possible to single out specific foods with protective qualities, a review of about 200 worldwide studies found overwhelming evidence indicating that just by having a high intake of fruit and vegetables, the risk of developing cancer is approximately halved.[23] Some individual studies found an even more marked protective effect from vegetables. Greek research showed low vegetable consumers to have ten times more risk of developing breast cancer than women with a high vegetable intake.[24]

Considerable interest has been given to the possibility that increasing specific nutrients, especially the anti-oxidants, may be even more protective. The anti-oxidants, vitamin A, C and E, beta-carotene and selenium, are known to block various phases of cancer development. As well, anti-oxidants act synergistically with each other and with dietary components to exert a protective effect.[25]

Vitamin C and E, for example, can change the potential carcinogen, nitrosamine (a compound made from nitrites in foods), into less harmful compounds in the stomach before it has been absorbed; selenium and beta-carotene can also restrict carcinogen formation in the gut. But the main protective effects of the anti-oxidants occur during the initiation and activation phases of cellular change—in other words, the anti-oxidants protect individual groups of cells from carcinogens which have managed to by-pass the usual defences.

All of the anti-oxidants are potentially protective at this point, but some seem to be particularly protective to some tissues. For example, cervical cancer incidence is lower when women have better intakes of the carotenoids, especially beta-carotene;[26] and a low beta-carotene intake has also been associated with breast cancer.[27] But despite the link with specific nutrients, there is a recurring suggestion that foods contain many different protective compounds which play an important role, and that it is the vegetables in their entirety, rather than individual components, that are protective.

Some vegetables and fruits which seem to be particularly useful will be discussed separately, but it is probably sufficient to simply eat as wide a range as possible. Some of these should be raw, but it is not necessary to eat a wholly raw vegetable and fruit diet.

Cabbage family

A high consumption of vegetables from the cabbage family, primarily cabbage, broccoli and brussels sprouts, is associated with a reduced incidence of cancer of the lung,[28] bowel,[29] and pancreas.[30] Of particular interest to women is the observation that some components in these vegetables increase the metabolism and excretion of oestrogens, which has raised the possibility of a positive protective effect against oestrogen-dependent cancers,[31] particularly breast and uterine cancer. So far, the only research has been conducted on animals,[32] and it is too early to make any firm statements about the positive effects for women.

Onions and garlic

Interest in garlic and onion in relation to cancer prevention is two-fold. Firstly, a number of researchers have noted a positive association between garlic consumption (in particular) and reduced risk of cancer,[33] and secondly, garlic contains high levels of naturally occurring selenium (a mineral with powerful anti-oxidant properties). Considerable effort has gone into identifying those agricultural practices which will enhance the selenium content of garlic,[34] because naturally occurring selenium seems to have less potential toxicity at high doses than selenium given as a supplement.[35]

At the moment, however, a statement that 'garlic reduces cancer risk' is just not possible. Researchers are in agreement that there is evidence of a positive effect from eating garlic, but not on what that effect might be. For instance, although there has been indications in animal research that garlic can reduce the incidence of breast cancer,[36] this has not been borne out by studies of large numbers of women who eat garlic regularly.[37]

At this stage it seems that garlic reduces the incidence of cancers in the gastrointestinal tract, primarily the stomach, colon, liver and oesophagus. There is a possible reduction in breast cancer risk, but as yet this has been only shown experimentally. Another role for garlic, along with cucumber, onion and tomato, is to reduce the mutagenic effects of chemotherapy, according to research in China. This research may be used in the future to design diets to prevent the return of cancer.[38]

Raw garlic is probably most protective, but the tradition to eat it cooked in food is much more acceptable to those who worry about the 'social' aspects of garlic. Add a few more cloves or a little more onion than recipes suggest.

Red, yellow and orange vegetables and fruits
The red, yellow and orange vegetables and fruits often contain high levels of beta-carotene. This red pigment is a precursor to vitamin A in humans and is one of the major anti-oxidants and cancer-preventative food components. It is found in high levels in carrots, sweet potato, pumpkin and in cantaloupe, papaya, oranges, apricots and peaches. Dark green leafy vegetables also contain high levels of beta-carotene.

Beta-carotene intake is associated with a lower level of cancer in many studies, and it may be one of the major food components responsible for the reduced cancer risk seen with a high level of fruit and vegetable intake.

Tomatoes are low in beta-carotene, but contain lycopene, another carotenoid with anti-oxidant properties. Tomato consumption is linked to a lower incidence of digestive tract cancers, particularly in Mediterranean populations where it is a major food component.[39] Lycopenes are also found in other red-skinned fruits and vegetables such as berries.

Beetroot is commonly self-prescribed by cancer patients in Germany and Switzerland.[40] In the 1950s, doctors who were working with cancer found that beetroot seemed to slow or stop cancer growth. They prescribed 200–250 grams of finely grated beetroot daily and found that, in many cases, the progression of cancer was halted. It is unknown whether beetroot contains agents which can inhibit the initiation or promotion stages of cancer.

A daily intake of several yellow, orange or red vegetables, as well as one or two pieces of yellow or orange fruit is advisable. A serve of dark green leafy vegetables, either as a salad or cooked will also increase beta-carotene intake, and provide a good source of other nutrients.

Citrus fruits
Citrus fruits are associated with a lower incidence of both cancers of the gastrointestinal tract and the breast.[41] There are likely to be different mechanisms for these protective effects: the vitamin C is most likely to be responsible for the reduction in cancers of the stomach (see pickled and cured food); the pectin fraction is more likely to be involved in breast cancer reduction.

Soya products
In countries where soya intake is high, there is a lower incidence of breast, colon, and prostate cancers. This is believed to be related to the presence of phyto-oestrogens (which act as anti-oestrogens), however, some of the studies also showed a lowered risk of non-hormonal cancers, indicating that soya products may have other protective constituents.[42]

In fact, five other naturally occurring components in soya beans have been shown to individually inhibit cancer cell formation. (These are the proteases, fibre, saponins, sterols, and phytic acid.) In comparison to other foods, soya products have relatively high levels of all of these components, which may work synergistically as protective agents.

The common types of soya products are tofu, miso, soya milk, soya flour, soya grits and textured soy protein. Of these foods, the most consistent protective effects are seen with the non-fermented products (the soya milk, flour, grits; tofu and textured protein), but not with miso.[43]

Green tea

Green tea consumption is strongly associated with a lower cancer risk in the gastrointestinal tract. It can reduce the risk of cancer of the oesophagus, stomach and large intestine; especially in countries where large amounts of pickled or preserved foods are eaten.[44] It reduces liver cancer risk[45] and returns liver enzymes to normal.[46] Green tea also seems to reduce the incidence of skin cancer (in mice) caused by ultra-violet radiation[47]—but don't try it as an alternative to sun-block creams! There may also be positive effects against breast cancer.[48]

Green tea also improves cholesterol levels and increases the levels of HDL (helpful) cholesterol[49]. Drinking too much tea may be a problem, though. More than five cups per day increased the risk of pancreatic cancer in one study,[50] and increased the incidence of lung cancer in another.[51]

Fibre and cereal grains

Dietary fibre is well known for its ability to reduce the risk of colon cancer. Fibre increases the production of the short chain fatty acids which protect the bowel wall from abnormal cell change. Fibre intake is specifically important for women because it reduces the risk of oestrogen-dependent cancers, including breast cancer.

The best way to safely include fibre in the diet is to eat it as part of whole foods. Fibre from different sources has different effects on the bowel wall and not enough information is available to confidently predict which type of fibre gives the greatest protection against colon cancer.[52] At any rate, there are other positive effects when foods are eaten whole, including the phyto-oestrogens, trace minerals and vitamin content,[53] and so whole grains and cereal products should be favoured over fibre-only cereals and supplements. Psyllium is also highly protective, and wheat and psyllium together have better effects than either alone.[54] A list of high fibre foods and cereals (chosen because they are low in fat and salt) are included on page 303.

Yoghurt and fermented milk products

Fermented milk products have been linked to a lower incidence of cancer of the breast,[55] and stomach;[56] and to a limited degree, to a reduced incidence of bowel cancer.[57] There is also evidence that the bacteria normally found in yoghurts and fermented milks can inactivate carcinogens in the bowel.[58]

A Dutch study which looked at a combination of factors associated with a lower incidence of breast cancer found that the most beneficial dietary combination consisted of a low fat, high fibre diet with a high intake of fermented milk products.[59] There is some suggestion that the lower incidence of colon cancer may also be related to the calcium in milk products.[60]

Foods to reduce or avoid

Fats

The relationship between fat in the diet and cancer incidence is unclear. Breast cancer and fat had been linked because of the observation that Western women had a higher incidence of breast cancer than Asian women who ate much less fat. But over the past ten or fifteen years the significance of a high fat intake has been questioned because a number of studies have found little association between breast cancer risk and fat intake.[61]

However, a review of the research data from 20 countries on cancer of the breast, cervix, lung and colon in women, *did* find a relationship between fat intake and risk. Saturated fats were particularly implicated and were associated with increased risk of breast and colon cancer. The polyunsaturated fats were also associated with breast cancer risk, but the fish oils (omega-3 polyunsaturated fatty acids) slightly reduced risk. The mono-unsaturated fats did not have any effect at any cancer site.[62]

In summary, fat is less of a problem than it was initially supposed to be, but certain fats are associated with increasing risk, particularly of breast cancer. Women are advised to eat as little saturated (animal) fat as possible; reduce polyunsaturated fats; buy good quality oils and store them correctly to prevent rancidity; use the monounsaturated fats for salads and cooking; eat plenty of fish; and generally keep fat and oil in the diet to a minimum. Additional information on fats and oils is included on pages 281–7.

Alcohol

There is evidence linking alcohol consumption to an increased breast cancer risk,[63] however alcohol consumption is associated with a lower risk of cardiovascular disease. It may be wise for women with a high risk of breast cancer, but a low risk of heart disease to abstain from alcohol.[64] Alcohol also seems to increase the incidence of colon cancer, particularly beer drinking.[65]

Coffee

Excess consumption of coffee has been linked to the development of bladder cancer,[66] but there is very little evidence that it has any effect on other cancers. In fact, in some studies, coffee consumption was associated with a lower risk of bowel cancer.[67] Other (adverse) effects of coffee are discussed on pages 293–4. Its consumption to excess is not recommended.

Many women are worried about coffee consumption and an increased risk of breast cancer or benign breast disease, but this has not been borne out by the research either,[68] and in one study, coffee seemed to reduce the breast cancer risk of lean women, but—'might have the opposite effect in relatively obese women'.[69]

Restricting kilojoules
An overall increase in risk is seen with increasing body weight above normal, particularly in relation to breast cancer. Women with high kilojoule intake, and those who don't exercise also have an increased risk.[79] The best advice is to eat a varied diet in moderation and exercise regularly.

THE DAILY DIET

Include these food groups every day

Fresh vegetables
A minimum of seven different vegetables daily; comprising as many different colours as possible.

Fresh fruit
Fresh, seasonal fruits, three pieces daily.

Whole grains and beans/legumes
Include four to five serves of grains such as rice, corn, millet (should be hulled); and/or beans such as chickpeas, lentils, red kidney beans, lima beans, soya beans and products. A serve is equivalent to a slice of bread or one cup of cooked grain or beans. Potatoes are also included in the complex carbohydrate category. One medium-sized to large potato equals one serve.

Seeds and nuts
• Seeds: linseeds, sesame seeds, sunflower seeds, pumpkin seeds.
• Nuts: almonds, hazelnuts, walnuts, pecans, cashews, pine nuts and peanuts.

Nuts and seeds have a high ratio of oils and should be kept to a maximum of half a cup daily when excess weight gain is a consideration.

Yoghurt and cultured milks
Include at least one cup of low-fat yoghurt or buttermilk daily. If sensitive to cows' milk, include soya, goat's or sheep's yoghurt instead. Yoghurts should contain live cultures.

Fibre
Fibre should come from whole foods such as grains, nuts, seeds, fruit and vegetables and not from fibre-only breakfast cereals (All Bran™, Bran Flakes™, etc.).

Fats and oils

Include three teaspoons of seed oils in the diet daily. Try a mix of safflower, sunflower, linseed (flaxseed) or canola oils. Cook with monounsaturated oils, preferably olive or canola oil. To make 'better butter' mix equal quantities by weight of a good quality olive oil and butter. Keep refrigerated.

Protein

Protein is found in meat, fish, eggs, dairy products and properly combined vegetable proteins. Some protein should be taken with every meal.

Meal suggestions

Commence the day with one of the following
- the juice of a lemon diluted in a glass of warm water
- $\frac{1}{2}$ a grapefruit
- citrus juice
- a whole piece of fruit

Breakfast
- Homemade muesli: raw oatmeal, rice flakes, puffed millet, sunflower seeds, linseeds, sultanas, chopped almonds or cashews, dried paw paw, coconut and chopped pumpkin seeds. Add low-fat cows milk, yoghurt or soya milk, and chopped fresh fruit.
- Fresh fruit in season with yoghurt and seeds or chopped nuts.
- Wholegrain bread, toasted, with nut butter, hoummos, low fat cheese, miso, with or without sprouts. Avoid the usual sweet spreads such as honey or jams. Butter is not necessary.
- Cooked cereal such as oatmeal, millet meal, brown rice or buckwheat, with added seeds or soya grits as desired or suggested. Add milk of choice and fruit or a little honey.
- Energy drink: Blend together low-fat yoghurt with either fresh fruit of your choice or fruit juice (about 50:50), and add seeds and rice bran e.g. linseeds, almond meal, wheatgerm, sunflower seeds, 1 teaspoon of each.

Lunch
- Wholegrain bread sandwich with a mixture of salad vegetables. Include a little protein such as tuna, salmon, egg, low-fat cheese, hoummos.
- Salad of mixed vegetables such as lettuce salad, coleslaw, tabouli salad, grated beetroot, tomatoes, carrot or celery. Protein should be included either in the form of correctly combined vegetable proteins or animal proteins as above.
- Soup with the addition of beans and grains, a little yoghurt or parmesan cheese.
- Any of the dinner choices or the energy drink.

Dinner

The evening meal is usually extremely varied, being only limited by the imagination. It should contain: at least three different vegetables, cooked or raw depending on season and preference; some protein; and a serve of complex carbohydrate e.g. rice, root vegetables, beans, pasta.

To keep animal protein to a minimum, combine meat with grain or bean dishes. Examples might be lamb and chickpea casserole, or similar combination, common in the Middle East and the Southeast European countries; pasta and tomato sauce with tuna; stir-fry vegetables with a little meat, and served with rice, common in Asia.

Other examples for the evening meal:

- vegetables with rice and tofu
- stir-fry beef and vegetables with rice
- vegetables with lentils and rice
- fish with vegetables or salad
- minestrone soup with beans and parmesan cheese

Fluids

- Limit caffeine-containing beverages to two cups of coffee or four cups of tea (not strong!).
- Drink at least two to three glasses of plain water daily.
- Restrict alcohol to two glasses every three days.

HIGH-FIBRE DIETS

Fibre is sometimes included in therapeutic diets to achieve a specific outcome such as lowering of blood fats (cholesterol) and oestrogens; to reduce the incidence of gall bladder disease and colon cancer; for weight loss; or control of constipation.

The recommended daily intake for fibre is 30 g from whole foods and not as fibre-only breakfast cereals.

Table 17.2 gives the amounts of foods that need to be eaten to obtain 10g of fibre. Obviously no-one wants to eat eight cups of rice or 5 slices of bread at a sitting, and so the way to use this table is to select foods to make up between 10 and 15 g from cereal and grain categories; another 15 g from vegetables and legumes; 3–5 g from fruit; and a small optional portion from nuts and seeds. For example,

- 1 cup Kellogg's Just Right and 2 slices multigrain bread is equivalent to 10 g.
- 1 cup cooked beans as a salad for lunch and an evening meal comprised of 1 potato, ½ cup spinach, ½ cup cooked carrot and ½ cup cooked broccoli is easily equivalent to 15 g.
- 3 pieces of fruit and a small handful of seeds and nuts equals 5 g.

Table 17.2 Amounts of common foods providing 10 g fibre

Grains

2 cups cooked rolled oats
¾ cup whole cooked barley
2 cobs sweet corn
3 slices whole rye bread
3 slices bran-enriched bread
5 slices wholemeal bread
4 slices multi-grain bread
⅔ cup oat bran

½ cup natural bran
3½ cups cooked brown rice
8 cups cooked white rice

Legumes

1 cup cooked mixed beans
1 cup cooked peas
1 cup baked beans
800 milligrams tofu

Nuts and seeds

90 grams almonds
1 cup peanuts
100 grams pistachio nuts
¾ cup pecans
¾ cup sunflower seeds

Breakfast cereals

Uncle Toby's Vitabrits 85 grams or 5½ biscuits
Kellogg's Just Right 100 grams or 2 cups
Uncle Toby's Fibre Plus 65 grams
Kellogg's Sustain 136 grams or 2½ cups
Kellogg's Puffed Wheat 115 grams or 5½ cups
Sanitarium Weet-Bix 90 grams or 6 biscuits
Sanitarium Weet-Bix Hi Bran 50 grams or 2.5 biscuits
Sanitarium Lite Bix 85 grams or 5½ biscuits
Uncle Toby's Crunchy Oat Bran Cereal 65 grams
Uncle Toby's Crunchy Oat Bran Cereal with Fruit 75 grams
Willow Valley Oat Bran Breakfast Cereal 70 grams or 1 cup
Willow Valley Oat Bran and Fruit Cereal 120 grams
Purina Muesli Flakes 135 grams
Kellogg's Komplete Oven-Baked Muesli 130 grams or 13 tablespoons
Uncle Toby's Muesli Flakes 105 gram
Uncle Toby's Natural Swiss Formula Muesli 80 gram

Vegetables

3 cups steamed mixed vegetables
2 cups cooked carrots
2 cups cooked cabbage
3 cups cooked broccoli
1 cup steamed spinach
2 cups cooked sweet potato
2–3 medium steamed potatoes with skin

Fruit

3½ medium apples
3 oranges
100 grams dried figs
10 dried apricots
3½ bananas
2 passionfruit
400 grams blueberries
4 kiwi fruit peeled
6–7 nectarines
2½ pears
20 grams prunes

* These cereals have been chosen because they have a low salt and fat content and a high fibre content.

Source: 'Modern Nutrition in Health and Disease; and 'Food for Health'[71]

18

Phyto-oestrogens

Key words

beta-sitosterol
biochanin A
competitive inhibition
coumestans
coumestrol
daidzein
endogenous oestrogen
enterodiol
enterolactone
equol
follicular stimulating
  hormone (FSH)
formononetin
genistein
isoflavonoid

lignan
luteinising hormone
  (LH)
oestradiol
oestrogen receptor
phyto-oestrogen
phytosterol
resorcylic acid lactones
SHBG
steroidal saponin
terminal phenolic
  group
triterpenoid saponin
zearalenone

One of the first indications that plants produced compounds which might affect mammals and humans came from the discovery that plant oestrogens in clover were responsible for infertility in sheep.[1] Gradually it became apparent that these plant 'oestrogens' occurred widely throughout the plant community and that their regular consumption could affect human health.[2]

The term phyto-oestrogen, literally an oestrogen-like substance produced by a plant, was coined to describe this group of plant components. Some writers include only those plant oestrogens from one group—the isoflavonoids—but in this chapter, phyto-oestrogen can be taken to indicate any of the plant substances which possess oestrogenic activity. All of the phyto-oestrogens are naturally occurring compounds found in a large range of grains, seeds, legumes and medicinal plants, as well as some other commonly eaten foods.

Phyto-oestrogens are particularly important for women and are known to influence the menstrual cycle;[3] to reduce the incidence of oestrogen-responsive cancers;[4] and to decrease the frequency and severity of menopausal symptoms.[5] Asian women who eat a traditional diet, excrete higher amounts of oestrogen than Western women, a factor which some researchers believe may contribute to their lower risk of breast cancer.[6] Soya products consumed regularly in Asian countries contain high levels of phyto-oestrogens, and are said to be responsible for these and other positive effects[7] (although other factors, including genetics have also been identified).

The levels of phyto-oestrogens in plants change as the plant grows and matures—very early plant growth, such as when seeds first sprout, is associated with high levels of phyto-oestrogens. Levels also increase when a plant is producing seeds or when it is stressed by drought or insect attack.

The drought-related increases in phyto-oestrogens seem to reduce the fertility of grazing animals by acting as a type of contraceptive. The result is fewer animals to eat the plant, which improves plant survival.[8]

There are six main types of phyto-oestrogens consumed by humans which are known to influence health. These are the isoflavones, coumestans and lignans, which occur in a number of commonly eaten foods; the triterpenoid and steroidal saponins; the phytosterols; and a sixth group known as the resorcylic acid lactones, of which zearalenone is the most important.

Phyto-oestrogens share many of the same biological activities with oestrogens produced in the body (endogenous oestrogens)—probably because phyto-oestrogens and endogenous oestrogens have structural similarities, and both have the ability to interact with oestrogen receptors. Although the plant oestrogens have an order of oestrogenic activity that is many times weaker than that of the endogenous oestrogens, oestrogen-like effects are apparent after the consumption of phyto-oestrogens in many, if not all of the oestrogen-receptive tissues.

Triggering the oestrogen-like response

Both phyto-oestrogens and endogenous oestrogens are transported to oestrogen-receptive tissues in the blood and there, they dock to the oestrogen receptors which are inside the cell. The capacity to bind to a receptor does not confer automatic oestrogenic potential—some types of compounds can trigger an oestrogenic effect, others can reduce or block one.

Unlike the endogenous oestrogen oestradiol, none of the phyto-oestrogens can trigger the full range of oestrogenic potential. So for example, physical maturation—ovulation and menstruation—cannot occur because of a phyto-oestrogenic effect. Phyto-oestrogens have a much more limited role and are capable of initiating only some of the changes associated with oestrogens—such as changes in vaginal cytology.

There are a number of tests used to assess a plant's oestrogenic potential. The oestrogenic effect of a substance can be measured in experimental animals by testing whether it causes uterine enlargement or the usual oestrogenic changes in cells of the vagina. Thus, the ability of each plant oestrogen to increase the size of the uterus, in say a mouse, or change the cells in its vagina, is used as an indicator of oestrogenicity.

Using these types of tests, the oestrogenic effect of a phyto-oestrogen is estimated to range from around 160 to many thousands of times weaker than oestradiol.

Another method is to determine the ability of phyto-oestrogens to bind to oestrogen receptors, known as the oestrogen-binding affinity. This laboratory procedure gives an indication of relative binding capacity and determines to some degree, the pro- or anti-oestrogenic activity of the phyto-oestrogen. Both of these methods have many flaws and can give misleading results—for instance mice do not menstruate—but are still used as the main methods for testing oestrogenic potential in the absence of a more accurate test.

Isoflavonoids and lignans

The isoflavonoids and lignans are important components of many foods and have been shown to have many beneficial effects for women. They have an active chemical group at one end of their molecular structure known as the terminal phenolic group which is similar to that found on an oestrogen molecule. This allows them to bind to oestrogen receptor sites.

Isoflavonoids are a large group of about 700 different substances. The most biologically active in terms of oestrogen-like potential are the coumestans, and the isoflavones genistein, daidzein, biochanin A and formononetin.

- Coumestans
  Of the coumestans, coumestrol is the most important. It is found in many foods such as soya products, peas, beans and other legumes. The highest levels occur in sprouted legumes such as soya beans and alfalfa. See Table 18.1. Compared to the endogenous oestrogens, the oestrogenic potential of coumestrol is rather weak, and has been estimated at about 160 times less powerful than oestradiol,[9] but approximately 30–100 times stronger than the isoflavones.[10]

Table 18.1 Coumestrol content of foods (mcg per 100 g dry weight)

Sprouted soya beans	7110
Sprouted alfalfa	500
Dry soya beans	120
Frozen green beans	100
Frozen green peas	40
Frozen Brussels sprouts	40

- Isoflavones

  Of the many different isoflavones now identified, the most important in terms of their oestrogenic potential are formononetin, genistein, daidzein and biochanin A. These phyto-oestrogens are found in soya products and other legumes.

  Formononetin is converted to daidzein by the plant, but once eaten, is changed by bacteria in the intestine into an even more active substance known as equol. Although it is not possible to make precise statements about any of the phyto-oestrogens, equol is considered to be the most oestrogenic of the isoflavones, but is still very weak, about 1000 times weaker than oestradiol.

  Of the other oestrogenic isoflavones, biochanin A is converted to the very weak phyto-oestrogen called genistein, believed to be about 100 000 times less active than oestradiol. Genistein, daidzein and equol are all weakly oestrogenic, and act as anti-oestrogens in pre-menopausal women by blocking endogenous oestrogen from interacting with cell receptors.

- Phyto-oestrogenic medicinal plants

  Medicago sativa (alfalfa/lucerne)

  Medicago is an important stock feed, and has also been introduced into the human diet in the form of sprouts. Medicinally, *Medicago* as a tea or extract is prescribed for convalescence or vitamin deficiency because it contains high levels of vitamins A, C, E and K. The presence of iodothyromines also make *Medicago sativa* a useful remedy for mild hypothyroidism.[11]

  Medicago also contains significant amounts of phyto-oestrogens including genistein, daidzein, and coumestrol, and some practitioners now recommend this herb post-menopausally when endogenous oestrogen levels are low, or even for pre-menopausal women with oestrogen-dependent conditions. No tradition exists to justify this practice, which seems to be based on an extrapolation of the benefits of *dietary* phyto-oestrogens to extracts and teas. See the caution on long-term use of phyto-oestrogens to follow.

  Trifolium pratense (Red clover)

  Trifolium has been used for centuries as a 'blood cleanser' for psoriasis and eczema; as a poultice for acne and ulcers; and irritable coughs, bronchitis and whooping cough.[12] It has also been used as part of cancer therapy—the flowers were applied to breast lesions, some of which were presumably cancerous,[13] while the leaves, flowers and roots were also taken internally as medicine.

Trifolium is an important phyto-oestrogenic plant containing biochanin A, a potent inhibitor of the carcinogen benzo[a]pyrene in cells.[14] This ability to inhibit carcinogen activation suggests that biochanin A is a potential chemoprotective agent[15] and seems to validate the traditional use of the plant.

Infertility in sheep grazing on clover may be due to the isoflavones in the foliage which cause a non-responsiveness in the uterus, cervix and vagina to endogenous oestrogen.[16] Despite this apparently potent oestrogenic effect, and a lack of traditional information on the long-term internal use of the herbaceous part of the plant (which has significantly more isoflavones than the flower), *Trifolium pratense* is also increasingly used as a phyto-oestrogen for post-menopausal women. Caution is warranted, however, until further information is available.

- Lignans
  The plant lignans are found in fibre-rich foods like seeds, grains and beans—linseeds are a particularly rich source. Like the isoflavone daidzein, the lignans need to be modified in the bowel by bacteria before they can have an oestrogenic effect in the body. Once modified they are referred to as 'mammalian lignans'. The most important mammalian lignans are enterolactone and enterodiol.

Reduced risk of hormone-related disease
Lignans and isoflavonoids have subtly different effects from each other which result from their interaction with oestrogen-sensitive cells in, for example, the breast, uterus and ovary, and the hypothalamic-pituitary unit. The changes brought about by these hormone-like effects seems to depend on the relative potency of the phyto-oestrogen in question; its availability; the activity of intestinal bacteria; and whether the woman is pre- or post-menopausal.

When a woman is pre-menopausal, her endogenous oestrogens bind to receptors causing cell proliferation (multiplication) which leads to an escalating number of cells and hence receptor sites. When phyto-oestrogens are available, they compete with the endogenous oestrogens for the same binding sites—the more phyto-oestrogens available, the weaker the endogenous oestrogenic effect.[17] This 'anti-oestrogenic' action of the phyto-oestrogens is termed 'competitive inhibition' and is believed to reduce the incidence of oestrogen-dependent conditions such as breast cancer by balancing the growth-promoting effects of the endogenous oestrogens.[18] Tamoxifen, a drug which is used to treat breast cancer, is structurally related to the phyto-oestrogens.[19]

The regular consumption of soya products in the diet seems to lower the risk of developing breast cancer. This may be related to the phyto-oestrogens, however, a number of other compounds, perhaps acting synergistically, have also been identified (see pages 297–8). The medicinal plant *Trifolium pratense*, traditionally used for the treatment of breast cancer, likewise contains phyto-oestrogens. One of these, biochanin A, inhibits carcinogen activation in cells. While abundant evidence for the role of phyto-oestrogens in cancer *prevention* can be documented, the position for women *with* oestrogen-responsive breast cancer is less clear. Phyto-oestrogens can reduce receptor site availability and therefore block endogenous oestrogen, a mechanism which is likely to confer protection to pre-menopausal women[20] and obese post-menopausal women who have high circulating endogenous oestrogens because of the peripheral conversion of androgens in fatty tissue.[21] Long-term studies which specifically investigate survival rates of post-menopausal women with breast cancer who consume high levels of dietary phyto-oestrogens are needed to determine whether phyto-oestrogens can be safely recommended for women of all ages with oestrogen-responsive breast cancers.

The isoflavonoids and lignans also stimulate liver production of SHBG.[22] SHBG binds to the sex hormones, especially androgens and oestrogens, and acts as a carrier protein. When the major portion of these hormones are bound to SHBG in the blood, they are less available to bind to hormone-sensitive tissues. This is believed to be another mechanism whereby phyto-oestrogens lower the incidence of hormone-related diseases.[23]

The symptoms of excess androgen production seen in polycystic ovarian disease and familial androgen disorders may be reduced by phyto-oestrogens because of the increase in SHBG seen when the diet contains high levels of phyto-oestrogens. SHBG reduces the availability of androgens and may limit their masculinising effects.

The phyto-oestrogens are also capable of slowing down the production of non-ovarian oestrogen (the oestrogen produced in the fat). The aromatase enzyme which normally converts androgens in fatty tissue into oestrogen, is inhibited by phyto-oestrogens.[24] Inhibition can range from moderate to weak, depending on which of the plant oestrogens are tested and results in a reduction of the production and availability of non-ovarian endogenous oestrogen.

Periods
Other more immediate benefits from dietary phyto-oestrogens include lighter periods and longer menstrual cycles.[25] Including phyto-oestrogens in the diet, especially lignans, may also reduce the risk of endometrial hyperplasia by improving ovulation and oestrogen:progesterone ratios.[26]

Bone density
A new area of research is the potential for the phyto-oestrogens to improve bone density. At the moment, investigation is in its early stages. Soya beans, possibly due to the isoflavones, reduced bone loss in rats.[27]

Coumestrol[28] has been shown to inhibit bone resorption and, at the same time, increase bone mineralisation in *in vitro* experiments.

Post-menopausal complaints

The role of the phyto-oestrogens in a relatively oestrogen-poor environment, such as after the menopause, is quite different to that seen in pre-menopausal women. The phyto-oestrogens bind to receptor sites and cause a weak oestrogen-like response which can reduce some of the symptoms of menopause such as hot flushes and vaginal dryness.

Recently Australian researchers decided to test just exactly how effective the phyto-oestrogens were for hot flushes by giving dietary supplements of either 45 g of soya flour or wheat flour. Both of these foods contain phyto-oestrogens, but the plant oestrogens in soya flour are more potent than those in wheat. As was expected, the soya flour decreased hot flushes by a larger margin: 40 per cent compared to 25 per cent in the wheat flour group.[29]

One cup of soya beans is reported to contain about 300 mg isoflavone.[30] Assuming that the oestrogenic activity of the isoflavones is about 0.1 per cent of oestrogen preparations used for menopausal women, this is equivalent to about 0.45 milligrams of conjugated oestrogens. The dose of Premarin tablets, a common form of hormone replacement therapy, ranges from 0.3 mg to 0.625 mg.

Increasing soya intake can be as easy as substituting soya for ordinary milk and using soya flour in cooking. As little as 100 g per day of tofu can reduce hot flushes and vaginal dryness. Dried or fresh (frozen) soya beans can be added to soups and bean dishes. As little as 25 g or about 2 heaped dessertspoons of ground linseeds per day can help to reduce symptoms associated with low oestrogen levels, including vaginal dryness.[31] Linseeds contain lignans and can be used in cooking or ground and added to drinks or breakfast cereals.

The lignans and some of the isoflavones require normal levels of bowel bacteria and women who have taken, or who are taking antibiotics can be expected to gain less benefit. Yoghurt may help restore these necessary bacterial colonies.

Research into the effectiveness of phyto-oestrogens for menopausal women is continuing all over the world. While the researchers are to be applauded for investigating the positive effects of plant medicines, it is possible that this type of research will eventually lead to the production of a 'natural' oestrogen which will be marketed as the safe 'alternative' to HRT. And here there is need for some caution.

Traditionally these plants were never used like HRT. When oestrogenic herbs were prescribed for menopausal complaints, they were used only while symptoms persisted. There is no herbal tradition to prescribe phyto-oestrogens for long periods to prevent bone density loss, breast cancer or cardiovascular disease. When herbalists use plant oestrogens, the herbs they usually prescribe belong to the steroidal saponin group.

The length of time a herb is prescribed should be in accordance with traditional guidelines. Women who self-prescribe, and doctors who suggest herbs, but are not trained herbalists, may not be aware of these important restrictions.

An ongoing concern for many herbalists is the prevailing view, usually expressed by the general public, that if it's natural, it's safe. Many herbs are very safe in the short term, but long-term administration is another matter. When herbs are neatly packaged in tablet form, and are readily available all year round (which would never have been the case in the past), there is the potential that they can be taken in large doses and for long periods.

A prudent question to ask is what will happen to endometrial cells when menstruation has stopped and the cells are subjected to prolonged stimulation by plant oestrogens in a herbal preparation. Numerous animal studies using aqueous, alcoholic and ether extracts of plants in an otherwise oestrogen-free environment, have shown phyto-oestrogens to be capable of changes in endometrial cells and to cause an increase in uterine weight after relatively short administration.[32]

Some herbs have relatively high levels of plant oestrogens, but that doesn't mean they will be necessarily useful for menopausal women in the long term. Alfalfa and red clover, for example, have very high levels of phyto-oestrogens, but have been associated with infertility in sheep. This suggests a very powerful oestrogenic effect. People don't eat as much alfalfa or clover as sheep, of course, but the effects of plant oestrogens taken over long periods is as yet unknown in menopausal women.

In countries where positive effects have been seen with phyto-oestrogen-rich foods, the foods, such as soya beans, are eaten as part of the normal diet—not prescribed as extra supplements. My advice is—think twice before taking anything long term (more than three months), or ask for advice from a trained herbalist. Otherwise, stick to the plant oestrogens found in foods until more information is available on the long-term effects of herbal preparations. After all, it's the foods that have been shown to have the positive effects with long-term use.

Saponins

The saponins have a similar structure to the steroidal hormones oestrogen, progesterone, the androgens and the corticosteroids which have cholesterol as their starting compound. This structural similarity has meant that pharmaceutical companies can use the saponin-containing plants to manufacture steroid hormones, especially progesterone and cortisone.

Saponins, when present in large amounts, can cause an unpleasant irritating sensation on contact with the mucus membranes (saponins are 'soaps'). This is usually experienced as an irritation of the back of the throat and can make these herbs somewhat difficult to take. Traditionally, they were indicated for menstrual irregularity, abnormal bleeding patterns, infertility, menstrual pain and menopausal symptoms. Some like *Chamaelirium luteum*, were not to be used when women were unmarried because of an observed increase in fertility (and presumably libido as well!).

The saponins are divided into two groups depending on their structures—the steroidal saponins and the triterpenoid saponins. Only some of the saponins from either group are capable of eliciting an 'oestrogenic' response. Medicinal plants which contain saponins known to be 'oestrogenic' belong to the hormone regulatory or tonic categories of herbs and are prescribed for conditions associated with infertility, erratic or heavy bleeding patterns, and for menopausal complaints.

- Triterpenoid saponins

Some triterpenoid saponins found in medicinal plants can have steroid-like structures. Oestrogen-like effects have been observed after administration of some of these plants, especially *Cimicifuga racemosa*, *Panax ginseng* and *Glycyrrhiza glabra*.

The triterpenoids do not seem to elicit direct oestrogenic effects, but cause secondary changes in the reproductive tract through stimulation or modification of the function of the hypothalamus and pituitary glands.[33] *Cimicifuga racemosa* has been shown experimentally to reduce the levels of LH, an affect attributed to the triterpenoids. *Cimicifuga racemosa* also contains the isoflavone formononetin, however its effect on LH release is very slight.[34] This herb can be used to improve the symptoms of menopause,[35] and is also useful for menstrual disorders associated with an elevated LH, such as polycystic ovarian disease.

There are numerous reported oestrogenic effects of *Panax ginseng*, a well-known tonic herb. Effects on the gonadotrophin release combined with a local oestrogen-like response have been suggested.[36] Isolated medical reports have shown changes in vaginal and cervical cytology;[37] abnormal vaginal bleeding;[38] as well as breast pain and lumpiness[39] consistent with an oestrogenic effect amongst post-menopausal women who took prolonged doses of ginseng. The triterpenoid saponins (ginsenosides) are widely reported to possess these qualities. Properly prescribed, *Panax ginseng* is a herb with low toxicity and is beneficial for all women, particularly during times when the body is adapting to physical changes.

Glycyrrhizin, a triterpenoid from *Glycyrrhiza glabra*, has a weak affinity for oestrogen and androgen receptors, and for SHBG; but has no affinity for progesterone receptors.[40] Compared to oestradiol, its oestrogenic effect is weak.[41] Glycyrrhetinic acid, which is metabolised from glycyrrhizin in the bowel, reduces the synthesis of testosterone from androstenedione;[42] and the whole herb reduces prolactin secretion.[43] These two different hormonal effects result in increased fertility by improving ovulation rates. This *outcome* has been traditionally described by herbalists as 'oestrogenic'. Steroidal saponin-containing herbs have also been referred to as oestrogenic for these and other reasons.

- Steroidal saponins

Steroidal saponins are found in varying amounts in a number of commonly eaten foods such as root vegetables like carrots and yams; the deadly nightshade family, especially potato; asparagus and grains. Many of the important medicinal plants used for gynaecological complaints also contain steroidal saponins, usually in larger quantities than in foods, including *Chamaelirium luteum*, *Dioscorea villosa* and *Aletris farinosa*.

Steroidal saponins probably need to be acted upon by bacteria in the bowel before they can be absorbed and initiate oestrogenic activity. In the bowel, bacteria cleave a sugar molecule from the steroidal saponin which then becomes a sapogenin. One of the important sapogenins, diosgenin, is produced in this way from the herbs *Chamaelirium luteum*, *Trillium erectum*, *Trigonella foenum-graecum*, *Dioscorea villosa* and *Aletris farinosa*. Because diosgenin is the pharmacological constituent common to all of these medicinal plants, some of their biological effects are similar.

Considerable confusion surrounds these plant components. Media reports have erroneously claimed that plants containing steroidal saponins have an hormonal effect which is 'stronger than the Pill'—claims recognised as absolute nonsense by anyone with even a rudimentary understanding of plant pharmacology. Others claim that these plants contain 'natural progesterone' (see following) because they contain dioscin, which can be converted in the test tube into progesterone. There is no evidence that dioscin can be changed into progesterone in the body.

There is also some related confusion amongst herbalists concerning the use of the steroidal saponin-containing herbs. Traditional use of these herbs (often referred to as women's tonics, especially *Chamaelirium luteum* and *Aletris farinosa*) is to improve fertility. This has earned these herbs the reputation of being 'oestrogenic'. Because of this some herbalists ignore traditional indications and won't use these herbs for conditions associated with oestrogen excess—endometriosis and fibroids, for example—believing the herbs to be capable of mimicking the effects of oestrogens.

Once converted from steroidal saponins, sapogenins can bind to the receptor sites like the isoflavones, coumestans and lignans, but their binding capacity (and therefore potency) is very weak. So it seems unlikely that the observed effects of the sapogenins are due to a direct interaction with oestrogen receptor sites. A more probable explanation of the consequences of giving these and the closely related triterpenoids is that they interact with hypothalamic and pituitary hormones and have an indirect effect on the body's production of oestrogens by initiating ovulation.

Conditions like endometriosis, which are believed to be exacerbated by excessive exposure to oestrogens, are associated with a shorter follicular phase, reduced oestrogen *clearance* (not excess oestrogen production) and an inadequate luteal phase with poor progesterone production. Herbs which can stimulate ovulation frequently, normalise the length of the follicular phase and can also improve the balance between oestrogen and progesterone levels by regulating ovulation. The use of the steroidal saponin-containing herbs for conditions associated with oestrogen excess, can be expected to normalise the luteal phase and provided that they are prescribed according to the traditional indications, they should be beneficial rather than harmful. These conditions include menstrual irregularity, abnormal bleeding, infertility caused by failure to ovulate, and pain.

Research on diosgenin, shows that it has a weak oestrogenic effect, but is devoid of progesterogenic activity.[44] In Europe, *Tribulus terrestris*, a herb with high levels of diosgenin, has been synthesised into a drug known as Tribestan. Tribestan increases FSH and oestradiol in premenopausal women; improves fertility; and reduces hot flushes without increasing oestradiol levels in post-menopausal women.[45] This implies that the primary site of action of steroidal saponins is the hypothalamus.

'Natural' progesterone and wild yam creams

The progesterone molecule is a unique substance that is synthesised in the body, but progesterone (exactly the same form as made in the body) can also be manufactured commercially. Unhelpfully, some manufacturers and books refer to both kinds as 'natural progesterone'.

This term has been coined to differentiate 'progesterone' from the 'progestogens'—drugs, also manufactured commercially—that have a progesterone-like effect. Of the two types of progesterone manufactured commercially, one is structurally the same as the progesterone synthesised in the body, the other is a group of chemical substances known as the progestogens which are sold under brand names such as Provera, Primolut N and Micronor. The progestogens have the advantage, unlike progesterone, of remaining biologically active after oral ingestion.

Confusion arises when *herbal* creams are said to contain natural progesterone or plant-based progesterone. Naturally occurring progesterone is *not* known to exist in plants at biologically active levels, and even though some popular writers claim that plants such as wild yam and mistletoe contain progesterone, there is no scientific evidence to confirm this.

Wild yam creams are popularly recommended for their 'progesterogenic' effects to treat a range of premenstrual and menopausal disorders. Users of these creams, however, report quite varied responses in effectiveness—some claim they are absolutely useless (and expensive as well); others cite miraculous results for complaints like premenstrual breast soreness. Wild yam creams *may* have therapeutic effects, but the actual mechanism for this is not yet known, and there have been no independent trials to ascertain who will respond best to these products.

Other herbalists and manufacturers suggest that the progesterogenic action of wild yam creams is due to the transdermal up-take of steroidal saponin, dioscin, which is converted into progesterone in the body. Chemically, this assumption is quite illogical, especially considering that the starting compound for progesterone in the body is cholesterol. In fact, if transdermal applications of a starting compound could be reasonably expected to produce progesterone, rubbing the body with butter should have a greater (and far cheaper) effect on progesterone levels.

It is also unreasonable to assume that the application of a wild yam cream would in some way favour the *in vivo* production of one steroid hormone—progesterone—over others, corticosteroids or androgens, for instance.

Dioscin has been used for many years as a starting material for the commercial production of a number of steroidal drugs, including progesterone and cortisone. For dioscin to become progesterone, a carefully controlled series of chemical steps are performed in a factory—the same process does not occur in the body when substances like wild yam are applied to the skin or taken orally. When a salivary analysis of progesterone levels was performed on women using wild yam creams and compared to that of non-users, no differences in salivary progesterone levels were found.[46]

The traditional uses for wild yam (*Dioscorea villosa*) include bilious colic, colitis, dysmenorrhoea, prevention of miscarriage, arthritic complaints, diverticulitis and appendicitis. It can also be used for nausea in pregnancy in small but frequent doses. The dose range is 6–10 mL daily, taken orally.

Very little is known about the therapeutic effects of saponins such as dioscin. They are converted to sapogenins before absorption from the gut and therefore, much of the interest has focused on the biological activity of the sapogenins, in this case, diosgenin. Research on animals shows oestrogenic changes in tissues after administration of diosgenin, but no progesterogenic activity. Transdermal applications of wild yam bypass this important saponin-to-sapogenin step meaning that wild yam applied to the skin can be expected to have quite different effects and indications to wild yam taken orally.

Saponins are known to cause haemolysis (break down of red blood cells) if injected into the blood stream, but their biological effects when absorbed transdermally remain obscure. It is not known whether the effect of dioscin is similar to diosgenin, that is weakly oestrogenic, or whether it may be capable, like diosgenin, of increasing endogenous progesterone production via an effect on the hypothalamic–pituitary unit. This may explain the lack of effect with wild yam creams, commonly seen in post-menopausal women who have stopped ovulation and therefore, progesterone production.

Progesterone receptors are more selective than oestrogen receptors— near enough is not good enough. They will only allow progesterone and the commercially synthesised progestogens to exert a progesterogenic effect. Natural progesterone does not occur in plants in appreciable amounts, and the progesterone precursors found in plants, such as diosgenin, must be commercially processed before they can behave like progesterone. In fact, there is only one 'natural progesterone'—the one made in the body.

Phytosterols

Of the phytosterols, beta-sitosterol is the most significant and has oestrogenic activity.[48] This compound is ubiquitous in the plant kingdom and when isolated from *Glycyrrhiza glabra*, beta-sitosterol was shown to possess oestrogenic activity 400 times weaker than oestradiol.[49] However, only small fractions are absorbed,[50] and so its oestrogenic potential from food is almost inconsequential.

The major role for the phytosterols is in the intestine where they compete with cholesterol for absorption, leading to lower cholesterol levels.[51] Phytosterols have also been shown to experimentally inhibit the development of colon cancer.[52] High levels of phytosterols are found in all edible oils, but corn, rice bran, sesame seed and wheatgerm oils contain the highest levels.[53]

Table 18.2 Edible plants with recognised oestrogenically-active compounds[55]

Isoflavones	Coumestans	Resorcylic acid lactones	Lignans	Steroidal saponins	Others
soya bean*	alfalfa	oats	linseed*	liquorice*	fennel
chick pea	soya sprouts*	barley	rye	potato	carrot
cherry	cow pea	rye	buckwheat		aniseed
alfalfa	green bean	sesame seed	millet		hops
parsley	kidney beans	wheat	sesame and sunflower seeds		cabbage family
liquorice	split peas	peas	legumes and beans		sage
whole grains	mung beans	corn	whole grains		rhubarb
mung bean	olives	rice			beetroot
					yeast
					plum
					garlic

* Contains high levels of phyto-oestrogen.

Zearalenone

Zearalenone, unlike the other phyto-oestrogens, is not produced in the plant itself, but by moulds which contaminate poorly stored cereal crops.

It is reported to be 80 times less active than oestradiol in primates, however, the effects of zearalenone are known to vary widely amongst other animal species. Isolated zearalenone (as a drug) has been used for post-menopausal symptoms and as a contraceptive Pill in doses which suggest agreement with the potency of this phyto-oestrogen in primates.[54]

19

Herbs

Key words

abortifacient
anti-haemorrhagic
anti-spasmodic
aromatase
astringent
carminative
dysmenorrhia
emmenagogue
haemostatic
incoordinate uterine
   action
ischaemia
latent
   hyperprolactinaemia

leucorrhoea
menorrhagia
nervine
partus praeparator
photosensitivity
polysaccharide
prostaglandin
sapogenin
saponin
spasmolytic
thromboxane
trimester
uterine tonic

One of the fundamental tenets of herbalism is that the body is a self-repairing organism that almost always seeks to return to a state of equilibrium. Herbs are ideal agents to support healing and the return of normal function because they are gentle and effective.

Women and herbs have had a strong association throughout recorded history and a complex understanding of the causes and treatment of many gynaecological complaints has developed over the centuries. Modern science has, by and large, only supported and extended these understandings.

This chapter describes the traditional and contemporary use of a group of herbs used commonly in the treatment of women's complaints. It is not intended as a manual for the untrained, but as an overview of the scientific and traditional uses of these herbs in the treatment of gynaecological complaints.

HERBS WHICH AFFECT THE UTERINE MUSCLE: THE TONICS, SPASMOLYTICS AND EMMENAGOGUES

There are a number of herbs that can affect the activity of the uterine muscle. These herbs can be thought of as lying somewhere along an imaginary spectrum of action—from the relaxant and anti-spasmodic group of herbs called spasmolytics, to the herbs which can increase spasm and initiate muscular contraction.

When muscular activity is increased in hollow organs such as the uterus or bowel, expulsion of the contents of the organ will be the result. In the uterus this may bring on a period or cause a miscarriage; in the bowel, these herbs can stimulate peristalsis and effect the regularity of the bowel movements. Those herbs which increase muscular activity in the uterus are termed emmenagogues.

In addition to the spasmolytics and emmenagogues, another group of herbs also effect the uterine muscle. These herbs improve uterine muscle tone and are called the uterine tonics.

The grossly oversimplified indications for herbs influencing uterine muscle are: spasmolytics for pain, emmenagogues after childbirth or to initiate menstrual flow, and uterine tonics to regulate the activity of the uterus. Experimentally, it can be shown that the tonics, spasmolytics and emmenagogues initiate a number of different effects on uterine muscle which can be summarised as follows:

* Tonics *increase the tone* in the muscle and improve the overall strength of the organ. (Tone is assessed while a muscle is at rest and is the 'resistance to passive elongation or stretch'.)[1]
* Spasmolytics *slow the rate and decrease the amplitude* of uterine contractions. This will effect the number of contractions in the uterine muscle per unit of time.
* Emmenagogues *increase the amplitude* of the contraction and therefore effect the expulsive activity of the uterus.

THE UTERINE TONICS

Uterine tonics are key herbs in gynaecology. They have a normalising effect on the uterus and assist with normal uterine function. The uterine tonics have a pivotal role in herbal prescriptions and are usually prescribed as part of a formula if a complaint involves the uterus. The primary aim of the herbalist is to restore homeostasis—to support normal function and the inherent capacity of the body to self-regulate and repair. Tonics are central to this aim and are used to achieve a 'balanced' effect from a formula. If an emmenagogue is used to increase the expulsive capacity of the uterus, a tonic is added to moderate this effect. If a spasmolytic is used to relax, the addition of a tonic will maintain uterine tone.

Each of the uterine tonics has specific indications which are described in the section dealing with that herb. As a group, the uterine tonics are prescribed:

- for all conditions where uterine pain is a feature;
- for all complaints associated with abnormal bleeding patterns;
- for all conditions associated with prolapse, malposition or enlargement of the uterus;
- as *partus praeparators*. These formulas for pregnancy are used to regulate uterine tone until labour commences, assist with a smooth delivery and regular contractions during labour, and help with involution of the uterus after birth.
- as herbs to improve fertility. Some of the uterine tonics (and a number of other common gynaecological herbs) contain various chemical compounds which have hormonal effects. These effects may account for some of the fertility-enhancing and regulatory actions of these herbs.

THE UTERINE TONICS

Angelica sinensis (Dang Gui)
Aletris farinosa (true unicorn root)
Caulophyllum thalictroides (blue cohosh)

Chamaelirium luteum
  (helonias or false unicorn root)
Rubus idaeus (raspberry leaves)

Rubus idaeus/strigosus (Red raspberry leaf)

Rubus idaeus, the red raspberry, is a native of Europe, North America, and Asia. The roots were once eaten like turnips;[2] the fruit contains vitamins A, B, C, and E, pectin, ferric citrate (a type of iron)[3] and calcium, and is useful to prevent anaemia;[4] and the leaf is used medicinally. The active constituents of *Rubus idaeus* leaves are largely unknown, however flavonoids, unspecified polypeptides and tannins have been described.[5] The leaves also contain the compound known as fragarine which is responsible for the uterine tonic effect.[6]

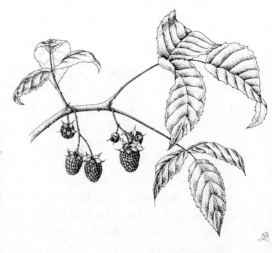

Uterine tonic effects

Rubus idaeus has been used for centuries as a popular uterine tonic and a *partus praeparator*. Traditionally, the herb was drunk as a tea for period pain and heavy periods, as well as before and during pregnancy to prevent or relieve nausea, to ease labour and to assist with breast milk production.[7] The active constituents of raspberry leaves seem to possess contradictory effects—on one hand relaxing the uterine muscle and on another initiating contractions. This has confounded researchers, but confirmed herbalists' belief in raspberry leaves as a uterine tonic.

In 1941, several constituents collectively named 'fragarine' were discovered in the leaf. These constituents were shown to have a relaxing effect on the pregnant uterus. Contractions were diminished in force and frequency, and occurred at evenly spaced intervals. Secondary contractions were eliminated.[8] In addition to these effects, other researchers found that if the muscle was relaxed, the herb *induced* contractions.[9]

But how, if the effect of raspberry leaves was primarily to relax the uterus, could the herb assist with labour? Or as the researchers put it: 'It is difficult to understand how uterine relaxation should assist parturition [labour]; rather it would be thought to delay it by diminishing the force available to bring about the birth of the child'.[10]

Yet another team of researchers isolated several constituents from raspberry leaves, some of which increased uterine contractions, while others relaxed the uterus. They concluded that although raspberry leaves contain a powerful 'spasmolytic', the overall effect was to stimulate the uterine muscle. This, they said, made the traditional use of *Rubus* 'difficult to assess . . .'.[11]

It wasn't until 1970, when the leaf (as opposed to its isolated constituents) was tested on uterine muscle, that a reason for the beneficial effect of raspberry leaf was proposed. These later researchers suggested that *Rubus* would prevent or reduce the risk of incoordinate uterine action (a common cause of difficulty and failure to progress in labour), by regulating the action of the uterine muscle.[12]

Raspberry leaves (and all other uterine tonics) should be used with care in the first trimester of pregnancy because of a slight possibility of miscarriage. It is unwise to use *any* medication during the first three months of pregnancy unless absolutely necessary. When trained herbalists use raspberry leaf for nausea in pregnancy or threatened miscarriage, it is usually prescribed with other herbs which offset this possibility. To improve labour, there seems to be no additional benefit in starting the herb earlier than the eighteenth week.

There is some confusion about the use of raspberry leaves for conditions that are not associated with pregnancy. Experimentally, *Rubus* has not been shown to affect the non-pregnant uterus,[13] despite its historical and current use for period pain and heavy bleeding. *Rubus* contains tannins, but tannins are usually not absorbed in any quantity from the gut. Any therapeutic effect, then, must be due to other constituents in the herb.

Raspberry leaves have very high levels of manganese, moderate levels of iron, calcium and selenium, and the vitamins A and C. Perhaps this breakdown of nutritional components gives the best clue to the reported effectiveness of *Rubus* in heavy menstruation. Vitamin C and iron can both improve menorrhagia. For dysmenorrhoea, it is seldom useful alone.

Gynaecological indications for *Rubus* can be summarised as follows:

- As a *partus* in the latter 5 months of pregnancy.
- To aid in involution of the uterus after delivery.
- To aid with production and maintenance of breast milk.
- As an adjunctive treatment for menorrhagia.
- As a general and uterine tonic following surgery to the uterus, for example, the removal of fibroids, termination of pregnancy or a curette.

Additional effects

Raspberry leaves are astringent because of the tannin content, and are used to treat diarrhoea and inflammation of the throat and eyes. Garden and wild varieties have similar therapeutic properties.[14]

Raspberry leaves taste pleasantly aromatic with a slight bitterness. They are Cool and Dry.

Dose

Fluid extract: 2–10 mL, or dried leaf 2–8 g, three times daily.

One recipe for raspberry leaf tea follows: Make a strong cup of raspberry leaf tea and squeeze into it the juice of an orange. Take 3 cups of this mixture daily in the last months of pregnancy.

Rubus in the form of dried leaf is very bulky and fluffy. Prescriptions of 1 tsp per cup three times daily results in low doses which may not be therapeutically active.

Angelica sinensis (Dang Gui)

Dang gui is another of the important tonic herbs for the uterus. It shares a general tonic effect with the other uterine tonics, *Aletris farinosa* and *Chamaelirium luteum*. These three herbs have a number of similar actions and can be used interchangeably in some instances, but the unique combination of indications for *Angelica sinensis* have secured it a prominent place in herbal medicine.

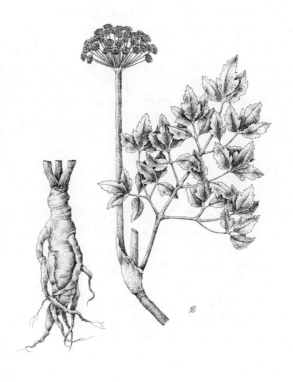

Dang Gui has been the subject of a great deal of research. The herb or its active constituents have liver-cell protective effects against a variety of poisons including carbon tetrachloride,[15] paracetamol[16] and aflatoxins.[17] Dang Gui also slows the heartbeat, increases coronary circulation, controls various types of arrhythmia, reduces blood pressure, and improves blood flow to the periphery.[18] It also has a blood cholesterol-lowering effect, a property it has in common with other herbs which contain beta-sitosterol. When given *Angelica sinensis*, irradiated mice had longer survival times and adult female mice maintained a higher fertility rate;[19] the latter effect is thought to be related to a protective effect on ovarian tissue.

Angelica sinensis also regulates prostaglandins synthesis and can regulate experimentally induced inflammatory responses caused by prostaglandins release.[20] Thromboxane A2, which is a member of the prostaglandins family, increases blood viscosity and promotes blood clotting. Its activity is regulated by *Angelica sinensis*. This may form the basis of the observed improvement of blood circulation by this herb.[21]

In traditional Chinese medicine, *Angelica sinensis* is referred to as a *blood tonic*, and has general and non-specific affects on the blood and circulation.[22] *Blood tonics* are prescribed for pallor, weakness, dizziness, dry skin, late or absent periods, pale menstrual flow, weakness after the period, after giving birth, or while breast feeding. *Angelica sinensis* has been shown to improve red blood cell counts,[23] and a number of theories have been proposed to explain the observed *blood tonification* properties. Although some writers report the presence of B_{12},[24] the validity of this must be queried on the grounds that it is highly unlikely that plants manufacture B_{12} in large quantities, or at all. Other investigations have shown polysaccharides to be responsible for the *blood tonification*,[25] however, they do not survive digestion, and it is likely that other factors are yet to be discovered which may more fully explain the effects of *Angelica sinensis* on blood quality.

Angelica sinensis is also used for constipation associated with debility and (often) old age. Symptoms include sluggishness of the bowel due to debility and dry, hard or pebble-like stools.[26] Another traditional use is for the treatment of coughs and shortness of breath. Researchers found that the herb relaxed bronchial smooth muscle and had an anti-asthmatic effect.[27]

Uterine tonic effects

Dang Gui is frequently used in a wide range of gynaecological conditions—amenorrhoea, dysmenorrhoea, irregular menstruation, and leucorrhoea. It is primarily a herb for the uterus and for improving the quality and circulatory dynamics of the blood. It is said to potentiate the action of vitamin E, a property which may explain its popular use at the time of menopause.

One of its most important effects is the effect on the uterus. As with *Rubus*, *Angelica sinensis* appears to contain a number of components which can increase tone, stengthen contractions, improve the orderly rhythm of contractions and relax the uterine muscle. A controversial point is whether *Angelica sinensis* is 'oestrogenic'. Mice given *Angelica sinensis* were reported to exhibit oestrogenic effects,[28] but this is often disputed.

The essential oil ligustilide[29] and ferulic acid[30] seem to be the major components with the uterine spasmolytic effect. Other components, some not identified, have an excitatory effect on uterine muscle. The sum total of all components is a slight increase in uterine activity—a mild emmenagogic effect, but which also seems to cause the contractions to become more orderly.[31] This herb should not be used in the first trimester of pregnancy unless prescribed by a trained herbalist as part of a traditional formula.

Herbs which have a spasmolytic effect on the uterus and improve the circulation are particularly indicated in the treatment of dysmenorrhoea. Apart from normalising uterine activity, they ease and, in some instances, increase the pelvic blood flow, which in turn relieves pelvic congestion and pain. Traditionally and experimentally, *Angelica sinensis* in combination with *Paeonia lactiflora*[32] and *Ligusticum wallichii*[33] is superior to *Angelica sinensis* alone. For menstrual pain that becomes worse with cold and is associated with a slow start to menstruation, *Angelica sinensis* is prescribed with *Cinnamomum*.

Traditionally, *Angelica sinensis* is also used as a *blood tonic* to regulate the period and to enhance the fertility of women who are *blood deficient*. It is usually prescribed with other herbs during the follicular phase of the cycle. It is sometimes poorly tolerated by those with weak digestion, and may need to be combined with *Zingiber*, *Cinnamomum* or bitters.

Dose

3–30 g dried herb or 2–4 mL fluid extract three times daily.
It is Warming and Moistening.[34]

Chamaelirium luteum (False unicorn root or Helonias)

Helonias dioica was the early name for *Chamaelirium luteum*, the false unicorn root, which has a reputation as a uterine and ovarian tonic. It has been used historically for a wide variety of gynaecological complaints from amenorrhoea and menorrhagia to irregular menstruation and period pain. It is also used as a bitter tonic to improve digestion, and to assist women with poor stamina and low spirits.

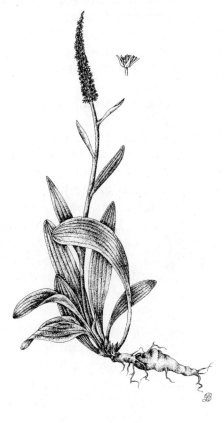

Although it is usually described as a uterine tonic, early research on its ability to affect muscle tone and rate or amplitude of contractions were consistently negative.[35] It is still recommended however as a herb to prevent miscarriage.[36] Another far more interesting traditional use is to regulate ovarian function and problems which originate 'in the first half of the cycle'.[37]

Chamaelirium is often referred to as an amphoteric to the ovary—as having the ability to regulate and normalise ovarian function.[38] Research on this herb is scarce and certainly nothing as elaborate as an investigation into the effects on the ovary have been performed. However, *Chamaelirium* does contain diosgenin, a steroidal saponin which has been shown to have possible effects on ovarian function via its action on the hypothalamic–pituitary unit (see pages 313–14).

Chamaelirium is threatened in the wild because of the increasing demands for collection and so its use should be restricted. *Paeonia lactiflora* or *Aletris farinosa* may prove to be suitable substitutes.

Dose

1–2 mL of fluid extract, three times daily.

Aletris farinosa (True unicorn root)

Aletris farinosa, commonly known as
the true unicorn root, is a member of
the lily family. It has a long history of
use as a uterine tonic, first by native
Americans, then by the early American
settlers, and now by many herbalists
worldwide. The part used is the dried
rhizome and root.

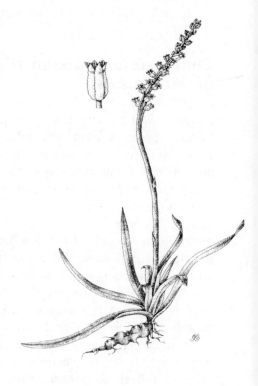

Uterine tonic effects

Aletris was popularised by Ellingwood,
one of the early American herbalists,
who claimed that it should be given to
tired, overworked and anaemic women
who were suffering from the consequences of giving birth too frequently.
He and others found it especially helpful for anaemia, constipation or
leucorrhoea of peri-menopausal
women.[39] Good results are also
achieved with pelvic floor weakness
and prolapse, particularly in older women with low back pain.[40]

This is one of the best uterine tonics for women with a sense of
pelvic heaviness or congestion, and seems to be especially beneficial for
women in their forties and fifties. *Aletris* can be taken by women of
any age however, for conditions which are accompanied by a sense of
pelvic discomfort, heaviness, a dragging sensation, or a feeling 'as
though everything might fall out'.

In the past, the true unicorn root, *Aletris farinosa* and the false
unicorn root, *Chamaelirium luteum*, were frequently substituted for one
another. Both were used to regulate the activity of the menstrual cycle
and as women's tonics, presumably because both (and many other plants
besides) yield the steroidal sapogenin, diosgenin, which has a mild
'oestrogenic' effect.[41]

Early animal experiments revealed that *Aletris* can have contradictory effects on uterine muscle, and can exert the entire spectrum of
effects from relaxation to stimulation in the same animal species and

between different animal species.[42] In most experiments, however, *Aletris* reduced the amplitude of uterine contractions which may explain its historical use, in combination with spasmolytic herbs for the prevention of miscarriage. Because of the conflicting reports on its actions, and because it needs to be used in combination with other herbs, its use by the untrained, especially during pregnancy, is unwise.

As is common with all uterine tonics, *Aletris* is recommended for the whole spectrum of gynaecological disorders, from light or absent periods, to periods which are too heavy or too frequent; for period pain and infertility; for the symptoms associated with a retroverted uterus and for leucorrhoea. This property is shared by all tonic herbal remedies—they are seen to regulate irrespective of the problem. The additional herbs in the formula direct the therapeutic effect toward the desired outcome.

Additional effects

The bitter and spasmolytic properties of *Aletris* are responsible for its effects in the gastrointestinal tract. It can be prescribed as a digestive tonic for loss of appetite arising from inadequate digestion; for flatulent colic or for nervous dyspepsia. The bitter principle in this herb also imparts a mild laxative effect.

Like all bitter tonics, it is strongly indicated during convalescence and is especially for debilitated women who are recovering from surgery or childbirth. Recovery from hysterectomy, particularly in the first weeks post-operatively when constipation, flatulence, pelvic discomfort and debility are common complaints, is one of the modern indications for this herb.

Dose

1–2 mL, three times daily.

It is Warming and tastes sweet, then bitter and soapy.[43]

Caulophyllum thalictroides (Blue cohosh)

Caulophyllum, an important remedy for female complaints, has come to us from the native Americans. Historically it was used to prepare the uterus for labour (*partus praeparator*), for period pain and for various 'inflammations' of the uterus. It is generally classed as a uterine tonic.

Like other uterine tonics, *Caulophyllum* seems to possess constituents with contradictory actions and it is also recommended for the usual contradictory array of complaints. Early research showed that the alcoholic extract of the whole herb increased uterine tone, but decreased the rate and amplitude of contractions.[44] The saponin fraction, however, seems to increase the amplitude of the contraction and cause a small increase in rate.[45]

It is ideal as a uterine tonic for the last six weeks of pregnancy to improve the normal function of the uterus during labour. On the other hand, it is recommended to prevent miscarriages.[46] The therapeutic effect is in part dependent on the other herbs it is combined with—as a *partus praeparator* it can be combined with *Mentha pule-gium*; to relax uterine muscle, for example from period pain, or to prevent a miscarriage, it is recommended with *Viburnum prunifolium*.

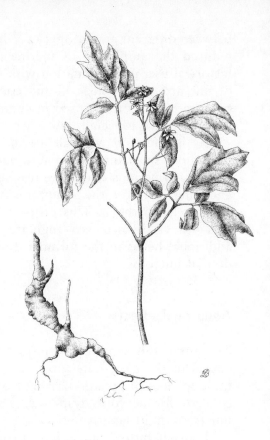

Dose

0.5–1 mL three times daily; not more than 0.25–0.5 mL in the first trimester of pregnancy, and always with *Viburnum prunifolium*. This herb should only be prescribed for pregnancy-related complaints by a trained herbalist.

SPASMOLYTICS

The spasmolytics or antispasmodic herbs have a relaxing effect on the smooth muscle and can slow or regulate the rate of contractions, both in the case of the uterus and in peristalsis in the bowel. Spasmolytics are frequently used to alleviate organ pain caused by excessive muscle contraction. When muscle spasm is severe, the blood flow and oxygen supply to the organ is impaired (ischaemia), resulting in pain. Relaxation of the affected muscle brings relief.

Included in this section are the spasmolytics *Viburnum opulus* and *prunifolium*, and *Ligusticum wallichii* from the Chinese pharmacopoeia. Other spasmolytics (discussed elsewhere) are *Dioscorea villosa*, *Paeonia lactiflora* with *Glycyrrhiza glabra*, and *Leonurus cardiaca*.

Specific uses in gynaecology

Spasmolytics reduce spasm and calm uterine activity:
- They are specifically indicated when the pain is colicky, crampy or contraction-like.
- They are used to calm the uterus in pregnancy and as an aid to the prevention of miscarriage and early labour.

Viburnum opulus and *v. prunifolium*

Viburnum opulus (cramp bark) and *Viburnum prunifolium* (black haw) are often discussed and prescribed interchangeably, having very similar therapeutic effects; however individual herbalists may show a particular preference for one or the other, and some texts describe slightly different indications.

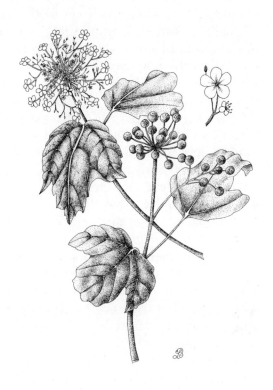

Native Americans used a decoction of the bark of *Viburnum opulus* for swollen glands, mumps and eye disorders;[47] as a diuretic; or as a tea and tobacco substitute.[48] *Viburnum prunifolium* has been extensively used to treat spasmodic dysmenorrhoea— one writer in 1877 reporting it to be superior to any other remedy for this problem. It is also used to prevent miscarriage;[49] to prevent cramps from hysterics(!) and to tone the uterus after fibroid removal.[50]

Both *Viburnum* spp. have been the subject of considerable controversy as to their efficacy. Studies between 1910 and 1920 found *Viburnum* spp. to have no significant action on the uterus,[51] while later research showed *Viburnum prunifolium* root bark to relax the uterus.[52] Several reasons for these inconsistencies have been suggested. The uterine strips tested may have been from different parts of the uterus—from the upper or lower segments which have different contractile characteristics; or they may have been taken from uteri at different times in the menstrual cycle (the uterine muscle is much less irritable just after the period).

However, much of the problem seems to have arisen because of frequent substitution, usually with *Acer spicatum* (mountain maple)[53] instead of *Viburnum*. In 1939 up to fifteen different plants were being sold instead of *Viburnum prunifolium*.[54] Samples also varied widely in their physical state, often being contaminated with plant parts devoid of therapeutic effect.[55]

Despite this, both *Viburnum prunifolium* and *V. opulus* have been the subject of a considerable amount of research. A patent formula containing *Viburnum prunifolium* extract was trialled in 1932 on 100 patients with primary dysmenorrhoea with excellent results. In 1940, it was concluded that *Viburnum* spp. had a sedative action on the uterus based on experiments in which tracings of uterine muscle activity were obtained by placing a balloon in the uterus of women![56]

The constituents responsible for the uterine sedative action are non-toxic and cause sedation of involuntary muscle, which is associated with a decrease in blood pressure,[57] however, exactly what these constituents are is still the subject of some dispute. Three components are reported to be uterine relaxants which act directly on the muscle'. Scopoletin (a coumarin)[58,59] has long been suggested as important; as well as viopudial, a non-alkaloid material, which is also strongly antispasmodic.[60] The glucoside salicin which is converted into salicylic acid in the gut has also been suggested as possessing uterine sedative properties;[61] however, its presence in *Viburnum opulus* is not always confirmed[62] and the levels are very low.

This is an important herb in gynaecology and obstetrics. When the correct herb is available, it can be expected to relax the uterus and help to relieve dysmenorrhoea. Its use in pregnancy should be left strictly to trained herbalists, but it is useful to prevent uterine overactivity at any stage of pregnancy, and has a place in the prevention of miscarriage where a viable pregnancy has been identified (with ultrasound imaging) and the cervix is closed.

Other observed effects of *Viburnum* relate to its effect on the blood pressure. In anaesthetised dogs, it has been shown to lower blood pressure, slow the heartbeat and decrease myocardial contractility. The proposed mode of action is a potentiation of acetylcholine.[63] The leaves also contain varying amounts of arbutin, a urinary antiseptic also found in *Arctostaphylos uva-ursi* (bearberry). Some species (*Viburnum phlebotrichum*) contain very high levels and may have been substituted for *uva-ursi* leaves as a urinary anti-infective. The leaves need to be treated with hot steam while fresh otherwise arbutin degrades rapidly.[64]

Dose

The dose of *Viburnum prunifolium* is 4–8 mL three times daily; and of *Viburnum opulus*, 2–4 mL three times daily. Viburnin, a bitter glycoside, is responsible in part for the distinctive bitter taste of these two herbs and the upper end of the dose range is likely to cause nausea and occasionally vomiting. These herbs are rarely prescribed alone and are best combined with *Cinnamomum* or *Zingiber* to offset this possibility.

Ligusticum wallichii (Cnidium or Chuan Xiong)

Ligusticum wallichii is from the Chinese pharmacopoeia and is used primarily for its ability to relax smooth muscle. Angina pectoris, stroke, menstrual pain and uterine overactivity have all been treated with this herb. An active, short-acting substance—tetramethylpyrazine—has been shown to improve coronary blood flow (probably through non-specific depression of smooth muscle) and to relax uterine muscle. Tetramethylpyrazine is under investigation as an isolated agent to be used to reduce uterine contractions in pregnant women at term.[65]

Ligusticum is commonly used in *blood tonics* in Chinese medicine, combined with other herbs such as *Angelica sinensis* and *Paeonia lactiflora*. It is often assumed that the term *blood tonic* refers to a herb with the ability to improve blood parameters as measured by blood tests. However, in this instance, the improvement is in both quality and regularity of menstrual blood flow and not in quantifiable blood test results. *Ligusticum* may have a hormonal action, but much of the outcome is related to the spasmolytic effect on the uterus.

Both *Ligusticum wallichii* and *Angelica sinensis* also contain ferulic acid, and both herbs have an inhibitory effect on uterine contraction in rats when given intravenously and orally. Tetramethylpyrazine and ferulic acid, given in combination at doses individually insufficient to inhibit uterine contraction, act synergistically.[66] Traditionally these two herbs are combined to treat menstrual disorders and coronary insufficiency leading to chest pain.

Ligusticum is also part of a traditional formula used in the treatment of anxiety, insomnia and related symptoms.[67] It has been shown to have a mild sedative action, but the effects of the whole formula (Suan Zao Ren Tang or Zizyphus Combination) are much stronger.

Dose

Ligusticum is acrid and Warm and as a fluid extract (1:2) can be given in doses 2–6 mL, one to three times daily.

THE EMMENAGOGUES OR UTERINE STIMULANTS

Emmenagogues are used when there is a need to increase the strength of uterine contractions, usually so that the uterine contents can be efficiently expelled. They are usually prescribed when the period is slow or delayed (for example by shock), and can be used to initiate menstruation caused by hormonal irregularities. Traditionally, they have also been prescribed to bring on a late period due to pregnancy, but this is dangerous, illegal and frequently unsuccessful. Additionally, almost all of the information on the correct dose, timing and route of administration for an abortifacient effect has been lost or forgotten.

Emmenagogues can also be prescribed for certain conditions which are associated with excessive bleeding, historically referred to as 'poor uterine tone'. This is characterised by symptoms of heavy flow, little or no pain and large clots. These symptoms may be inherited; due to poor diet or lack of exercise; or conditions such as fibroids or a prolapse which prevent the uterine muscle from behaving normally. In such cases, complex differentiation and treatment of the causes is required.

After a miscarriage, a useful combination is an emmenagogue with a uterine tonic. The expulsive activity of the emmenagogue aids removal of retained tissue and the uterine tonic assists with healing and regeneration of the uterine lining. Following childbirth, emmenagogues can be used to assist with normal involution and to reduce bleeding after delivery caused by a 'relaxed' uterus. They can also minimise the risk of intra-uterine infection by expelling any retained placenta or membranes after delivery.

They are also indicated after a termination of pregnancy (TOP), especially when a suction curette has been performed and there is a possibility of tissue remnants which may later cause a pelvic infection. The combination of emmenagogues and bacteriostatic herbs for women who have refused to take antibiotics (commonly prescribed after this procedure as a prophylactic measure) reduce the risk of a pelvic infection.

Heavy menstrual flow caused by lack of tone and following repeated pregnancies can respond well to the stimulant action of the emmenagogues, however, as usual, herbs which are both tonic and stimulant herbs are most suitable. Long-term treatment is usually required.

Emmenagogues should only be used by trained herbalists. Their indications are complex and they are difficult to prescribe, needing appropriate dosage, duration of use and combinations with other herbs. As Hoffmann points out: 'These [emmenagogues] are quite powerful herbs that have a specific stimulating action on the womb. This is not necessarily all that healing and they can be very irritating and potentially dangerous in too high a dose.'[68]

Ruta graveolens (Rue)

Ruta has been called the 'herb of grace' and was once believed to possess metaphysical powers. Both Leonardo da Vinci and Michelangelo claimed that *Ruta* had improved their eyesight and their creative inner vision. Reported uses include as an insect repellent (leaves contain a powerful insecticide), to increase the appetite, to treat hysteria and epilepsy, and as a homoeopathic for rheumatism, arthritis and neuralgia.[69] It is also used for bronchial and croupy conditions and for amenorrhoea where pregnancy has been excluded.[70]

Ruta is also used for strained eyes and headaches from eye strain; as a tea to expel worms; to strengthen fragile blood vessels; and as an ointment for sprains, gout and rheumatic pains. It contains coumarins which may cause photosensitivity and a skin rash on contact.[71]

Ruta is a traditional remedy for the treatment of convulsions by Amazonian rural populations.[72] Studies have shown *Ruta* to have a variety of anti-spasmodic effects. Anti-convulsant effects have been observed in mice;[73] and the alkaloids possess a definite spasmolytic character in the gastrointestinal tract,[74] indicating that *Ruta* is suitable for the alleviation of some intestinal spastic disorders such as gall bladder colic. *Ruta* also exhibits an anti-spasmodic action on heart muscle and its action has been compared to known coronary vasodilators.[75]

According to oral reports from Chile, clinically verified cases of multiple sclerosis (MS) have been improved for indefinite periods by long-term use of *Ruta* tea. Nine of these patients were examined for the effects of the tea on lesions in their visual pathways and of these, five showed improvements.[76] In another report, MS patients noticed improvement in vision and considerably decreased spasticity after drinking *Ruta* tea, lasting for about a day. No unwanted side effects were reported.[77]

Use in gynaecology

Ruta has been used for centuries as an abortifacient worldwide and many early references to its use can be found. Soranus, a gynecologist in the second century AD, used *Ruta* in one of his four recipes for oral contraceptives and abortifaciens; Dioscorides said that *Ruta* 'extracts the menses'. Another writer used a mixture of egg, *Ruta* and dill in a vaginal suppository as an abortifacient. In other early writings, emmenagogues and abortifaciens were listed according to their activity. *Ruta* was considered to be one of the extremely strong and dangerous drugs.[78]

Ruta is a traditional abortifacient among Hispanic people in New Mexico, and is used as a tea for abortion purposes throughout Latin America.[79] The activity of the herb is thought to be caused by a combination of the anti-oestrogen principles and other constituents which induce uterine muscle excitability.

Recent studies were performed on rats and hamsters to test for possible post-coital antifertility activity. *Ruta* was shown to inhibit implantation in rats, but not in hamsters. The difference in results between the species may be attributable to antagonism of the pre-implantation oestrogen surge which occurs in rats and not in hamsters, indicating that the anti-oestrogenic effects of rue extracts may not be strong enough for hamsters[80] (or humans).

An active constituent, chalepensin, has been isolated from *Ruta*, which may increase uterine muscle excitability and inhibit hormone production when given in the very early stages of conception (days one to four in rats).[81] An alkaloid, skimmianine, increases the spontaneous contractions of the guinea pig uterus.[82]

The safety and efficacy of *Ruta* as an abortifacient in humans is under review. It is wise to note that in rats, dosages which resulted in an anti-fertility rate of about 50 per cent, also killed about 10 per cent of the animals.[83] Until further information about this herb is available, the use of this herb for the termination of pregnancy is not only illegal, but dangerous.

Ruta is now mainly used in gynaecology to bring on delayed periods (due to shock, stress or other causes) in combination with the uterine tonics such as *Chamaelirium luteum*. Its use by the untrained is unwise.

Dose

It is Warming and Drying and the dose is 0.5–1 mL three times daily.

Artemesia vulgaris (Mugwort)

The Latin name of mugwort refers to Artemis, the goddess of hunting, young women, and of childbirth. All of the herbs from the *Artemesia* family help during and after childbirth, by regulating and strengthening contractions and aiding with the expulsion of the placenta.[84] Other historical and contemporary uses include the treatment of anorexia, atonic gastritis and worm infestations, brought about by a bitter effect which imparts stimulant and antiseptic effects to the digestive tract;[85] as a mild nervine which improves depression and tension; and in the past, the root was used for palsy, fits and epilepsy.[86]

Use in gynaecology

Artemesia vulgaris is used largely as a uterine stimulant to improve congestive dysmenorrhoea and to bring on a delayed period. Like *Ruta*, it is discussed extensively in early writings as an abortifacient. A poem known as the *Salernitan Regimen of Health,* of which there have been over 300 editions, names *Artemesia vulgaris* as the major abortifacient.[87] However, on the issue of safety and efficacy, there is the justifiable concern that '. . . many emmenagogue herbs damage the foetus rather than completely terminating the pregnancy'.[88]

In China, *Artemesia vulgaris* is used in combination with other herbs to prevent miscarriages associated with debility and *blood deficiency*. It is also used, with other herbs, to regulate the period and stop menstrual pain. Moxa, a form of *Artemesia vulgaris* often prepared as a long cigar-like stick, is burnt on the needles during acupuncture treatments for conditions associated with Cold and Damp.

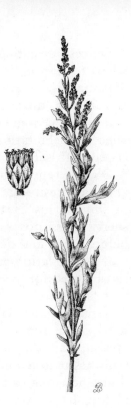

Dose

Artemesia vulgaris should be avoided during lactation and pregnancy. It is Cool and Dry. 0.5–2 mL three times daily.

Salvia officinalis (Sage)

Sage has antiseptic, gut-calming (carminative), drying, memory enhancing and uterine stimulant activities. Thujone, which comprises less than one per cent of the whole plant (30 per cent of the volatile oil content), is antiseptic and carminative, but is also relatively toxic. Sage is used as a mouthwash, gargle and/or taken internally for inflammations or infection of the mouth and throat, including gingivitis, glossitis, stomatiris, laryngitis, pharyngitis, tonsillitis and quinsy; and can also be taken internally to relieve bronchitis, asthma, catarrh and sinusitis. It can be used as an inhalant at first signs of acute respiratory infection to disinfect the airways.

As a compress it promotes the healing of wounds. The phenolic compounds in sage are anti-bacterial, especially to *Staphylococcus aureus*. Thujone is also a strong antiseptic, but is toxic and the tea should be taken only for a week or two at a time because of the potentially toxic effects. Thujone-containing herbs are contraindicated in epilepsy.

Excess sweating of any origin seems to respond to sage. It is traditionally used to improve circulation during convalescence and to reduce night sweats. A useful wine for debilitating sweating associated with serious illnesses such as AIDS, is reported to be 80–100 grams of fresh sage leaves to a litre of wine. This is to be taken by sherry glass doses (about 60 mL) before lunch and dinner.[89] Sage also reduces salivation and lactation and can be used for sweating associated with menopause.

Traditionally, sage tea has been used as a tonic to the nervous system, the thujone being potentially restorative and calming. Large doses, however, cause nervous excitability. It is excellent for nervous exhaustion and can be used to improve clarity of thought and vitality.

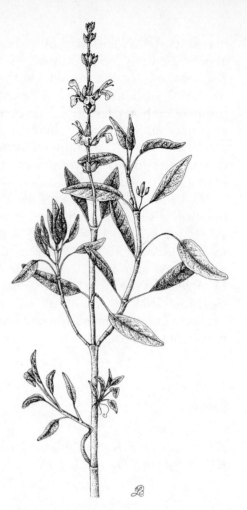

Use in gynaecology

Sage is another of the abortifacient herbs and should be avoided in pregnancy. It is often used for delayed or scanty periods; or for congestive period pain. It is also useful as a tonic in the last weeks of pregnancy and after childbirth to expel the placenta. Sage contains oestrogenic principles and is useful for menopausal problems, especially night sweats and hot flushes.

Dose

1–2 mL three times daily, not to be prescribed in pregnancy by the untrained.

Mentha pulegium (Pennyroyal)

The latin name for *Mentha pulegium* is derived from *pulex*, meaning flea, because of its ability to repel fleas and other insects. It is a popular remedy to promote sweating during colds, and is used for flatulence, dyspepsia and abdominal pain due to wind, an effect brought about by the volatile oils (mainly pulegone, and menthone).

Use in gynaecology

Mentha pulegium is another herb with a long tradition as an abortifacient. Its emmenagogic action was mentioned in plays and other writings in ancient Greece and in Europe in the Middle Ages; a picture in a thirteenth century herbal shows *Mentha pulegium* being used on a pregnant woman as an abortifacient; and Pliny (23–79AD) describes *Mentha pulegium* as an emmenagogue that also dispels a dead foetus.[90]

Again, there are safety issues. It is just as likely to damage the foetus as cause an abortion; the oil taken internally is highly toxic and there are a number of cases of the deaths of women who took the oil to induce abortions.

Mentha pulegium is used for insufficient and painful menstruation to strengthen uterine contractions; and for delayed periods (with *Tanacetum vulgare*).

Dose

Mentha pulegium is Warming and Drying and the dose is 1–4 mL, three times daily.

ANTI-HAEMORRHAGIC HERBS

The anti-haemorrhagics are 'astringent' herbs and are a large category of (usually) tannin-containing plants which reduce blood loss. This effect is seen on the stomach lining, the bowel wall, on the skin, and in the urinary, respiratory and reproductive tract. Almost all tannin-containing plants are Drying and leave a 'drying' and 'puckering' sensation in the mouth. Thus, astringency is experienced as something like the sensation felt after drinking strong black tea and may have been one of the properties early herbalists used to identify this class of herbs.

The haemostatic (haemorrhage-arresting) affect of astringents is brought about by the 'curdling' of proteins when tannins are in direct contact with bleeding tissues, such as on the skin or in the gut. Because of this effect in the gastrointestinal tract, long-term administration of tannin-rich plants can reduce the uptake of nutrients. They should, therefore, only be prescribed for short periods of time.

Tannins are poorly absorbed, but those that are broken down and absorbed into the bloodstream, have little appreciable astringent action on internal organs or tissues. In the reproductive tract, the anti-haemorrhagic herbs used to correct bleeding of uterine origin are often high in tannins, however, they contain other components which are responsible for the reduction in bleeding.

Achillea millefolium (Yarrow)

Historically, *Achillea millefolium* gained its notoriety as a plant with the ability to stop the bleeding of wounds, a reputation which soon spread to include bleeding anywhere in the body. *Achillea* contains the tannins usual in astringent herbs, but its ability to stop gynaecological bleeding is considered to be related to other constituents, notably the flavonoids and the alkaloid achilleine.[91]

Achillea is used for a wide range of complaints worldwide, some of them apparently contradictory.[92] For example, it might be used by one culture for amenorrhoea and by another for abnormally heavy bleeding; or for constipation in one place and to stop diarrhoea elsewhere. Its use in gynaecology can be variable too—in some areas it was used frequently and for a wide range of complaints, but in others no use was found for it at all. One aspect of its use which is agreed upon by all is that it is safe for long-term use.

Some of the apparent discrepancies in the traditional use of *Achillea* can be explained by the different levels of the volatile oils in plants from different areas. For example, the American and eastern European species are azulene-rich, while *Achillea* from western Europe and England is azulene-free. Azulene, the brilliant blue compound found in the volatile oil of a number of plants, has an anti-inflammatory effect, and is particularly useful as a topical application to treat skin disorders. The native North Americans (azulene-rich area) used *Achillea* as a dermatological agent for inflamed and itching skin as well as for bleeding, but did not use it as an emmenagogue, which was common in other parts of the world.

Achillea has traditionally been used to promote sweating during colds, for bleeding haemorrhoids, for menstrual irregularities,[93] as a bitter digestive and for spasmodic bowel pain.[94] The flavonoid apigenin exerts anti-platelet activity and can reduce the incidence of thrombosis while at the same time being anti-inflammatory and spasmolytic.[95] The actions of *Achillea* in reducing the tendency to clot formation and also having the ability to stop abnormal bleeding, are an example of the complexity to be found in plant medicines.

Use in gynaecology

Achillea has been referred to as 'a balanced and amphoterically acting emmenogogue.'[96] The stimulating effect of the thujone and the spasmolytic effect of the various flavonoids are responsible for the apparently contradictory effects on the uterine muscle, the sum total of which results in uterine stimulation without excessive spasm. The flavonoids also posses haemostatic effects due to a decrease in capillary fragility and permeability. The bioflavonoid, rutin, is in part responsible.[97]

The constituents in *Achillea* explain some of the wide range of uses for the plant in gynaecology, from assisting with cases of amenorrhoea to relieving menorrhagia; and acting as a uterine relaxant to relieve pain and a uterine stimulant to increase muscular tone and initiate menstrual flow.

Dose

Achillea tea is prepared by covering 15 g of the dried herb with boiling water and infusing overnight. After straining, the tea is taken in divided doses over the next day during times of heavy menstruation. It is described as Drying (Culpeper). The dose of fluid extract is 2–4 mL three times daily.

Alchemilla vulgaris (Ladies' mantle)

At various times in history *Alchemilla* seems to have excited much interest. The alchemists are reported to have used the dew droplets that formed on its leaves as part of their tonics for longevity (and gave it the name *Alchemilla*); and its common name is attributed to its suggested resemblance to the Virgin Mary's cloak.

Alchemilla is useful for skin complaints and wounds, and has nervine, astringent and anti-inflammatory effects. It can be used for insomnia, diarrhoea and to reduce inflammation associated with rashes. Its astringency makes it useful as a suppository for controlling the severity of haemorrhoids.[98] Flavonoids in ladies' mantle can reduce capillary permeability and may protect connective and elastic tissues from degradation.[99]

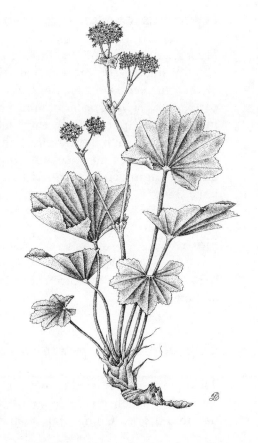

Use in gynaecology

Although little is known about its actions, *Alchemilla* has been used in traditional and folk medicine for women's complaints, including menorrhagia, leucorrhoea, as an emmenagogue and to promote contractions during labour. It can also be used to treat period pain and regulate the menstrual cycle.

It is popular in Europe for menorrhagia around adolescence. In one trial, 341 young women between eleven and seventeen were given *Alchemilla* for ten to fifteen days before the expected next period. The flow was reduced, the cycle shortened and premenstrual administration prevented the menorrhagia from recurring.[100] It is also recommended for heavy bleeding around menopause,[101] and for urinary incontinence in post-menopausal women.[102]

Dose

Alchemilla is Drying and Cooling. The dose is 2–4 mL of the fluid extract three times daily.

Hydrastis canadensis (Golden seal)

Hydrastis is a useful haemostatic herb which has very slight oxytocic activity due to the presence of trace amounts of hydrastinine. Its main effect on excessive bleeding is believed to be due to its effect on the capillaries. *Hydrastis* is commonly used with other herbs in a mix for menorrhagia, particularly the uterine tonics as well as the tannin-containing herbs such as *Achillea* and *Geranium maculatum*. It is bitter and Cold and makes an excellent choice for bleeding associated with Heat, either from infection or due to pent-up emotions (Liverishness). See also page 380.

Dose

0.25–1 mL of the tincture three times daily. *Hydrastis* is contraindicated in pregnancy.

Capsella bursa pastoris (Shepherd's purse)

The common shepherd's purse, *Capsella bursa pastoris*, named after its seed pods which resemble small purses, has a long history of medicinal use in Europe, China, Japan and Arabic countries. In Asia it is also eaten as a food (it is a member of the cabbage family and has the usual acrid taste). The plant has diuretic, anti-inflammatory, anti-ulcer, oxytocic and anti-haemorrhagic actions.[103] Tumour-inhibiting,[104] and antimicrobial[105] effects have also been identified.

Use in gynaecology

Capsella is indicated for menorrhagia of practically any origin (but differentiation of the causes must always precede treatment). It has Drying and Cooling properties and can be used for uterine bleeding accompanying pelvic infection. It combines well with *Trillium* and *Hydrastis*, but this combination is only for the brave because of the very strong taste.

At one time *Capsella* was injected for the treatment of haemorrhages,[106] however, little is known of the active constituents that impart anti-haemorrhagic effect. There is some suggestion that they may be related to a white fungus that resides on the plant[107] which may explain some of the inconsistencies noted in clinical use, since the fungus may not always be present.

It should be taken as an extract because of the production of toxic agents (nitriles) when the plant is subjected to water temperatures above 45° C and is contraindicated in cases associated with hypothyroidism.[108]

Dose

The usual dose is 1–4 mL of the extract.

Lamium album (White deadnettle)

The white deadnettle epitomises one of the common incongruities of herbal medicine. While there is popular and continued use, especially in Europe, as well as clinical evidence of the plant's effectiveness, very little research into the efficacy or even the active constituents has been undertaken. One herbalist sums up the situation thus: 'Popular medicine has become firmly attached to this drug, which is in contrast to the lack of information on its efficacy. No gynaecological trials have been done . . . Yet women keep asking for the drug and using it.'[109]

Lamium is a bitter digestive with abundant amounts of trace minerals. It is described as Hot and Drying (Culpeper), Warming (Hildegard of Bingen), Cooling, astringent and pungent (Holmes).[110] The differences may point to the use of different parts of the plant. In Germany, there are two officially recognised forms, the flowers and the aerial parts.[111] It is possible that Holmes, in describing *Lamium* as Cooling, is describing the properties of the whole plant. (He lists the whole plant as the part used in his text.)

Use in gynaecology

Lamium is a tannin-containing herb, but its anti-haemorrhagic action in the reproductive tract is almost definitely explained by other constituents, similar to those found in *Capsella bursa-pastoris*, namely histamine, choline and tyramine, which may explain the common actions of both of these plants.[112] *Lamium* also contains flavonols, which may be responsible for some of the haemostatic properties.

Lamium is useful for many different types of menstrual complaints associated with bleeding irregularities. Examples are late, irregular and light periods related to weakness, nutritional deficiencies and overwork; late and heavy periods caused by stress or nervous tension; heavy periods associated with a lack of uterine tone; and bleeding between periods associated with hormonal irregularities. As always, a diagnosis must be sought before treatment is started for any of these complaints.

Dose

2–4 mL three times daily.

Panax notoginseng (Tienchi ginseng)

Panax notoginseng is a valuable herb. It has been used to stop bleeding in China for centuries, but also became famous as a component of the patent medicine *Yunnan Bai Yao*. During the Second World War, American pilots (the Flying Tigers) followed the example set by the Chinese army and carried *Yunnan Bai Yao* in case of traumatic injury and haemorrhage.[113] It can also be used as a poultice for external bleeding.

In Chinese medicine it is considered to be a very safe anti-haemorrhagic agent because '. . . it can stop bleeding without causing congealed blood . . .'.

Many of the active constituents in *Panax notoginseng* have been isolated and studied, particularly those that have an effect on the heart and blood. It shortens coagulation time (the time taken for a blood clot to form);[114] and reduces the deleterious effects of shock from severe blood loss;[115] but also prevents platelets from clumping.[116]

The sum total of these effects seems to be completely contradictory, however *Panax notoginseng* can be relied upon to stop haem-

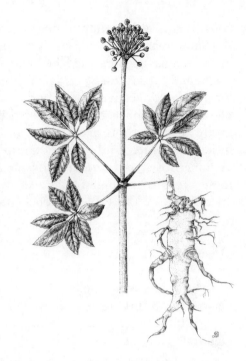

orrhage and improve circulation. It can be used for conditions associated with increased capillary permeability, bleeding associated with idiopathic thrombocytopaenia (ITP), trauma, nose bleeds or menorrhagia.

Panax notoginseng has been investigated as an effective treatment for cardiovascular disorders.[117] It has been shown to relieve the symptoms of angina pectoris and also reduces high blood pressure.[118] It also lowers serum cholesterol levels[119] and as part of a traditional formula (containing *Ligusticum wallichii*, *Carthamus tinctorius* and *Salvia miltiorrhiza*) can reduce damage to brain tissue caused by lack of blood supply (ischaemia) after a stroke (in rats).[120] In other research, it was shown to increase cerebral circulation in rats and rabbits[121] and to improve memory in mice.[122]

Use in gynaecology

The obvious application for *Panax notoginseng* is for menorrhagia caused by conditions such as fibroids, dysfunctional bleeding and heavy bleeding after the birth of a child. It is an acute remedy and is usually prescribed at the time of bleeding only. Traditionally, *Panax notoginseng* is contra-indicated during pregnancy because it '*promotes the circulation of blood*', but the exact pharmacological reasons for this precaution are unclear.

To stop bleeding, *Panax notoginseng* is traditionally given as a tablet, and this may be a wise practice to continue to ensure the active constituents are available. Because it is so effective at stopping bleeding (but not treating the cause), it is absolutely essential that the reason for menorrhagia be identified before treatment is commenced.

Panax notoginseng is also useful for conditions associated with localised, congestive pain; and heavy and/or dark clotted menstrual blood, which may be accompanied by immobile abdominal masses. This group of symptoms are known as *blood stagnation* in traditional Chinese medicine, and can accompany complaints such as fibroids, endometriosis and primary dysmenorrhoea with congestive pain. For these types of complaints, *Panax notoginseng* should be prescribed as an extract, or the tablets (tienchi tablets) should be taken with wine.

Dose

This herb is sweet, slightly bitter and slightly Warm. The usual dose is between 1–3 mL three times daily for *stagnant blood* symptoms, or one 500 milligram capsule or tablet every two to four hours for menorrhagia.

Trillium erectum (Beth root)

Trillium extract contains agents which are so strongly acrid that compliance is usually very poor unless it is administered in tablet form. As its common name suggests, *Trillium* is used as an aid to labour and as an anti-haemorrhagic to be used in and after the third stage of a birth. It is also used in any situation where abnormal bleeding is a feature of a gynaecological complaint.

Trillium contains the steroidal saponin trillarin;[123] and yields the sapogenins diosgenin, bethogenin and trillogenin;[124] as well as pennogenin, nologenin, and fesogenin.[125] Diosgenins are discussed elsewhere (see pages 313–14) and seem to be capable of interacting with the receptor sites for hormones in the hypothalamic–pituitary unit. The other sapogenins may also play a role, but have not been investigated. These steroidal substances

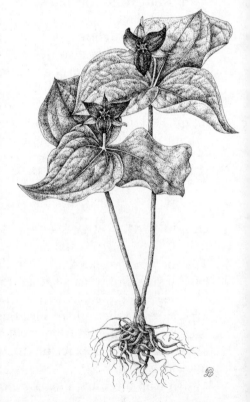

provide a possible explanation of the hormone-regulating effect and perhaps even the anti-haemorrhagic effects of the herb.

Trillium is possibly the best herb for women with menorrhagia between 30–50 years because of its range of functions. Long-term administration is usually required, however the tannin fraction should inspire caution and symptoms such as constipation may indicate adverse effects from tannins on the gut wall.

Dose

Trillium is Drying and usually prescribed in doses of 0.5–2 mL three times daily, or as a tablet (follow manufacturer's recommendations as these are usually compound formulations).

HERBS WITH AN INFLUENCE ON THE HYPOTHALAMIC–PITUITARY UNIT

A number of herbs are used for menstrual disorders which are associated with a disturbance of the hypothalamic–pituitary unit (sometimes also referred to as the central control mechanism, or simply as the central control). These disorders can manifest in many ways and sometimes cause a wide range of seemingly contradictory complaints including heavy periods or no periods at all, to irregular cycles and premenstrual syndrome (PMS).

Many herbs and some foods are known to influence pituitary hormones—luteinising hormone (LH), follicle-stimulating hormone (FSH) and prolactin. Soy products for instance, which contain phyto-oestrogens, can depress mid-cycle surges of both LH and FSH[126] and lead to longer menstrual cycles. Herbs containing the steroidal sapogenin, diosgenin (see pages 313–14), also seem to influence these hormones; and beer can increase prolactin levels.

The principal herbs used by herbalists in the treatment of hormonal imbalance are *Vitex agnus castus* (chaste tree berries), *Paeonia lactiflora* (peony) and *Cimicifuga racemosa* (black cohosh). Each has a range of effects which are now known to be brought about by their ability to influence the activity of the hypothalamic–pituitary hormones.

Vitex agnus castus (chaste tree berries)

Vitex has been used as a medicinal plant for centuries. Hippocrates (450 BC) suggested it be used to treat injuries, inflammations, enlargement of the spleen and to help the uterus expel the afterbirth; others around

this time used it to reduce headache, fever and stimulate
perspiration; to dispel wind and
flatulence and check diarrhoea.
Dioscorides (50 AD) recommended *Vitex* for inflammation of
the uterus; in Persia, it was used
to cure insanity, madness and epilepsy; and Pliny, first century AD,
used the berries to promote menstruation, reduce fever and
headaches, stimulate perspiration
and to promote lactation in new
mothers.

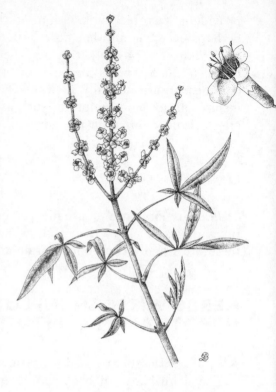

   Vitex was also used 'to cool
passions'—some said it was
infallible, others claimed it had a
very stimulating property, but this
may have depended on gender
(and many of the old herbals were
lacking in information on this
point). The dried fruits have a
peppery taste and were used in
monasteries as a condiment, supposedly to suppress libido. A common
name for *Vitex* even today is monk's pepper. In Rome, the Vestal Virgins
carried twigs of it as a symbol of chastity. The eclectics in the nineteenth
century used a tincture of berries for impotence and 'sexual melancholia', but whether this was for men, women or both sexes is unclear.

Use in gynaecology

Vitex is said to be a herb for the luteal phase and can be useful for a
large number of gynaecological complaints, especially those that occur
or worsen premenstrually. Positive effects have been noted in acne,[127]
post-traumatic epilepsy,[128] mouth ulcers,[129] and herpes simplex (cold
sores and genital herpes)[130] which worsen before the period. As well,
many of the common premenstrual symptoms, such as fluid retention[131]
and breast soreness,[132] improve with *Vitex*. These complaints may be
caused by latent hyperprolactinaemia.

   Latent hyperprolactinaemia is a syndrome characterised by lower
than normal progesterone secretion and normal to mildly elevated
prolactin levels. It is thought to cause a spectrum of menstrual disorders
which can range from the usual symptoms of PMS, to altered menstrual
cycle lengths, to complete absence of ovulation and menstruation. Its
causative factors are not entirely understood, but seem to be in part

related to stress leading to an alteration of the activity of the hypothalamic–pituitary unit.

Vitex seems to be capable of improving amenorrhoea,[133] menstrual irregularities,[134] and especially cyclic changes associated with latent hyperprolactinaemia.[135] In one trial, thirteen women with elevated prolactin levels and irregular cycles were given Mastodynon N (a German herbal preparation containing *Vitex* extract). Following a decrease in prolactin levels, normal cycle(s) returned in all cases.[136]

In another study, 52 women with luteal phase defects due to latent hyperprolactinaemia took part in a randomised double blind versus placebo study. They were given a daily dose of 20 milligrams of *Vitex*. Prolactin levels were normalised after three months, and deficits in the luteal progesterone production were eliminated. There were no side effects and two of the women treated with *Vitex* became pregnant.[137]

Rats have been used to identify the mechanism of action. An active dopamine-like principle in *Vitex* binds to the lactotrope cell in rat pituitary cells, inhibiting prolactin release.[138]

Although some types of infertility respond to *Vitex*, especially when associated with elevated prolactin levels, self treatment should not be undertaken. An article in a British medical journal reported that a woman on her fourth cycle of a drug-free in vitro fertilisation (IVF) program, who self-administered *Vitex* (dose not stated), produced increased numbers of ovarian follicles and developed symptoms suggestive of mild ovarian hyperstimulation (symptoms not stated).[139] *Vitex* is a complex herb and the correct dose and timing of administration are essential.

Vitex can also be used to promote the secretion of breast milk (as a galactogogue), especially in the first ten days after delivery. In one controlled trial of 817 patients, milk production tripled in 20 days.[140]

How *Vitex* improves breast milk production is unknown, and seems particularly curious in the light of recent findings that *Vitex* lowers prolactin levels (prolactin is necessary for the initiation of normal milk production after delivery). It may be that the effect of *Vitex* on prolactin secretion is dose dependent. In the studies of breast milk production, a low dose homoeopathic preparation of *Vitex* (mother tincture) which is about ten times weaker than the usual herbal preparations was used. A clinical study involving men showed that lower doses caused a rise in prolactin and higher doses a much reduced secretion.[141]

During the peri-menopausal phase, *Vitex* can be used to regulate the menstrual cycle by initiating regular ovulation. It is very useful for peri-menopausal women with menstrual irregularities as well as premenstrual symptoms, and in some cases, normalises elevated FSH levels once menstruation recommences.

Vitex affects the hypothalamic–pituitary unit. As such, it should be prescribed by a trained practitioner familar with its actions and contraindications. It should be started in the early part of the cycle, preferably prior to ovulation, and is usually given as a single dose in the morning. Dosage is important—doses which are too high or too low may worsen some conditions, and should be adjusted according to the problem treated, any additional symptoms, and the age of the woman.

Vitex should not be prescribed when hormonal preparations are used, including the Pill, HRT, or any of the commonly prescribed progestogen drugs such as Provera, Primolut, Duphaston and danazol. It should be prescribed cautiously (and only by a practitioner) for young women (under 20) for whom the hypothalamic–pituitary–ovarian interplay is still fragile and easily disrupted.

For full benefit, *Vitex* is usually prescribed for between three and nine months. Longer-term administration is necessary in some cases and there are reports of women taking *Vitex* for up to sixteen years without ill-effect.[142] Positive changes to the menstrual cycle are usually evident in the first month; however, some women report longer or shorter cycles than usual initially, until stabilisation occurs.

Dose

Dose of fluid extract 1:2: 1–4 mL daily; tablets or capsules 500–1000 mg per day.

The German preparation, Agnolyt, contains 9 gram of *Vitex* fruit tincture (1:5) per 100 g extract, and is prescribed at a dose of 40 drops per day.

Paeonia lactiflora (Peony, *bai shao*)

Paeonia lactiflora is an important herb from the Chinese pharmacopoeia. In Traditional Chinese Medicine (TCM) three different types of peony are used—the white peony (*Paeonia lactiflora*), red peony (also usually from *Paeonia lactiflora*, but collected from wild plants and known as *chi shao*), and peony bark from *Paeonia suffruticosa* (*mu dan pi*). 'Peony' without specific reference to the type, indicates white peony/*bai shao*.

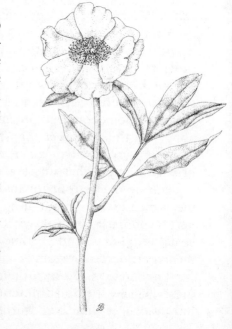

In TCM, *Paeonia lactiflora* is commonly used in combination with *Bupleurum falcatum*, *Ligusticum wallichii* and/or *Angelica sinensis* for a wide range of gynaecological problems; or combined with liquorice for muscle spasm and inflammation. It is said to 'calm the foetus' (which may allude more to an effect on the uterine muscle than the foetus) and is considered to be safe in pregnancy.

Gynaecological disorders

Paeonia lactiflora is effective in the treatment of PMS, polycystic ovarian disease (PCOD), hyperprolactinaemia, ovulatory failure, infertility, endometriosis and adenomyosis, androgen excess, mastalgia and menopausal symptoms. These conditions have at their core various hormonal irregularities, including elevated androgens, low progesterone, high or low oestrogen, and elevated prolactin, all of which peony has been shown to influence. Menstrual pain and uterine overactivity during pregnancy also respond to peony.

In China and Japan, where peony has been widely researched, much of the experimental work has been performed using traditional Chinese formulas which contain varying numbers of different herbs. It is sometimes, therefore, not possible to draw firm conclusions about the action of peony *per se*, however many of the biological effects seem to be due to paeoniflorin, a monoterpene glycoside which is the major active constituent.

In vitro experiments showed that paeoniflorin effected the ovarian follicles through its action on aromatase enzyme.[143] Aromatase is widely distributed throughout the body, including the ovaries, the liver, and fatty tissue. It plays an important role in the development of the follicle and the biosynthesis of steroid hormones; the functioning of the corpus luteum and ovulation; and the conversion of androgens to oestrogens in both the fatty tissue and the ovary. Prolactin, GnRH and the glucocorticoids all inhibit the activity of aromatase.

Inhibition of aromatase activity can lead to low oestrogen levels and erratic ovulation. Peony-containing formulas seem to reverse these effects and can also increase progesterone levels. Interestingly, herb formulas containing peony will normalise ovarian function when the activity of aromatase is inhibited, but do not increase hormonal activity above normal or lead to the development of multiple ovarian follicles.[144]

Paeoniflorin reduces the production of the androgens in a dose-dependent manner through its effect on aromatase which promotes the synthesis of oestradiol from testosterone.[145] Elevated androgen levels, which can be associated with hirsutism, androgenic hair loss, acne, and infertility, are seen in PCOD and obesity, and can occur after the menopause.

In menopausal women, aromatase increases the peripheral conversion (in the fatty tissue) of androgens to oestrogen and seems to reduce the incidence of hot flushes especially when used with *Angelica sinensis*. *Paeonia lactiflora* can also be used for post-menopausal symptoms associated with androgen excess such as androgenic alopecia, although treatment needs to be continued for many months.

Peony-containing formulas can also be used to treat lowered rates of fertility due to androgen excess. The two herb formula, Liquorice and Peony Combination, reduces testosterone levels in women with PCOD and improves pregnancy rates.[146] The LH to FSH ratio is also normalised. The same formula is also useful for the treatment of hyperprolactinaemia via an effect on dopamine receptors in the pituitary, although the lowering of prolactin levels seems to be related to a synergistic reaction between the liquorice and peony and not due to the peony alone.[147]

Conditions believed to be associated with relative oestrogen excess in relation to progesterone also respond well to peony-containing formulations, including adenomyosis and endometriosis,[148] uterine fibroids[149] and mastalgia.[150] The formula which has been the subject of most research is Cinnamon and Hoelen Combination which contains both *Paeonia lactiflora* and *Paeonia suffruticosa*, as well as *Cinnamomum cassia*, *Prunus persica* (peach kernels) and *Poria cocos* (hoelen).

This formula is believed to act either as a GnRH antagonist, reducing levels of LH, FSH and oestrogen, or as a weak anti-oestrogen by competing with oestrogen in uterine or breast tissue.[151] The exact mechanism of action of this formula is unknown, however, and it is most likely that the beneficial effects arise from a synergistic action between all herbs in the formula rather than from *Paeonia lactiflora* or paeoniflorin alone.

Paeoniflorin can counteract the oxytocic effect of some drugs[152] and has been experimentally shown to have sedating, antispasmodic and anti-inflammatory effects.[153] It is used in association with liquorice, for any condition characterised by abdominal pain associated with muscle spasm. Dysmenorrhoea and overactive uterine activity during pregnancy respond to *Paeonia lactiflora*. (Any condition associated with pregnancy must be treated by a trained herbalist with experience in this area.)

Dose

1:2 Fluid extract: 1.5–3 mLs per dose TDS.

Cimicifuga racemosa (Black cohosh)

Traditional uses of this plant include a large range of gynaecological complaints, sore throats, bronchitis and rheumatic conditions. A vascular antispasmodic, *Cimicifuga* is also recommended for hypertension, owing to the blood pressure-lowering effect of one of its constituents, acteine.[154]

Use in gynaecology

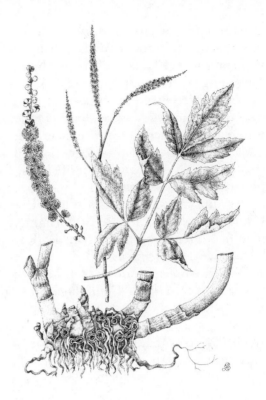

Cimicifuga is considered to be specific for the treatment of musculo-skeletal disorders which may accompany menopause, and for the treatment of hot flushes.[155] It can also be used during adolescence for delayed menstruation caused by hormonal imbalance, especially when associated with stress and emotional factors.[156]

Recent research has shown *Cimicifuga* to contain three types of hormonally active substances, one of which suppresses luteinising hormone (LH) secretion after prolonged administration, and another two of which have weak oestrogen-like effects. LH surges are thought to cause flushing, and the suppression of this hormone by *Cimicifuga* is thought to control the symptom.[157] *Cimicifuga* has also been studied for its effect on the vaginal cells of menopausal women. It is found both topically and orally to favourably alter the cells and reduce symptoms of vaginal dryness and irritation, and although this is not achieved rapidly, it has been shown to be as effective as synthetic oestrogen.[158]

Numerous clinical trials in Germany have attested to the efficacy of *Cimicifuga* for menopausal complaints. Thirty-six women treated in one trial reported significant improvements in hot flushes, sweating, insomnia, nervousness, irritability and depressive psychosis after 4 weeks of treatment, and highly significant improvements after 12 weeks.[159] Another very similar study of 50 women, 39 of whom could not take hormone therapy, also showed highly significant results. Symptoms improved after 4 and 12 weeks, with dramatic changes in mood profiles, a decrease in depression, tiredness and dejection, as well as increased activity.[160]

A double blind study compared low dose oestrogen therapy to *Cimicifuga* therapy in 80 women with menopausal symptoms. After three months, the women on the herb had significantly improved—the daily dose of oestrogen (0.625 mg conjugated oestrogens) was considered to be too low to have any effect.[161]

The effectiveness of *Cimicifuga* for younger women complaining of menopausal symptoms due to surgery has also been assessed. Sixty women under 40 years old, who had had a hysterectomy, and had one remaining ovary each, were tested in a controlled study for the effects of four different treatments—estriol, conjugated oestrogens, combined oestrogens and gestagens, and *Cimicifuga*. There was no significant differences between groups concerning therapy success.[162]

Cimicifuga can be used instead of HRT, as well as HRT, or as a treatment to 'wean' a woman off HRT. Remifemin™, a common German preparation, was used in 1738 menopausal patients, with only 20 per cent requiring additional hormone therapy. When combining HRT and *Cimicifuga* a smaller dose of hormone is required.[163] Half of all women who had already been prescribed HRT no longer needed hormones after being given *Cimicifuga*.[164]

When women want to stop hormone replacement therapy (HRT), it is usual to take both *Cimicifuga* and HRT together until the herb has taken effect (usually 6–8 weeks), then stop the HRT. The advantages of *Cimicifuga* are '. . . its outstanding sphere of action in the climacteric syndrome, the absence of toxic side effects and thus the possibility of long term therapy'.[165]

Dose

The usual dose of *Cimicifuga* is between 0.5–2 mL, two to three times daily. It is Cool and Dry.

WARMING HERBS

When herbalists consider the manifestation of a particular illness in a particular individual, two important differentiations must be made—whether the person is constitutionally Hot or Cold; and whether the condition is Hot or Cold. Warming herbs play a part in Cold conditions such as cramping and in the early stage of a fever, where chills are common. They render Cold people more Warm, helping to support digestion and blood flow and thus increasing vitality and the ability to respond to illness more appropriately.

Zingiber officinale (Ginger)

The common culinary herb *Zingiber officinale* is also a very important medicinal herb. Traditionally used for its Warming properties, *Zingiber* has now been found to have an astonishing array of additional uses.

It is an important herb in the first stage of acute infectious illness where it is traditionally used in conjunction with other herbs to facilitate a sweat. The outcome of using *Zingiber* is to cause a lowering of the temperature, an effect similar to that of aspirin.[166] It is possible that the observed benefits are also related to an anti-infective effect, as some components are known to have activity against the rhinoviruses which are implicated in the common cold.[167]

Zingiber is a valuable herb for nausea, especially when associated with pregnancy,[168] motion sickness,[169] and following surgery.[170] It also increases gastric motility (improves stomach emptying);[171] and experimentally reduces the incidence of gastric ulcers in animals.[172] In addition, it seems to lower cholesterol levels, at least in rats.[173]

Lately, research has also shown that *Zingiber* reduces platelet stickiness by inhibiting thromboxane synthesis;[174] reduces the risk of blood clots (again, similar in effect to aspirin);[175] and has prostaglandin-inhibiting effects,[176] which make it useful as a preventative against cardiovascular disease. Inflammatory conditions such as arthritis and rheumatism also improve with *Zingiber*,[177] as may migraine headaches,[178] but the herb should be taken preventatively. In research conducted in India, *Zingiber* is shown to be theoretically useful in the prevention of cancer, due to its induction of certain hepatic microsomal enzymes.[179]

Use in gynaecology

The Warming properties of *Zingiber* make it useful for period pain that is improved by the application of heat or warm drinks. It is not only the Warming qualities that improve pain, however. The pungent components have analgesic effects,[180] and the prostaglandin-inhibiting actions can be assumed to also play a role (although there are no specific studies that look at the anti-prostaglandin effect of *Zingiber* in period pain). *Zingiber* is also useful for the many women who experience nausea and vomiting with their period.

Premenstrual and menstrual migraines can be helped by *Zingiber*, but not when these occur around the menopause as *Zingiber* often aggravates flushing.

Dose

The taste is pungent; the quality Hot. *Zingiber* can be taken as a fresh herb, grated as a tea; as tablets; or as an extract. Tablet doses up to one gram are usually effective, between four and eight hourly. The extract (tincture) dose is between 0.25–3 mL depending on strength. During pregnancy, lower doses are advisable.

Cinnamomum zeylanicum (Cinnamon)

As well known as *Zingiber*, this Warming herb is the dried bark of a tropical evergreen tree. *Cinnamomum* is a common culinary herb known to stimulate appetite and digestion and is classed as a carminative which means it can help reduce the discomfort of intestinal griping. It is also used as an astringent, and has been used to reduce diarrhoea, through a combination of antimicrobial and astringent effects.[181] *Cinnamomum* can be useful during the first stages of a cold, when drunk as an infusion with such herbs as *Achillea*, *Sambucus*, *Mentha* spp. and *Zingiber*.

Use in gynaecology

Cinnamomum is commonly used in traditional Chinese medicine for 'Cold' period pain or pain related to *stagnant blood* (a constellation of symptoms including localised pain, dark clotted menstrual blood and immobile masses). It is often combined with *Angelica sinensis*, *Ligusticum wallichii* and/or *Paeonia lactiflora*. *Cinnamomum* can also reduce excessive menstrual bleeding.[182]

Dose

It is Hot and aromatic, and is taken at a dose of up to 1 g three times a day as an infusion, or as part of a herbal formula at a dose of between 2–4 mL, three times daily.

ANODYNES

Herbalists have always used pain-reducing medicines—known as anodynes in herbal medicine—to reduce suffering from pain. One of the earliest, and still most effective, was the opium poppy, now pharmaceutically manufactured as morphine, codeine and pethidine. In situations where individuals suffer from recurrent and non life-threatening painful complaints—period pain for example—the modern-day herbalist places less emphasis on reducing pain, and instead favours remedies that treat the underlying causes. Those anodynes still in use play a secondary role in these types of treatments.

Corydalis ambigua (Corydalis)

Corydalis ambigua is a herb from the Chinese pharmacopoeia and is prescribed for the treatment of pain anywhere in the body. This herb is one of the strongest anodynes used in herbal medicine and has an analgesic affect estimated to be one per cent that of opium. It is more effective if used as an alcoholic or acetic acid extract, but is never used alone—one writer comments 'This herb is very widely used in the treatment of pain. It may be used for any type of pain, if combined with appropriate herbs.'

This herb also has nervine effects and can be used as a hypnotic and sedative; it relaxes muscles and is used for skeletal muscle spasm; it is also cardio-tonic and can be used for cardiac arrhythmias, and with *Panax notoginseng* for angina pectoris. For migraines, *Corydalis* can be used with *Tanacetum parthenium*, *Zingiber* or *Cinnamomum* (Cold migraines), bitters (Hot migraines), or with *Cimicifuga racemosa* for peri-menopausal migraines.

Specific uses in gynaecology

Corydalis is used to treat dysmenorrhoea with either congestive or crampy pain. In Chinese herbal medicine one of the traditional combinations is with *Angelica sinensis* and *Cinnamomum*; Western herbalists use the anti-spasmodics *Viburnum opulus* and *V. prunifolium* combined with uterine tonic herbs. *Corydalis* is also reported to stop excessive bleeding and is indicated for severe pain with menorrhagia. The mechanism for this action is unknown.

Dose

It is acrid, bitter and Warm. Fluid extract (1:2) 1–3 mL, three times per day. *Corydalis* is contraindicated in pregnancy.

Piscidia erythrina (Jamaican dogwood)

The medicinal part of *Piscidia erythrina* or *Piscidia piscipula* is the outer bark of the root. This plant, often found in 'women's tonics',[183] is a mild sedative and relaxes smooth muscle. Traditionally, *Piscidia* has been used as an analgesic and narcotic for neuralgias; and as a fish poison (fish poisons from plants are not toxic to humans unless they are injected).[184] Its official indications today are as a sedative; to stop coughing, especially of whooping cough and asthma; as an anti-spasmodic and an anti-inflammatory.[185]

Specific uses in gynaecology

The anti-spasmodic and sedative effects are responsible for this herb's efficacy for period pain. As early as 1916, research showed *Piscidia* to have strong anti-spasmodic effects on isolated strips of uterine muscle.[186] Doses of between three and five millilitres were later shown to be effective antispasmodics in cats and monkeys.[187] Piscidia has a very low toxicity, even at high doses, but is contraindicated in pregnancy.[188]

Dose

This herb is Cooling and is prescribed at a dose of between 2–8 mL, three times per day.

Anemone pulsatilla (Pulsatilla)

Anemone pulsatilla is an anti-spasmodic, sedative and central nervous system depressant with a specificity for painful and spasmodic complaints of the genito-urinary tract. The traditional indications for this plant were for complaints associated with 'nervousness'—for conditions caused or accompanied by worry, a gloomy mentality, depression, a brooding disposition, or the tendency to look on the dark side of life.

This herb must always be prescribed by a trained herbalist—given in the wrong dose it can cause severe inflammation of the stomach and vomiting. The fresh plant is poisonous. *Anemone pulsatilla* is an emmenagogue (stimulates uterine contractions), and is contraindicated in pregnancy and while women are breast feeding.

Specific uses in gynaecology

Painful and spasmodic conditions of the uterus, such as spasmodic period pain, and inflamed conditions of the genito-urinary tract including the pain of pelvic inflammatory disease (PID) and interstitial cystitis, all repond well to this herb: 'Many unpleasant conditions of the urinary apparatus are relieved by pulsatilla, as frequent but ineffectual attempts at urination, the bladder giving a sensation as if bloated . . .'[189]

Anemone pulsatilla can be used for amenorrhoea caused by nervousness or stress. For period pain it is frequently combined with *Viburnum opulus* or *V. prunifolium*.

Dose

The herb is described as Warm with a Cooling potential. The standard dose is 1–2 mL of the tincture (dried plant), daily.

Tanacetum parthenium (Feverfew)

Tanacetum parthenium was historically used to treat fever, headache and migraine; to regulate menstruation; for difficulties during labour; for minor skin irritations; and for toothache.[190] It has been called the herbal aspirin, partly because, as a tea, it will increase perspiration and reduce fever. Its most common usage today, however, is for the treatment of migraine headaches and arthritic complaints. It also has a role in the control of menstrual pain.

Some of the positive actions of feverfew are brought about by the effect on prostaglandin synthesis. *Tanacetum parthenium* blocks the enzymes necessary for the production of PGE 2 from arachidonic acid[191] (the actions of PGE 2 in the reproductive tract are discussed on page 78) which may in part explain its anti-inflammatory and muscle-relaxing effects.

Tanacetum parthenium also blocks the release of the inflammatory mediators (serotonin and histamine, for example) which, among other actions, cause vasodilation of blood vessels in the meninges.[192] Dilation of blood vessels is believed to be the precursor to the development of migraines and a number of common drugs (such as the ergot alkaloids) as well as feverfew seem to be capable of interfering with this response. Parthenolide, a sesquiterpene lactone in the fresh plant, has been shown to be one of the active components.[193]

Another as yet unidentified substance found in the dried leaf, which has a different mode of action, has also been found to cause vasoconstriction.[194] This indicates that two different mechanisms are operating to bring about migraine relief and prevention. Two clinical trials for migraine prophylaxis have confirmed that it is an effective remedy.[195] Researchers have also found that *Tanacetum parthenium* can inhibit the release of inflammatory substances found in the synovial fluid of rheumatoid arthritis sufferers. The extent of inhibition was greater than that achieved with the use of non-steroidal anti-inflammatory drugs (NSAIDs).[196]

Specific uses in gynaecology

Tanacetum parthenium can be used for women of all ages, and has been traditionally used as an emmenagogue to bring on delayed periods. Recurrent premenstrual, mid-cycle or peri-menopausal migraines, which are believed to be caused by oestrogen fluctuations, also respond well. It must be used all month as a preventative for best results. Except in exceptional circumstances, it is not wise to use *Tanacetum parthenium* for the prevention of migraines associated with the use of the Pill. Stopping or changing the Pill is a much better option.

It is a bitter herb and can be used to treat 'liverish' premenstrual symptoms (or for that matter, liverish symptoms at any time) such as irritability, lethargy, headaches, constipation and digestive disturbances. During labour, it is said to increase the frequency and regularity of contractions and is reported to relax a rigid cervix.[197]

Women taking *Tanacetum parthenium* for migraines have reported both a reduction and an increase[198] in period pain while taking the herb. *In vitro* research has shown different effects with fresh and dried plant products. Researchers investigating the effects on smooth muscle found that the fresh plant inhibited muscle spasm, while the dried plant increased it.[199] Although *in vitro* research does not always equate well with therapeutic outcomes, it may be that women with period pain will benefit more from use of the fresh plant or fresh plant extracts.

Dose

The effective dose of feverfew can be quite low at 50–100 mg per day, although doses of around 200 mg twice daily are often recommended. Doses up to 400 mg per day should be safe, but should only be prescribed by a trained herbalist.

An oft-repeated caution in the media that *Tanacetum parthenium* causes mouth ulcers is not related to the taking of tablets or extracts, but to the chewing of the fresh leaf which may cause a type of contact dermatitis in susceptible individuals.[200]

Given as a 1:5 tincture, the dose is 0.25–0.5 mL, three times daily. *Tanacetum parthenium* is Cooling and bitter. It should be used cautiously during pregnancy, and only by a trained herbalist.

OTHER IMPORTANT HERBS USED FOR GYNAECOLOGICAL COMPLAINTS

Nervines

At some stage in their lives, nearly everyone will experience symptoms associated with anxiety or depression. Herbal medicines, known as nervines, can be used as a gentle and effective means of controlling symptoms while addressing some of the underlying causes. Nervines can be divided into several classes—the nervine tonics which can be used for either anxiety or depression and are seen to have a 'balancing effect'; the nervine sedatives which are calming; and the nervine stimulants, a common example of which is coffee. Nervines find a particular role in gynaecology in the treatment of premenstrual and peri-menopausal complaints; and as adjuncts to the treatment of period pain.

Hypericum perforatum (St John's Wort)

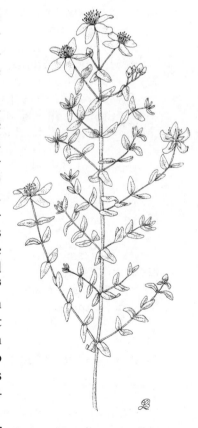

Hypericum is possibly the most important nervine tonic in herbal medicine. It is specifically indicated for the treatment of mild to moderate anxiety depression.[201] Herbalists consider *Hypericum* to be especially useful during menopause,[202] but it is known as *the* herb to reduce anxiety or stress during any transition period.

Hypericum has been the subject of a number of clinical trials in Germany but the mode of action remains unclear. Early research suggested that hypericin, one of the active constituents, was a monoamine oxidase (MAO) inhibitor, however this has not been confirmed. A meta-analysis of 23 randomised trials involving 1757 outpatients concluded that 'there is evidence that extracts of *Hypericum* are more effective than placebo for the treatment of mild to moderately severe depressive disorders'.[203] *Hypericum* was found to be more effective than placebo, as effective as standard anti-depressant treatment, and had far fewer side effects than standard anti-depressant treatment.[204] Also noteworthy is the statistic that German doctors prescribed 66 million daily doses of preparations containing *Hypericum* in one year.[205]

Combinations of *Hypericum* with other

herbs have also been successfully trialled. A combination of *Hypericum* and *Valeriana* was compared to the drug Tryptanol (amitryptyline).[206] The herbal combination was found to be of equivalent benefit but without the frequently observed side effects of lethargy and dry mouth. In an earlier double-blind trial, a *Hypericum* and *Valeriana* combination was shown to be more effective than Valium (diazepam).[207]

Mood-elevating effects may take up to four weeks to become apparent. When a more immediate effect is needed, *Hypericum* can be combined with other nervines such as *Piper methysticum*, *Valeriana* or *Scutellaria laterifolia*.

Hypericum has also been shown to contain substances (hypericin and pseudohypericin) that are active against enveloped viruses. These include the retroviruses (HIV); the Herpes viruses; hepatitis A and B; influenza A, B, and C; measles; and Rubella.[208]

Use in gynaecology

This herb is indicated in conditions where exhaustion and tension combine—a common finding in women who present with hormonal problems. *Hypericum* is particularly useful in menopausal and perimenopausal women and may have a hormonal effect.[209]

A combination of *Hypericum* and *Cimicifuga racemosa* was studied in 812 women suffering menopausal symptoms.[210] Symptoms such as reduced concentration and hot flushes were significantly reduced, with 79 per cent of subjects electing to continue treatment after the trial.

Hypericum extracts (infusions or fluid extracts) may produce photosensitisation and increased sensitivity to pain and thermal stimuli at the upper end of the dose range. It is prudent to recommend that those on high doses avoid excessive exposure to the sun, especially fair-skinnned individuals.

Dose

Doses can range from 2–8 mL per day of a 1:2 fluid extract containing between 0.4 and 1.0 mg per mL of total hypericins. Higher doses are recommended for acute viral infection (enveloped viruses); lower doses for long-term treatment of depression are from 2–4 mL per day.

Leonurus cardiaca (Motherwort)

Leonurus is a nervine with cardiotonic actions and can be used for palpitations associated with anxiety and excessive worry, especially when they are a feature of insomnia. Its effects are gentle and progressive and long-term administration is usually advisable. *Leonurus* is also a safe and effective treatment for mild hyperthyroidism,[211] and has mild anti-hypertensive properties.

Use in gynaecology

The spasmolytic, sedative, diuretic, hypotensive and cardiotonic actions of *Leonurus* have secured it a place in the treatment of women's complaints. It is also a mild emmenagogue and 'provokes women's courses' (brings on the period)[212] (but large doses are needed) possibly because of the alkaloids strachydrine and leonurine.[213] It is often used in the last weeks of pregnancy to facilitate labour, and following childbirth to minimise blood loss. With *Viburnum prunifolium* (a uterine sedative), it is also used to treat hypertension in pregnancy.

This is one of the many herbs which possess the apparently contradictory actions of relieving spasm and stimulating uterine activity—an effect which seems to be brought about by a reduction in the irritability (spasticity) of the uterine muscle. This allows contractions to be followed by an adequate rest period when blood can circulate through the uterine muscle again. The more orderly uterine contractions reduce the pain of dysmenorrhoea, and allow childbirth to proceed smoothly.

For peri-menopausal insomnia, night sweats and palpitations, *Leonurus* is used in conjunction with *Humulus lupulus* and *Cimicifuga racemosa* with excellent results.

Dose

Leonurus is Cooling and Drying and is used in doses of between 2–4 mL three times daily.

Humulus lupulus (Hops)

Humulus is mainly useful for symptoms of restlessness, anxiety and insomnia,[214] although the bitter and smooth muscle relaxing properties[215] also improve symptoms related to nervous indigestion, colon pain and spastic constipation. Irritable bowel syndrome, especially when triggered by episodes of stress, respond well to this herb. Its bitterness, however, makes it difficult to take as a tea.

Use in gynaecology

Before mechanisation, women hop-pickers regularly started to menstruate two days after commencing to pick the hops. This was thought to be related to an oestrogenic principle in the cone-like fruits (strobiles) and three different groups of investigators identified an oestrogen-like substance in relatively large amounts.[216] Subsequent research, however, has failed to find any oestrogenic activity in hops.[217] 'The medicinal use of hops has a long and romantic history . . .' the last group of researchers noted. Perhaps the reported hormonal effects were nothing more than an extension of folk legend?

But if it is legend, then it certainly has far-reaching effects. In addition to their sedative properties for insomnia, *Humulus* is used for 'sexual neuroses (wet dreams, premature ejaculation, and to reduce sexual appetite in men)'. If oestrogens are not responsible, could other hormonal substances, perhaps anti-androgens, be responsible for this effect?[218] More than a decade passed before another possible explanation for the hormonal effects of *Humulus* was discovered—they possess substances with an antigonadotrophic activity,[219] which suppress oestrogen, progesterone and luteinising hormone (LH) levels. These components could explain many of the observed actions of *Humulus*, from treating hot flushes and sexual neuroses, to improving menstrual regularity when women have polycystic ovarian disease (PCOD). The question of the hormonal activity of *Humulus* is far from resolved, however, and it may be that future research will discover oestrogenic effects.

Cimicifuga racemosa, which also suppresses LH levels, successfully treats hot flushes. *Humulus*, however, have the additional advantage of being sedative and are specifically indicated in the treatment of flushing that accompanies stress, worry or insomnia. *Humulus*, combined with *Cimicifuga*, is a useful treatment for PCOD. Only time will tell if this is purely an antigonadotrophic effect or if it is related to the speculated anti-androgenic effect as well. *Humulus* have also been shown to antagonise contractions induced by oxytocin (a spasmolytic effect),[220] which suggests a beneficial application for spasmodic dysmenorrhoea.

Dose

Humulus is Cold and Dry. A tea can be made by infusing 1–2 g in boiling water, however this is very bitter. The dose of the extract is 1–2 mL, two to three times daily.

Verbena officinalis (Vervain)

The medicinal uses of *Verbena* were first recorded in Dioscorides' *De Materia Medica* written around 78 BC. Before and since, *Verbena* has been regarded as a useful herb for the treatment of an astounding array of illnesses. These include rheumatism; in fever management as a diaphoretic;[221] as a mild sedative and mood elevator (thymoleptic) for depression or melancholia; as a galactagogue;[222] and in asthma or migraine as an antispasmodic.[223]

In Germany *Verbena* is used when there are liver or gall bladder symptoms[224] and in France, writers have extolled its usefulness in neuralgia, including trigeminal neuralgia, for migraine, and as an anti-fever agent superior to quinine.[225] It is a bitter digestive, which may account for many of its indications.

Some authors have described *Verbena* as having antithyrotropic activity, however, this was not confirmed in research.[226]

Use in gynaecology

Verbena potentiates the actions of prostaglandin E2 on uterine muscle and has been investigated as a potentiating agent for prostaglandins-induced abortions.[227] It may also exhibit weak androgenic activity,[228] as well as nervous tonic and milk-increasing properties. *Verbena* can be used to treat spasmodic dysmenorrhoea and delayed menstruation, and to reduce the impact of menopausal symptoms due to its nervine properties.

Valeriana officinalis/edulis (Valerian)

Valeriana is probably modern herbal medicine's best-known sedative. It has been a popular sleep aid since the 17th century, never more so than at present. *Valeriana* also finds applications in the treatment of anxiety, depression, neuroses, hypertension, some headaches, and smooth muscle spasm in the digestive or reproductive tract.

A large amount of research conducted over the last twenty years has extensively reviewed the chemistry and pharmacology of *Valeriana*[229] and it has been shown to be effective in a number of clinical trials as a mild sedative. It decreased the time taken to fall asleep and improved the quality of sleep in one trial;[230] in another, a blend of standardised active ingredients were successfully used to treat a group of 120 children with a range of psychosomatic and behavioural problems including hyperactivity, restlessness, sleeplessness, constipation, and headaches.[231]

Use in gynaecology

Valeriana finds one of its major applications in gynaecology as a herb to potentiate the action of the spasmolytic herbs used in the treatment of dysmenorrhoea.

Dose

Valeriana is Warming and slightly Drying. Doses of the extract range from 2–4 mL, three time daily. Up to 1 g of the dried root can be used as an infusion or decoction for a tea.

Zizyphus spinosa (Zizyphus)

Zizyphus, like *Valeriana*, has been extensively studied. It has been in use since at least the fifth century AD, mainly for the treatment of illnesses whose symptoms include neurasthenia, insomnia, forgetfulness, palpitations, excessive dreams and nightmares.[232]

More recently, it has been extensively trialled as part of a traditional formulation called Suan Zao Ren Tang or Zizyphus Combination for the treatment of anxiety,[233] and for insomnia.[234] This formula contains five herbs, and when each was tested for sedative activity, only *Zizyphus* and one other, *Ligusticum wallichii*, were found to possess any sedative activity. The other herbs exhibit synergistic activity, as the formula proved to be much more effective than any of the component herbs individually. Improvement in symptoms such as palpitations, chest pain and faintness were reported, and rather than a reduction in daytime performance and psychomotor skills as was seen in a comparative diazepam (Valium) group, the daytime performance and psychomotor skills of the Suanzaorentang group improved.[235] Reduction in aches and pains such as neck pain and lower back pain were also reported.[236]

Use in gynaecology

Zizyphus prevents abnormal sweating and has been traditionally used for spontaneous sweating and night sweats, especially when accompanied by anxiety, irritability, palpitations and insomnia. These symptoms can occur during the peri-menopausal years, as well as being common symptoms of nervous exhaustion.

Dose

Zizyphus is sweet, sour and neutral. The usual dose is between 1–3 mL, three times daily of the fluid extract, but can be up to 15 mL in total in any one day.

Piper methysticum (Kava-kava)

A plant from the pepper family, *Piper methysticum* is used in the Pacific region as part of religious ceremonies and in social settings, in kava bars, where it is used in a similar way to wine in southern Europe.[237] A kava-kava abuse syndrome has been reported in the Pacific region and in northern Australia,[238] but this is linked with intakes more than ten times the recommended therapeutic dose.

Piper methysticum has been in use in Europe for many years, mainly as a gentle tranquilliser. An official German Commission E monograph recommends its use in nervous anxiety, stress and unrest,[239] and a number of trials have shown beneficial effects from *Piper methysticum* or its constituents in the treatment of anxiety, and an improvement in physical and psychological symptoms.[240] Local anaesthetic and anti-microbial properties also make it a useful component of preparations for urinary tract infections.[241]

Use in gynaecology

Piper methysticum reduces the anxiety depression symptoms sometimes seen in association with menopause,[242] and can also be used for anxiety associated with PMS.

Dose

Dose of the dried root is 1–3 g per day; of the fluid extract 2–6 mL, containing up to 210 milligrams of kava lactones per day.

ADAPTOGENS

Adaptogens are a non-toxic group of herbs known to normalise physiological processes in times of increased stress. They help the body to *adapt*, having a 'sparing' effect on the adrenal glands and often normalise the activities of other organs, especially the liver and heart. Adaptogens are not used to treat specific illnesses (although some are used for certain sorts of depressions),[243] but are prescribed to enhance vitality and improve resistance to the vicissitudes of life, disease and pollution.

An adaptogen, therefore, is like an old-fashioned tonic and is often indicated at those times of life when stress is high, during convalescence after surgery or illness, or during potentially difficult periods of change.

For women, these events are common following childbirth, during lactation, or around menopause. Adaptogens prescribed at these times would tend to be combined with herbs that have additional effects—after childbirth, a uterine tonic would commonly be given; while breast feeding, nutritive tonics are indicated; and during menopause, herbs which have a regulating effect on hormone balance are useful.

After childbirth and while breast feeding, adaptogens (*qi* tonics) are often combined with *blood* tonics in Chinese medicine. One of the common formulas is Ba Zen Tang (also known as Women's Precious Pills in pill form) which combines *Codonopsis pilosula*, *Glycyrrhiza uralensis*, *Atractylodes macrocephala*, and *Poria cocos*, as the 'energy' or *qi* part of the tonic, with *Angelica sinensis*, *Ligusticum wallichii*, *Paeonia lactiflora* and prepared *Rehmannia glutinosa* as the 'nutritive' or 'blood' tonic.

Adaptogens commonly used during menopause are *Eleutherococcus senticosus*, *Panax ginseng* and *Glycyrrhiza glabra*. These herbs reduce menopausal symptoms, possibly by stabilising the body's hormone production, and helping the body to adapt during times of emotional or physical stress. They are often combined with the hormone regulatory herbs *Vitex agnus castus* or *Cimicifuga racemosa*, or with nutritive tonics (see Chinese blood tonics).

Eleutherococcus senticosus (Siberian ginseng)

Eleutherococcus has been extensively studied and found to be virtually non-toxic at any reasonable dose. Soviet research found that *Eleutherococcus* was useful for times when dramatic increases in physical stamina were required.[244] However, its main indication is during times of stress associated with a wide variety of conditions ranging from extremes in weather, to mental and physical stress, to exposure to drugs and chemicals.

Use in gynaecology

For women, *Eleutherococcus* is useful for any type of stress or during convalescence. It can be used for the symptoms of over-work or 'burning the candle at both ends', it can regulate stress-induced PMS symptoms; it is a useful general tonic after childbirth and following surgery; and it is one of the best adaptogens for the menopause, especially in combination with other herbs for low oestrogen symptoms.

Eleutherococcus is not known to interact with any drugs and its use is accompanied by few if any side effects. Rarely, some women find that it makes them feel more tense, especially if they drink coffee (excess coffee intake should be avoided when taking both *Eleutheroccocus* and *Panax ginseng*).

Dose

The dose range is usually between 1–3 mL of the extract, three times daily; and *Eleutheroccocus* can be taken for up to three months without a break—in fact, longer term (more than one month), low dose (around 1 mL or 1 g), twice daily is generally much more useful than higher doses for short periods.

Panax ginseng (Korean ginseng)

Panax ginseng is one of the most commonly used adaptogens for stress. It is believed to be more 'stimulating' and tends to have an uplifting effect which is usually noticed fairly quickly. It is mildly oestrogenic and anabolic (growth promoting) and, in some circles, is considered to be a 'male' herb. Women, however, can use *Panax* for stress, and particularly when there is a concurrent need for maintaining stamina under conditions of high physical output.

One series of controlled trials showed that *Panax* improved immune function,[245] and brain function (memory and performance).[246] It has also been shown to reduce the negative effects of the drugs used for chemotherapy, including improving stamina and the sense of well-being, and even normalising white blood cell levels.[247]

Panax should not be taken with herbs which contain large amounts of caffeine or by heavy coffee drinkers, because it can potentiate the undesirable effects of caffeine. It should not be taken by those with high blood pressure, acute asthma or acute infections, including viral infections. It is not known to interact with any drugs.

Use in gynaecology

Panax can be of benefit before and during menopause. It eliminates menopausal symptoms in a significant number of women, possibly because of an oestrogen-like effect or an indirect hypothalamic-pituitary response. Long-term unsupervised use, however, is unadvisable because there have been reports of changes in vaginal and cervical cytology;[248] abnormal vaginal bleeding;[249] as well as breast pain and cystic changes[250] among women taking prolonged doses of *Panax*.

Dose

Panax ginseng is sweet, slightly bitter and Warm. It can be used as a single herb at a dose of 3 mL daily, in the morning, for 2 weeks. A break for two weeks before having another course is advisable.

Codonopsis pilosula

Codonopsis pilosula is similar in action to *Eleutherococcus* and *Panax ginseng*, but is not as uplifting, or as expensive. It has the usual effects of the adaptogens—improving vitality and stamina; and in addition, stabilises the blood pressure.

Whereas *Panax* is indicated for more profound collapse or conditions associated with an acute onset—after physical exertion or a period of difficult and stressful work, for example—*Codonopsis* is more useful for conditions associated with chronic fatigue, especially of the variety that interferes with digestion and assimilation, or causes symptoms of shortness of breath and heaviness in the limbs.[251]

It is an excellent remedy for post-viral fatigue syndrome, chronic fatigue syndrome or post-operative fatigue. It provides support during convalescence and can be used to return vitality to pre-illness levels. For debility associated with anaemia, *Codonopsis* is traditionally combined with *Astragalus membranaceous* and *Angelica sinensis*. In China, it is used for 'wasting and thirsting syndrome'—diabetes.

Use in gynaecology

Codonopsis can be used for women who need an adaptogen, but for whom *Panax ginseng* may be too stimulating—for example, when anxiety is one of the predominant symptoms accompanying fatigue. In traditional Chinese medicine, *Codonopsis* is combined with *Bupleurum falcatum*, *Cimicifuga clahurica*, *Astragalus membranaceous* for prolapses.

Dose

Codonopsis is sweet and neutral (neither Hot nor Cold). It is always combined with other herbs; the dose of the fluid extract is between 1–4 mL, three times daily.

Glycyrrhiza glabra (Liquorice)

Like *Panax* and *Eleutherococcus*, *Glycyrrhiza* has been the subject of extensive research. It is an adrenal adaptogen with expectorant, antibacterial properties which make it useful for infections in the respiratory tract. The saponin, glycyrrhizinic acid, has anti-viral effects when applied topically and is available in a cream to prevent and treat herpes of the mouth and genitals. *Glycyrrhiza* is also soothing (demulcent) and antispasmodic and is effective in the prevention and treatment of gastritis and stomach ulcers.

The saponin aglycone, glycyrrhetinic acid is excreted via the liver and seems to exert an anti-oxidant (and protective) effect on liver cells prior to excretion in the bile. *Glycyrrhiza* mimics the action of cortico-steroid drugs, and there is a synergistic action between it and endogenous cortisol. *Glycyrrhiza* prolongs the biological activity of cortisol by retarding its breakdown and excretion.

Glycyrrhiza is one of the very few pleasant tasting herbs—glycyrrhizin is 50 to 100 times as sweet as sucrose—and is frequently self-prescribed. The cortisone-like effect, however, should inspire caution, and points to one of the possible dangers of prolonged administration of *Glycyrrhiza*. It can cause an elevation of the blood pressure, fluid retention and potassium depletion with prolonged use. Experienced practitioners offset this possibility by either restricting the duration of use or combining *Glycyrrhiza* with other herbs (*Taraxacum* leaf, for example). Those who self-administer are usually unaware of these cautions and practices.

Use in gynaecology

Glycyrrhiza has oestrogenic properties which are discussed in Chapter 18 'Phyto-oestrogens'. Many women report (and some books recommend) that they take *Glycyrrhiza* as tea for menopausal symptoms, however the possibility of side effects makes this a risky practice except in the short term.

Dose

Glycyrrhiza is sweet and Warm. It should not be taken by anyone with hypertension or impaired kidney or heart function, without strict supervision; and must be avoided when taking the drugs spironalactone or amiloride. Its use should be restricted to less than six weeks. The usual dose is between 0.5–1.5 mL, three times daily. Its use should be restricted to less than six weeks unless closely supervised.

THE BITTERS/LIVER HERBS

Bitters are a large and chemically diverse group of herbs. They are grouped together because they have a bitter taste, and it is the *taste* of bitterness that gives these herbs many of their therapeutic effects. The bitter taste on the tongue triggers a series of impulses which are carried by the nervous system and culminate in physiological and biochemical changes in the gastrointestinal tract, liver and pancreas.

Bitters medicine has the ability to generally and non-specifically improve the overall state by improving digestion, assimilation and evacuation. These effects are brought about by increases in bile production, dilution and excretion; improved digestive enzyme and gastric acid production; regulation of peristaltic action; repair of the gut wall lining; and a general improvement in the micro-environment in the bowel. It is not surprising then, that for many Western herbalists, the term 'bitter' is synonymous with 'tonic'.

Even after years of using bitters, the number of possible therapeutic applications still seems remarkable. They can be used for all types of digestive disorders, including indigestion, lack of appetite and constipation; to protect the liver from damage; to reduce the risk of, or treat gall bladder disease; to regulate blood sugar levels; to lower cholesterol levels; to regulate the excretion of hormones; to increase the uptake of nutrients (themselves being a rich source); and to exert a general tonic effect brought about through the culmination of all of these changes.

Of the countless bitter remedies, four are particularly useful. *Berberis vulgaris* has uterine stimulant properties and is anti-inflammatory; *Taraxacum officinale*, root and leaf, is safe and readily available for general use; *Silybum marianum* has protective and restorative effects on liver cells which makes it useful for women on hormonal preparations which affect the liver; and *Bupleurum chinensis*, the main 'liver' herb used in Chinese medicine, has additional calming effects, making it useful for PMS.

Herbalists consider bitters to be Cooling, and (almost always) Drying, and they are often recommended for conditions associated with Heat and excess Moistness.

Berberis vulgaris

Berberis vulgaris is a bitter 'liver' remedy which contains a number of alkaloids including berberine. Berberine-containing herbs are used for infections of the mucous membranes of the mouth, the throat, sinuses, eyes, lungs, genito-urinary tract and gastrointestinal tract, because of their antimicrobial,[252] anti-infective,[253] and immune-enhancing effects.[254]

This herb is said to improve anaemia and malnutrition, and is a tonic for the delicate. It contains high levels of calcium, iron and selenium.[255] American Indians used *Berberis vulgaris* with cayenne to enhance its liver stimulant properties. *Berberis vulgaris* is a strong bitter and at too high a dose it can cause diarrhoea or abdominal cramps. The bark from the stem and root is used for medicine.

Use in gynaecology

Berberis vulgaris is a very useful herb for women with congestive period pain where the flow is slow to start, or where the pain is relieved when the flow commences. This herb is not a pain-killer, but seems to influence the events associated with this type of period pain. The flow is easier, redder and usually starts quickly; the heavy dragging pain is diminished; and the overall volume of menstrual loss is reduced.

Berberine, an alkaloid in *Berberis vulgaris* increases the activity of macrophages[256] which may in part account for the positive effects seen when this herb is prescribed for endometriosis.

Dose

Berberis vulgaris is Cold, Drying and bitter.

Dose is 0.5–2 gms of dried bark or equivalent, three times daily, or 1–4 ml of a 1:2 tincture.

Taraxacum officinale (Dandelion root)

Taraxacum has been used medicinally since at least the tenth century AD. The whole plant is bitter, but the root is considered to have the major 'liver' and digestive effects. It is a gentle remedy suitable for long-term use, either self-administered as a beverage, or as a herbal extract.

The root stimulates appetite, increases bile production and excretion, and has mild laxative properties.[257] It can be used for indigestion, bloating and flatulence after eating, or signs of malabsorption such as light coloured, floating and strongly smelling stools, perhaps with signs of undigested food.

Taraxacum root is available in most health food shops and large supermarkets and is usually sold as *Taraxacum* 'coffee'. Coffee and *Taraxacum* root beverages bear no taste resemblance whatsoever, so to avoid disappointment it is best not to think of *Taraxacum* root as 'coffee'. Many of the commercially available dandelion beverages are also sweetened or may have chicory root added which reduces their therapeutic effect. *Taraxacum* leaf is also bitter and a diuretic, and is used mainly where there is a need for increased urinary output (see the following section on 'Diuretics').

Taraxacum has anti-inflammatory effects and is traditionally used as an anti-rheumatic agent and as a general tonic. The polysaccharides and aqueous extracts have anti-tumour activities in animals.[258]

Use in gynaecology

Taraxacum root is used as a general tonic after debilitating illness or surgery; to improve liver function generally, and especially in conditions associated with relative oestrogen excess such as endometriosis; or to protect the liver from the effects of hormonal preparations, including the Pill. It is also indicated as a gentle laxative to moisten the stool following childbirth and to increase milk flow if deficient.[259]

Taraxacum root is slightly bitter and Cooling, and makes a refreshing drink over summer; in winter it can be brewed with a little cinnamon and cardamom to make it more Warming. When *Taraxacum* root is prescribed by a herbalist, it will usually be in the form of an extract and be part of a mixture with a number of other herbs.

Dose

Dose of the liquid extract is 2–8 mL, three times per day; dried root needs 1–2 tspn in one cup of cold water brought gently to boil, then left to draw for ten minutes, three times a day.

Silybum marianum (Milk thistle or St Mary's thistle)

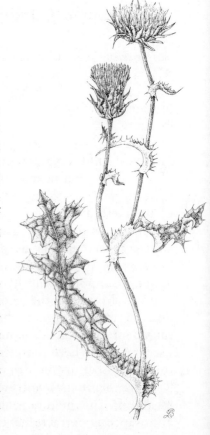

Culpeper said of *Silybum marianum* that 'the Germans were much fond of this remedy, but we find it to be of little use'.[260] How wrong he was! *Silybum marianum* seeds have been used therapeutically for at least two thousand years, especially in Europe.[261] They can protect liver cells from destruction by some of the most toxic substances known, including the death cap toadstool (*Amanita phalloides*) and carbon tetrachloride (drycleaning fluid).

Until recently it has been almost universally accepted that there was not and could not be any pharmacological treatment for liver diseases. Since the research on *Silybum marianum*, however, there is now a substantial body of evidence indicating that this herb, via its active constituents, can exert an almost specific influence on liver parenchyma (functional tissues of the liver).[262]

In liver disease, cells can be found in various states from undamaged, to degenerating or irreversibly damaged. Normal cells are protected by *Silybum marianum* and any cells not yet irreversibly damaged are stabilised. 'These now healthy cells are able to become centres for regeneration as a secondary action of silymarin on the nucleus of these cells stimulates them to produce polymerase A and therefore more protein and accelerated regeneration of liver tissue'.[263]

The protective compounds in *Silybum* are the flavonolignans, known collectively as silymarin, which protect the liver by stabilising liver cell membranes via non-competitive inhibition of lipoxygenase.[264] This anti-oxidant activity prevents or reduces the capacity of toxic agents to penetrate the cell, and reduces the damage done when they do enter the cell.[265] Herbal products are now available with standardised doses of silymarin.

Use in gynaecology

Silybum is useful at any time that a liver dysfunction is suspected of negatively influencing gynaecological problems, such as in cases of suspected relative oestrogen excess, where hepatic breakdown of oestrogen may be impaired. It is also a gentle laxative.

Dose

Research with silymarin suggests oral doses of 140 mg three times a day are safe and effective (this represents up to 10 ml of a 1:1 fluid extract three times a day, which may be excessively laxative).

Bupleurum falcatum

This is the most commonly used herb in Chinese medicine and is used in 80 per cent of all traditional formulas. Apart from 'bitter' effects, such as improving bile flow and excretion, increasing gastric acid levels, and peristalsis, *Bupleurum* also reduces fever especially when associated with influenza;[266] it also has analgesic and anti-convulsant properties.[267]

However, one of this herb's most interesting effects is its anti-inflammatory action. The major active components in *Bupleurum*, known as saikosaponins, seem to be capable of initiating anti-inflammatory effects,[268] while at the same time improving the endogenous (in the body) secretion of corticosteroids.[269] One study on rats showed that the anti-inflammatory result did not occur when the adrenal glands were removed, indicating a synergistic interaction between the corticosterone produced in the body and the anti-inflammatory effect induced by the saikosaponins in *Bupleurum*.[270]

The combined administration of saikosaponins and corticosterone increases the anti-inflammatory effects when compared to corticosterone alone;[271] and in some models, the anti-inflammatory effect can be compared to prednisolone.[272] The traditional use of *Bupleurum*-containing formulas for a wide variety of inflammatory complaints, such as gout, rheumatoid arthritis, osteoarthritis and intercostal neuralgia may be explained by these findings.

Bupleurum is also hepatoprotective against experimentally-induced liver damage[273] and is usually combined with liquorice for complaints associated with liver disorders. The traditional indications are for right-sided upper abdominal pain and tension or resistance along the costal margin. *Bupleurum* may also be useful in the treatment of chronic kidney disorders such as nephrotic syndrome, especially in combination with Western medicine. Relapses are less frequent amongst adults with nephrotic syndrome,[274] and a study conducted on children over a ten year period using a combination of prednisolone and *Bupleurum*-containing formulas led to improvements in protein loss and a reduction in cholesterol levels.[275]

Bupleurum has sedative and tranquillising effects and causes a slight decrease in blood pressure. A reduction in serum cholesterol levels is also observed. Nausea, diarrhoea or flatulence associated with prescriptions of *Bupleurum* may indicate that the dose is too high. Adjusting the dose or alternatively, adding liquorice, can help to prevent or relieve this symptom.[276]

Use in gynaecology

Traditionally, *Bupleurum* is prescribed for menstrual disorders associated with stress and worry, which culminate in amenorrhoea, irregular periods, dysmenorrhoea and premenstrual syndrome (PMS). For these complaints, *Bupleurum* is usually combined with *Paeonia lactiflora* and *Angelica sinensis*.

Taste is bitter, and it is slightly Cooling.

Dose

Dose for gynaecological complaints is 2–3 mL, three times daily. Higher doses are needed to reduce fever.

DIURETICS

A diuretic is any substance that increases urine output above current or normal levels. The diuretic activity of herbs has been questioned, probably because of the understandable confusion caused by those old herbals which describe any herb used in the urinary system as a diuretic. Of those herbs still used as diuretics, research has revealed variable results. Some are only effective if the patient has a diminished urine output, whereas in drug testing programs only healthy subjects are used; others are simply weak diuretics with limited application for increasing urinary output.

A number of different methods are used to improve diuresis in the body:

- Increasing blood flow to the kidney will increase glomerular filtration rate and therefore increase urine output. Xanthine-containing herbs, including *Coffea arabica* (coffee), are examples of this. Xanthines also decrease sodium and chloride reabsorption.
- Increasing sodium and chloride excretion (salidiuretics) will lead to increased urine output. Herbs with this property include *Taraxacum officinalis* (dandelion leaf) or *Betula pendula* (birch leaf). *Juniperus* (berries) are also known to increase chloride output in rats.[277]
- Ingesting substances that are not well reabsorbed, for example plants containing a high level of potassium such as dandelion leaf, corn silk, or sugars that are not metabolised such as sorbitol, mannitol and inositol, will cause an increase in osmotic pressure (osmotic diuresis).
- Ingesting substances that reduce the levels of, or interfere with anti-diuretic hormone (for example alcohol) will also improve diuresis.

Taraxacum officinale (Dandelion leaf)

Young dandelion leaves add a bitter freshness to summer salads and sandwiches, and are often an ingredient in European-style salad mixes. Their vitamin A content is higher than in carrots (14 000 IU per 100 grams),[278] which makes them a valuable addition to any diet.

Apart from their culinary advantages, dandelion leaf is a very safe and effective diuretic that, unlike most diuretics, adds to rather than depletes the body's stores of potassium. It is a rich source of potassium at 4.5 per cent dry weight.[279] The diuretic activity of dandelion has been questioned, however the poor results seen in these experiments can be explained by poor study design: where the herb was given in one or two doses; the incorrect plant part was used—the root instead of the leaf; or it was given in sub-therapeutic doses (one fifteenth of the usual dose).

The diuretic activity of dandelion leaf (given correctly) was compared to the drug Furosemide (Lasix) in mice and was found to be as potent, when tested over a month of daily administration.[280]

Use in gynaecology

Taraxacum leaf assists with the symptomatic relief of fluid retention common before menstruation. It is also useful for oedema and hypertension associated with pregnancy. The rich mineral content is also beneficial—*Taraxacum* leaf contains substantial amounts of many nutrients including potassium, calcium, magnesium and iron.

Dose

The usual dose of the dried leaf is 4–10 g by infusion (herbal tea) three times daily; of the fluid extract, 4–10 mL, three times daily; and of the fresh juice, 10–20 mL, three times daily.

Dandelion leaf is Cooling and Drying.

Juniperus communis (Juniper berries)

Juniperus has been a popular diuretic, anti-rheumatic and urinary antiseptic for generations in Europe. A blood sugar lowering effect has also been proven in animal studies,[281] which confirms the traditional use of *Juniperus* in diabetes mellitus.

For most of this century, *Juniperus* berries have been thought to contain an essential oil that was irritant to the kidneys and they have not been used when kidney infection or disease is a possibility. The oil of *Juniperus*, however, is not a renal irritant (in rats).[282] Adulteration with needles, branches and unripe berries (berries take 2–3 years to ripen) during distillation has been suggested as the cause for the higher levels of the urinary irritants alpha and beta pinene, which may have led to the unfair dismissal of this herb as dangerous.

Use in gynaecology

Juniperus has a reputation as a fertility control agent[283]—which has been confirmed, at least in rats.[284] Their main mode of action is to prevent implantation of the fertilised ovum at doses between 300 and 500 mg/kg however, an abortifacient action has also been confirmed.[285] This herb should not be used in pregnancy by the untrained and should be used very cautiously in large doses for any complaint. The injudicious use of juniper oil has caused death and the oil is therefore unavailable.

The mild diuretic activity of *Juniperus* makes it a suitable premenstrual remedy which is particularly suited to women who develop urinary irritation or symptoms of low-grade urinary tract infections prior to their period. The mild emmenagogic activity can also be useful to bring on a delayed period caused by hormonal irregularities, especially when associated with discomfort and bloating. However, the appropriate treatment of the cause of the hormone imbalance should always be given priority.

Dose

Juniperus is Warm and Dry and is given in doses of 5 g of dried berries two or three times daily as an infusion; or 2–4 mL of the fluid extract, three times daily. Juniper should not be used in the first trimester of pregnancy, and the daily dose should not exceed 3g or 6 mL.

Equisetum arvense (Horsetail)

Equisetum is a very primitive plant that makes an excellent diuretic with haemostatic, astringent and antiseptic effects. Of note is its high silica content (1.2–6.9 per cent), which may be extracted in hot water by simmering for around three hours over a low heat. For use as a diuretic, a simple infusion is all that is needed to extract the saponins that are the likely active ingredients.

Traditionally, *Equisetum* has been used for urethritis, cystitis with haematuria, enuresis and incontinence.[286] Mild kidney infections, urinary gravel and recurrent stones also respond to *Equisetum* and the therapeutic effect is aided by both its diuretic and antimicrobial properties. In the case of kidney stones, it has been suggested that the mucous membranes lining the urinary tract are protected from bacterial attack by *Equisetum*. This in turn aids the excretion of microscopic stones because they are less able to adhere to healthy epithelium.[287]

Other properties include a proposed connective tissue strengthening ability and a haemostatic action which is not due to vasoconstriction, and has no effect on blood pressure.[288] An anti-inflammatory action has also been identified which is related to the inhibition of an enzyme in the prostaglandins cascade (prostaglandin synthetase).[289] This may explain the traditional use of *Equisetum* for conditions associated with inflammation and swelling such as rheumatoid arthritis.[290]

Although many of the actions of *Equisetum* were once attributed to its high silica content, it now seems likely that the flavonoids and saponins are responsible for most of the therapeutic effects.[291] *Equisetum* contains antithiamine factors which should be noted before embarking on long-term therapy.[292]

Use in gynaecology

Equisetum is safe, gentle and well-tolerated, even at high doses and during long-term use. It is indicated for heavy menstruation, especially when accompanied by premenstrual fluid retention. It can be given throughout the cycle and not just during or prior to menstruation, and is a useful herb for any age group, although some say it is better suited to peri-menopausal women.[293]

The positive effects on menorrhagia seen with *Equisetum* may be due to the inhibition of prostaglandin synthetase[294] since it has been shown that an altered PGF 2α:PGE 2 ratio can be associated with excessive menstrual loss.[295] This is only speculative, since no research has ever been undertaken. *Equisetum* also contains the flavonoid luteolin (said to be found only in American and Asian plants),[296] which has been shown to have an affinity for oestrogen-binding sites in the rat uterus.[297] The significance of this in uterine bleeding is unclear.

Dose

Equisetum is Cold and Dry and given in doses of between 1–4 g as a decoction (see above); or between 2–4 mL of the fluid extract two to three times daily.

HERBS FOR INFECTION CONTROL

Herbalists are not really interested in killing bacteria or fungi as their primary way of controlling infection and the herbs used for infection control do not behave like conventional antibiotics. Instead, the focus of treatment is on the person with the infection—their immune responses and natural defenses. As such, many herbs improve the resistance to infections generally and non-specifically, and while they might have an antiseptic effect, this is seen as a bonus rather than their primary mode of action.

Of course, some infections are so extreme that antibiotics are necessary to save lives or prevent serious complications. Many infections, however, are trivial, while others, although more serious, are not life-threatening, and have nuisance value rather than causing grave harm to health and well-being. Included in this latter group are colds and flus, sinusitis, sore throats and low-grade vaginal infections. It is to these types of infections that the herbs in this section are directed.

Echinacea species

Echinacea is one of the best-known medicinal plants used in the West for infection control. In Germany, for example, over ten million units of various *Echinacea* products are sold annually, and an enormous weight of evidence suggests a high degree of safety and very low toxicity.

Echinacea can be invaluable as part of a long-term therapy to reduce susceptibility to and symptoms of various infections such as colds and influenza,[298] asthma and other inflammatory processes.[299] The three main *Echinacea* species have exhibited immune-enhancing activity in experimental models[300] including the stimulation of phagocytic activity (the ability of white blood cells to take in and destroy foreign bodies).[301]

Traditionally, *Echinacea* has been used for recurrent infections, colds and flus, boils and snake-bite. The native American use of *Echinacea* for snake-bite has been supported in part by modern research showing anti-hyaluronidase activity.[302] (Hyaluronidase is a substance in snake venom that enhances the spread of venom by loosening the 'glue' (hyaluronic acid) between the cells, allowing the venom to spread widely throughout the system.) This same activity makes the topical application of *Echinacea* useful for preventing the spread of bacteria and viruses into damaged flesh.

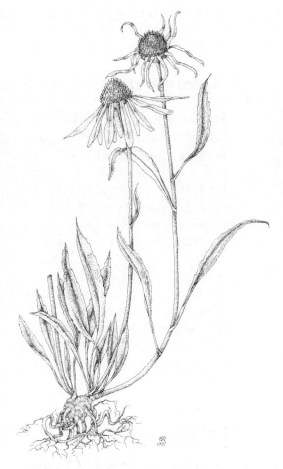

Use in gynaecology

Echinacea is a useful herb for the prevention of those chronic recurrent infections which occur in the premenstrual phase, such as recurrent sinusitis, genital herpes, acne and colds. It is also a useful adjunct to the treatment of pelvic inflammatory disease and can also be useful in the control of some of the common vaginal infections, in conjuction with other (often topical) treatments.

Dose

The dose of *Echinacea* can vary from between 1–5 mL, one to four times daily. In general, higher and more frequent doses are used in acute infections, while lower doses are indicated for prevention of infection. *Echinacea* is Cool and Dry.

Hydrastis canadensis (Golden seal)

Hydrastis has high levels of the antimicrobial alkaloid berberine, as well as a number of other alkaloids. It has a well-founded reputation as being the major herb for inflammatory, infective or catarrhal conditions of the mucous membranes, and is a major herb for the treatment of digestive underactivity.

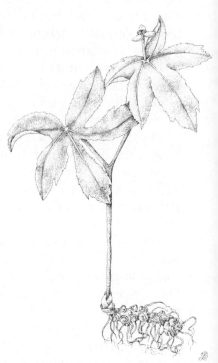

Its considerable antibiotic qualities are manifest against organisms as diverse as *Staphylococcus aureus* (golden staph), *Shigella boydii* (dysentery), *Candida albicans* (thrush) and *Mycobacterium tuberculosis* (TB).[303] *Hydrastis* also increases immune responses by increasing the activity of macrophages.[304]

Use in gynaecology

Hydrastis is a useful haemostatic herb which is also oxytocic. Its main effect on excessive bleeding is believed to be due to its effect on the capillaries, although the improvement of uterine tone also slows bleeding. *Hydrastis* is commonly used with other herbs in a mix for menorrhagia, particularly the tonics and tannin-containing herbs such as *Achillea millefolium*, *Trillium erectum* and *Geranium maculatum*.

It is bitter and Cold and is useful for infections associated with Heat, with signs of yellow discharge and fever. *Hydrastis*' considerable antimicrobial qualities make it useful for topical application for a host of gynaecological infections, for example, as a component of vaginal suppositories for the treatment of candidiasis, trichomonas and gardnerella.

Dose

The daily dose is between 0.5–2 mL, three times daily. *Hydrastis* is currently endangered due to extensive harvesting of wild plants and its use should be restricted until commercial crops are established.

Calendula officinalis (Marigold)

Extracts of the flowers of the *Calendula* (sometimes called pot marigold) have long been known to have topical anti-inflammatory and wound-healing activity;[305] as well as anti-tumour activity.[306] Like *Echinacea*, *Calendula* has been found to possess immuno-stimulating polysaccharides,[307] however these are probably not active once ingested.

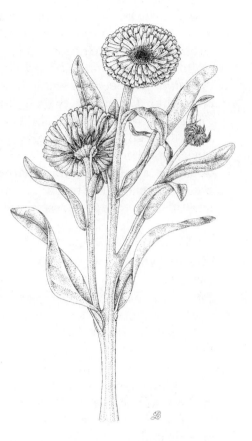

Calendula has an antimicrobial effect and is used to treat bacteria, viruses and fungal infections of the upper gastrointestinal tract and upper respiratory tract. Applied topically, the combination of antiseptic, astringent and wound-healing qualities make it the herb of choice for the first-aid treatment of cuts, abrasions and sores.

Use in gynaecology

Calendula can be taken internally for the treatment of excessive menstrual flow and seems to play a role in bringing on late periods. It is also a circulatory stimulant and reduces pelvic congestion, effects which when combined with the antimicrobial effects of *Calendula* make it ideal for pelvic infections and inflammation. It also has a reputation as a mild antispasmodic.[308]

Calendula can be applied locally as a wash, douche or lotion, or made into a vaginal pessary for the treatment of candidiasis (thrush), trichomonas, and gardnerella infections.

Dose

Calendula is bitter and Cold. It is prescribed as dried flowers—1–4 g three times daily as a tea; as a tincture (1:5) up to 1 mL, three times daily; or up to 2.5 mL, three times daily as a fluid extract.

Thuja occidentalis

Thuja, also known as *arbor vitae* or tree of life, has been a popular immune stimulant in Europe for many years.[309] There, it is widely available as a preparation called Esberitox, which also contains *Baptisia tinctoria* and *Echinacea purpurea*.

Thuja has been shown to stimulate the first phase of phagocytosis,[310] but unlike *Echinacea* (which stimulates later phases of phagocytosis), *Thuja* also improves the ability of lymphocytes (NK cells) to recognise and kill virally-infected T cells.[311] It also has antiviral activity against a range of other viral families.[312] Thus, *Thuja* is useful in the treatment of simple and genital warts either taken orally or applied locally. It is also used in the treatment of most common colds, acute conjunctivitis, hepatitis A and upper respiratory conditions.

Use in gynaecology

Thuja was used by the native inhabitants of the northern Americas as part of a treatment for uterine cancer, and has maintained a reputation for being useful in treating tissue growths such as nasal and uterine polyps.

Thuja has an emmenagogic action which means that it must not be used in pregnancy or whilst breast-feeding due to the presence of thujone in the plant; however, the same activity can be used to help bring on late periods when the reason for the lateness has been appropriately investigated.

Dose

It is important that the recommended dose not be exceeded. Dried herb: 1–2 g or by infusion; fluid extract: (1:1) 2 mL daily; tincture: (dried plant 1:5) 1 mL; tincture: (fresh plant 1:5) 2 mL daily. All doses are for three times daily administration.

Melaleuca alternifolia (Tea tree oil)

Tea tree oil is extracted from a shrub native to northern NSW. The essential oil is a powerful antimicrobial which is active against many common bacteria and fungi, including *Staphylococcus aureus* and *candidiasis*. It is a superb first-aid topical antiseptic, however it is best diluted because it can be irritating if applied as the pure oil. A cream or olive oil base is commonly used.

Use in gynaecology

May be included in vaginal suppositories for the treatment of thrush, trichomonas infections and gardnerella. It should not be taken internally.

20

Drugs and surgery

Key words

adenoma
adenomyosis
adhesions
amenorrhoea
androgenising drug
anti-oestrogen
chloasma
conjugated oestrogens
danazol
dydrogesterone
dysmenorrhoea
endometrium
ethinyl oestradiol
fibroadenoma

gonadotrophin-releasing
  hormone
HDL cholesterol
hormone replacement
  therapy (HRT)
hyperprolactinaemia
LDL cholesterol
medroxyprogesterone
melasma
menorrhagia
norethisterone
progestogen
prostaglandins
testosterone
thromboembolism

Not many of us relish the idea of having surgery or taking drugs, but sometimes they are necessary to adequately treat some gynaecological complaints or they may be necessary when natural therapies do not work effectively enough. The major drugs and surgical procedures mentioned in the previous sections are discussed in more detail in this part of the book.

Some natural therapies can help with preparation for or recovery from surgery. It is also possible to take vitamins, minerals or herbs to offset the side effects of some drugs or to improve their effectiveness.

DRUGS

Hormone preparations

Oral contraceptives (the Pill)

The side effects of oral contraceptives are well known and can include venous thromboembolism (blood clots), stroke, and heart attack especially for Pill users who also smoke. When taken correctly, the Pill is an effective contraceptive, but other benefits are less obvious to all but the researcher and scientist because they are largely related to prevention of conditions and are almost entirely determined by epidemiological studies. They include a reduced rate of ovarian and endometrial cancer, benign breast disease (not breast cancer), benign ovarian cysts, pelvic inflammatory disease, period pain, lighter periods and less anaemia.[1]

Today's low-dose oral contraceptives are much safer than the earlier, higher-dose Pills. However, there are still some problems. Menstrual changes such as breakthrough bleeding or spotting can occur, and some women experience androgenic effects, including weight gain and acne which are associated with the progestogen (synthetic progesterone) component of the Pill.[2] A small number of women develop long-term post-Pill amenorrhoea after coming off the Pill—estimated to be about one per cent after the first year.[3] Some women also report an increase in mood swings, depression and decreased libido (sex drive) while on the Pill.

These negative symptoms are more common when a woman first starts the Pill and may settle after two cycles, or they may necessitate a change to a different brand. Doctors usually advise waiting for two months before trying a new Pill. Pills which contain high oestrogen levels are more likely to be associated with depression—this can be reduced by taking a lower dose of oestrogen (30–35 mg)[4] and/or taking 50–100 mg vitamin B6 at the same time.[5]

Apart from its use as a contraceptive, the Pill can be prescribed for menorrhagia. It usually reduces bleeding by thinning the endometrial lining. The Pill can also be used for dysmenorrhoea, especially when a contraceptive is needed as well, or when prostaglandin inhibitors have not helped. The Pill improves dysmenorrhoea about 90 per cent of the time by preventing ovulation and reducing the production of the series 2 prostaglandins which cause muscle spasm.

The Pill improves PMS symptoms in some women, has no effect in others and makes some women worse. It is difficult to predict which women will respond well, although women eighteen years and less experienced much more tearfulness on the Pill in one study.[6] When effective, the Pill is believed to control the symptoms of PMS by superimposing a more balanced hormonal profile.

Pill regimes have been used to control the symptoms of premenstrual breast soreness and lumpiness. The rationale for these prescriptions is based on the observation that women on the Pill have a lower incidence of cyclic breast complaints including fibroadenoma and adenoma. Pills containing low doses of ethinyl oestrodiol and relatively potent progestogens (such as norethindrone acetate) are recommended. The ethinyl oestradiol reduces ovarian oestrogen secretion while the effects of oestrogens in breast tissue are modulated by the progesterone. Improvement is noted in up to 90 per cent of women, especially when oestrogen levels in the Pill are low.[7] Some doctors recommend that women 40 and over, or women with abnormal HDL: LDL cholesterol ratios should take 400–1200 IU vitamin E while on this regime to prevent progestogen-induced reduction in HDL and increase in LDL.[8]

Taking the Pill reduces the menstrual fluid volume and the risk of developing endometriosis.[9] The latest contraceptive pills have much lower levels of oestrogen and seem to reduce the amount of both normal endometrium *and* the amount of endometriosis. This is particularly the case when the Pill is used continuously (without a break for 'periods') to create a pseudo-pregnancy state.[10] The Pill compares favourably with other drug regimes for endometriosis that have more serious side-effects such as a decrease in bone density.[11]

However, the Pill is not as effective for advanced endometriosis and is not suitable for women who want to become pregnant. In one study, most women had a return of symptoms within six months of stopping the Pill.[12] The pregnancy rate of women who have endometriosis is also low following the use of the Pill, indicating that the Pill does not influence the severity of the endometriosis.[13]

All of the oral contraceptives listed in the Mims and PP Guide (medical books which describe the actions, indications and contraindications of drugs) warn that fibroids may grow with oestrogen use. However, it has been shown that fibroids do not necessarily increase in size when women take the Pill, that menstrual blood loss reduces significantly and that blood-iron levels increase.[14] A woman with fibroids should discuss the risks and benefits of oral contraceptives in her particular case with her doctor.

Significant numbers of different drugs interact with the Pill. These include some anti-epileptic drugs, some antibiotics and possibly the anti-fungal medication, Griseofulvin, which can all decrease the contraceptive effect of the Pill. Some drugs are cleared more slowly from the body when women are on the Pill. Theophylline, the anti-asthma drug, is one of these.

Paracetamol-containing pain-killers, such as Panadol, reduce the rate at which oestrogen is cleared from the body, leading to higher oestrogen levels than required for contraception. Women on thyroid hormones (Tertroxine) may need to increase their dose if they are also prescribed the Pill. Some sedatives, tranquillisers and anti-depressant drugs may not work as well; others show increased availability, such as the tri-cyclic anti-depressants Tofranil and Melipramine.[15] Women on the Pill should consult their doctor or pharmacist about the relevance of these and other possible drug interactions.

The Pill can cause increased pigmentation of the skin which is known as chloasma or melasma. This usually occurs on the face and becomes much darker with exposure to the sun. It is thought to be caused by oestrogen and can occur in pregnancy, or sometimes when women are neither pregnant nor on the Pill. Stopping the Pill does not necessarily mean that it will go away completely, although it does tend to fade. Sunblock is necessary, and skin creams or peels that contain glycolic acid can lighten the pigmentation. Doctors sometimes recommend creams containing hydroquinone or the acne treatment, isotretinoin (Roaccutane).

Symptoms or conditions which indicate that the Pill should be stopped immediately include blood clots, high blood pressure or serious headaches. Women who smoke should not take the Pill because of an increased risk of developing these complaints. Post-Pill amenorrhoea is not usually treated by doctors until a pregnancy is desired, when they will prescribe fertility drugs like Clomid. Until this time, the usual recommendation is for women to go back on the Pill to maintain their bone density.

There are many different types of oral contraceptives including ones with variable oestrogen and progestogen levels (Triphasil and Triquilar), or those with the same levels throughout the cycle (Brevinor, Microgynon). Some contain androgen-blocking agents (Diane) and are used for acne and excessive male-pattern hair growth; some are progestogen-only Pills (the mini Pills such as Micronor and Microlut). A lot of factors need to be considered when prescribing oral contraceptives and a doctor or gynaecologist skilled in this area should be consulted if difficulties are experienced.

Combined Pills containing oestrogen and progestogens influence a number of nutrients, some positively, others negatively. Requirements for vitamins B_2, B_3, B_6, folic acid and zinc increase, but the need for iron is reduced because of the smaller blood loss at the period. Calcium is retained in the bones more effectively when women take the Pill, but this does not indicate a lower requirement because most women do not get enough calcium in their diet anyway.

Blood levels of vitamin A increase while taking the Pill and so vitamin A supplements including cod liver oil, should never be taken with the Pill. The absorption of betacarotene (the precursor to vitamin A) from food, however, may be lower and so it is wise to eat plenty of orange or yellow vegetables such as carrots, pumpkin and sweet potato.

The serum copper level increases on the Pill and may be partly responsible for the mood changes. High copper levels can lead to a zinc deficiency and zinc supplements may be necessary especially for vegetarians and vegans. Information on zinc is included in Chapter 7 'Adolescence'. The usual dose of zinc is 15–30 mg per day.

Side effects, including mood changes and bloating are often associated with the progestogen component of the Pill. Taking vitamin B_6 50–100 mg or a B complex with 50 mg of B_6 in the week before the period can reduce these symptoms. Herbal diuretics, especially dandelion leaf tea, can help with fluid retention symptoms. One or two teaspoons per cup twice daily (but not before bed!) is the usual dose. Many women also report that evening primrose oil (between 1000 and 3000 mg per day) is useful for many of the symptoms they experience while taking the Pill.

Women who smoke and take the Pill may reduce their risk of blood clot formation if they take 100 IU of vitamin E every day. It is not advisable for women who have a pre-existing heart condition or high blood pressure to self-prescribe vitamin E and they should consult a practitioner first.

The progestogens

The commonly used progesterone-like drugs or 'progestogens' come from two classes—medroxyprogesterone acetate such as Provera, and norethisterone such as Primolut N. Both progestogens are used in the Pill, and are also prescribed for bleeding irregularities, endometriosis and for the menopause.

Progestogens can cause symptoms of nausea, bloating, acne, breast tenderness, weight gain and mood changes which may be related to the androgenising (male hormone) effects of the drugs. The medroxyprogesterones such as Provera have fewer androgenic effects and tend not to affect blood fats; Primolut N and other norethisterones have mild oestrogenic, anabolic (growth promoting) and androgenic effects, and can adversely alter blood lipid profiles with prolonged adminstration.

Progestogens are commonly prescribed for heavy periods, even though many women who have this problem do not have irregularities in progesterone production.[16] It causes complete shedding of the endometrium when it is stopped which often stops the abnormal bleeding.

These drugs need be given for about 21 days—usually from day five to day 25 of the menstrual cycle. They are usually prescribed for between one and three menstrual cycles, but sometimes longer administration is needed. The androgen-like side effects and blood lipid abnormalities associated with Primolut N and the norethisterones restrict their use to no more than 6–12 months.

Provera can be used to treat premenstrual breast pain. It is usually prescribed between day five to 25 to modulate the effects of oestrogen on breast tissue and to suppress pituitary–ovarian function. Although up to 80 per cent of women improve on Provera, many experience an initial worsening of their symptoms and up to 40 per cent will relapse after stopping the drug.

Provera and Duphaston (dydrogesterone) are the common progestogens used for endometriosis. These preparations can either be given in the last part of the cycle, but are frequently given continuously to create a pregnancy-like state with no period. About 30 per cent of women are troubled by spotting and break-through bleeding until the drug starts to work or the dose is adjusted. These drugs are relatively inexpensive (compared to some of the others used for endometriosis) and can give significant pain relief without serious long-term side effects.

On the downside, Duphaston can cause unpleasant side effects including increased hairiness, mood changes and a deeper voice. Fertility is not improved after using either of the progestogens. The return to a regular cycle may be delayed for many months and endometriosis may return after progestogen therapy.

For menopausal women taking oestrogens and who have not had a hysterectomy, progestogens are necessary. They can be given so that endometrial shedding (a 'period') occurs—often a medroxyprogesterone acetate such as Provera 10 mg is prescribed for ten to twelve days each month. Alternatively, a lower dose (5 mg) is given continually to shrink the endometrium and protect it from the over-stimulatory effects of oestrogen.

When side effects from progestogens are a problem, the B vitamins, herbal diuretics or evening primrose oil can sometimes reduce symptoms.

Danocrine (danazol)

Danazol is another progestogen which can cause pronounced androgenic effects such as male-pattern hair growth, deepening of the voice, weight gain, acne, and changes to the sexual organs such as atrophy of breast tissue, and hypertrophy of the clitoris. Severe and life-threatening strokes or thromboembolism (blood clots), and increased intercranial pressure have also been reported with the use of danazol; and long-term use may cause serious toxicity including jaundice and hepatitis.[17] Some women find it also causes severe mood changes and symptoms like premenstrual syndrome.

This drug needs to be carefully prescribed after due consideration of the risks and benefits for each woman. For endometriosis, danazol is prescribed in high doses (between 200–800 mg per day) to stop ovulation, suppress the period and cause the endometrium (both inside and out of the uterus) to shrink. Spotting can be a problem and is usually managed with a change in dose.

Danazol improves period pain and other pelvic pain, seems to have beneficial effects on the immune abnormalities,[18] is better than other progestogens in improving fertility, and does not have an adverse affect on bone density.

Danazol is sometimes used when abnormal bleeding has not responded to other treatments, but usually only when surgery is undesirable or not indicated, or when there are long waiting lists for hysterectomy. The dose is between 200–400 mg daily. It has also been used to treat breast tenderness and cystic breast changes, and to improve lethargy, anxiety and increased appetite associated with PMS.[19] For these conditions, it is used at doses of around 200 mg which cause less side effects and tend not to stop the period.

Side effects from danazol are difficult to control, especially at the higher doses required for the treatment of endometriosis. However, trying the supplements suggested for the Pill can sometimes make the difference between being able to stay on the medication comfortably and feeling really awful.

Progesterone

The hormone progesterone (not the progestogens, such as Provera and Primolut) has been used for some time for PMS. Progesterone cannot be given orally because it is rapidly broken down in the liver (it has a half-life—the time taken for half of a substance to be broken down—of only fifteen minutes) and must be administered as rectal suppository, vaginal pessary, a cream, an injection or an implant.

Progesterone has many enthusiastic supporters for the treatment of PMS and breast soreness,[20] even though many properly controlled trials fail to show a better than placebo effect.[21] It is most effective during cycles where the menstrual cycle has been disrupted, possibly because the progesterone is at a sufficient dose to stop ovulation. See also 'Natural progesterone and wild yam creams', page 314.

Hormone replacement therapy (HRT)

The accepted medical indications for HRT are for the treatment of hot flushes, vaginal dryness and for women who have an increased risk of developing osteoporosis or cardiovascular disease. Some doctors, however, prescribe HRT for *any* symptom experienced by menopausal women, including depression, mood swings, insomnia and migraines.

Australian women are amongst the highest users of HRT in the world,[22] despite the frequent and conflicting media coverage of risk versus benefit. Some of these issues are difficult to resolve as there simply is not enough information on the long-term use of some of the different types of HRT to confidently predict the cost-benefit ratio. That information will eventually come from the women who are (or are not) taking HRT now.

Breast cancer and HRT

For most women, the biggest concern about HRT is whether its use is associated with an increased breast cancer risk, however, it is very difficult for the average woman to understand the confusing and conflicting media coverage which usually falls short of reporting the full picture.

There appear to be four main factors which influence risk of breast cancer development when women take HRT.[23] First is the observation that breast cancer risk seems to increase with increasing duration of use of HRT.[24] In most cases, the increase is apparently small, but as one researcher points out: 'A relative risk as small as 1.2 increases a woman's chance of developing breast cancer each year from 1 in 250 to 1 in 200.'[25]

Another important issue is the type of oestrogen used. Synthetic oestrogens are associated with a statistically higher risk of developing breast cancer than the conjugated (more natural) forms of oestrogen.[26] A common form of ethyinyl oestradiol or 'synthetic' oestrogen is Estigyn (synthetic oestrogens are also used in the Pill); the most common form of conjugated oestrogen is Premarin. In Australia and America, conjugated oestrogens are used more often, in Europe, women are more frequently prescribed synthetic oestrogen. Studies from European countries which give statistics on breast cancer incidence do not truly reflect the Australian situation.

The jury is still out on whether there is an increased risk of developing breast cancer if a woman on HRT has pre-existing conditions which may predispose her to a higher risk anyway, such as a history of benign breast disease or a family history of breast cancer. At this stage researchers are unable to say either way, although some studies have showed an increase in risk in long-term users.

Another unresolved issue concerns long-term oestrogen and progestogens given together. Initially it was felt that progesterone would be protective to breast tissue in the same way that it is to endometrial tissue.[27] However, some researchers have suggested an increase in breast cancer rate with combined therapy.[28] It is estimated that after another decade oestrogen and progestogens will have been used together for long enough and by sufficient numbers of women to make a firmer statement on the combined effect.[29]

The Nurses' Health Study (a large American study of 121 700 registered nurses started in 1976) has shown a twofold increased risk of breast cancer for women who were currently on HRT,[30] but unlike other studies, no increased risk with increasing duration of use. The women between 60 and 65 were at most risk. Breast cancer incidence peaks at 80, and because many of the larger, long-term studies do not have an 80-year-old group, it is unlikely that we are seeing the entire picture yet. On a positive note, if a woman does develop breast cancer when she is on HRT, she is much less likely to die from it than a woman who either has stopped hormones or who has never taken them.[31]

Endometrial cancer and HRT

Endometrial cancer can occur when oestrogen is given without progesterone when a woman still has her uterus. The risk increases the longer the woman stays on the oestrogen-only regime, and remains elevated for five or more years after stopping the treatment.

Despite adequate medical guidelines, these potentially dangerous combinations of HRT may be given to women quite commonly. A recent survey of 2000 Melbourne women found that 26 per cent of women with an intact uterus were apparently given oestrogen without progestogen.[32]

There are two ways of prescribing the progestogens with oestrogen so that the endometrium is protected. Progestogens can be given for a short period of time and then stopped, causing a 'period'; or a low dose of progestogen can be given continuously which leads to endometrial 'shrinkage' and wasting.

Bones and HRT

Oestrogens, including the oral contraceptive pill,[33] have a positive effect on bone density, and long-term prescriptions of HRT can be used to prevent or treat osteoporosis. When HRT is given to comparatively young women (between 50 and 75) for ten to twenty years, the fracture rate is reduced by up to 50 per cent.

Women with substantial fracture risk should consider HRT, but be mindful that when they stop, any positive effect will be lost within a few years—and at a rate similar to that seen in the immediate post-menopausal years.[34] It would seem appropriate then for all women to protect their bones by taking up an exercise regime, staying a healthy weight, retaining agility and muscle strength, and eating a balanced diet.

Heart disease and HRT

Oestrogens reduce total levels of serum cholesterol, and increase levels of HDL ('helpful') cholesterol. These changes are associated with a reduced risk of heart disease. However, women who need to take progesterone may not receive the benefits seen with oestrogen alone. Some types of progestogen (norethisterone) can have negative effects on lipids and can elevate triglyceride levels.[35] So, while some researchers believe HRT reduces risk of heart disease,[36] others are not so sure and believe the issue requires further scrutiny.[37]

The risk factors for cardiovascular disease include poor physical fitness, high blood pressure, poor diet and obesity. Taking a tablet is easy, but falls a long way short of addressing all of these aspects of risk.

Gall bladder disease and HRT

Oestrogen changes the composition of bile and increases the amount of cholesterol in bile more than a dietary increase in cholesterol.[38] Because high levels of cholesterol in the bile are prone to precipitate out and form stones, women on the Pill and HRT are more prone to gall bladder disease than other women. To prevent this complication, an oestrogen patch is often suggested because the oestrogen is absorbed straight into the blood from the skin rather than having to pass through the liver first.

Types of HRT

HRT can be given as an oral medication of oestrogen with or without progesterone, as an oestrogen-impregnated patch, as a vaginal cream or pessary, or as an oestrogen (and sometimes testosterone) implant.

Tablets

Oestrogen only
The 'natural' oestrogens are favoured over the 'synthetic' because they cause fewer liver-related side effects, they are metabolised quickly and exert weaker oestrogen effects (and therefore are less of a problem for long-term use), and their use is associated with a lower incidence of breast cancer.

The 'protective dose' is the dose usually recommended to protect the bones and heart, but is included only as a guide since many factors will alter the dose needed by each individual.

- Premarin: a conjugated (natural) form of oestrogen synthesised from pregnant mares' urine. It is relatively potent and contains various different oestrogens including oestrone and smaller amounts of oestradiol.
  Dose range: 0.3–1.25 mg daily. Protective dose: 0.625 mg daily.
- Progynova: oestradiol valerate. This oestrogen is fairly rapidly broken down and excreted with less adverse affect on the liver than some forms of oestrogen. Oestradiol is the most potent form of oestrogen produced in the body.
  Dose range: 1.0 mg–4.0 mg daily. Protective dose: 2.0 mg.
- Ogen: piperazine oestrone sulphate. Oestrone is the second most potent form of oestrogen.

Dose range: 0.625 mg–2.5 mg. Protective dose: 1.25 mg.

- Ovestin: oestriol is the weakest form of oestrogen formed in the body. It needs to be given in large doses, but has very little effect on the endometrium and its use is associated with minimal vaginal bleeding.
  Dose range: 1.00 mg–4.00 mg. Protective dose: 2.0 mg.
- Estigyn: this is a manufactured (synthetic) form of oestrogen and is the most potent oestrogen. It is also used in the Pill.
  Dose range: 0.01 mg—0.03 mg. Protective dose: 0.02 mg.

Oestrogen and progesterone

- Trisequens: packaged like the Pill in a blister pack, the first group of tablets are oestrogen alone, the next are oestrogen and progesterone and the final group contain very low levels of oestrogen. Most women will have a 'period' while taking the low dose oestrogen tablets.

Progesterone (progestogens)

The progestogens are discussed on page 388 in this section.

Patches

Patches take advantage of the fact that oestrogen absorption through the skin is very efficient. They usually consist of a multi-layered, plastic-coated and adhesive patch which has an outer, impermeable layer; a drug reservoir containing the oestrogen; a semi-permeable inner membrane through which the drug is released; and then an adhesive coating. The patch is attached to the skin like a transparent band-aid and is usually applied to the buttocks or the abdomen.

Patches are usually changed every three or four days, and must be applied to a different area each time. They sometimes cause skin irritation which is reduced if the alcohol in the patch is allowed to evaporate prior to application (waving the patch around after removal of the adhesive cover is sufficient). Oestrogen absorption through patches is accelerated when body temperature rises and sweating occurs. It is advisable that the patch is removed during strenuous exercise or other activities that increase the skin temperature.

- Estraderm: oestradiol patch of different strengths (2 mg, 4 mg and 8 mg), which release 25 mcg, 50 mcg and 100 mcg respectively. The 50 mcg dose is equivalent to 0.625 mg of Premarin and is favoured as the protective dose.
  A new patch has been developed which lasts for seven days. It is called Climara and contains oestradiol.

Creams or pessaries

Vaginal creams or pessaries containing oestrogen are used for dryness, irritation and chronic, recurrent urinary symptoms associated with low oestrogen. The oestrogen in these creams is absorbed through the skin and causes blood oestrogen levels to rise. The newer creams are not often used with progesterone, because they contain oestrogens which are less likely to over-stimulate the endometrium.

Oestrogen creams and pessaries are usually recommended to be used every day for about three weeks then only about twice weekly. A break every three months for one month is usually recommended, or a progestogen (often Provera) is given for twelve to fourteen days every second month to induce endometrial shedding.

- Ovestin: available as a cream or pessaries and contains oestriol which is a relatively weak oestrogen. The cream or pessary is applied or inserted at night, while lying down, so that maximum absorption can occur. Ovestin is for mild to moderate oestrogen deficiency symptoms.
- Vagifem: this is a pessary which contains oestradiol, a stronger oestrogen. The treatment regime is similar to that described for Ovestin. Vagifem is used for moderate to severe oestrogen deficiency symptoms.

Implants

Implants are small 'tablets' of oestrogen which are injected under the skin with a special instrument. The oestrogen is gradually absorbed into the bloodstream and the implant needs replacing every four to eight months or when symptoms return. Women with a uterus require progesterone as well. The implants are usually oestrogen alone, but sometimes oestrogen and testosterone are used, especially if a woman complains of low libido.

Side effects from HRT

PMS-like symptoms such as breast soreness, pain or swelling can occur with combined oestrogen and progestogen treatment. Some women stop taking progesterone because of these symptoms, however, taking oestrogen alone is associated with an increased risk of endometrial cancer.

Rarely, blood pressure can increase after starting HRT and so a repeat visit to the doctor who prescribed the drug should be arranged several weeks after commencement. The incidence of gall bladder disease is higher when women take HRT, but usually takes months or years to develop. Both of these problems are associated with the impact of oestrogen on the liver and a change to patches is usually advised.

Oestrogen, either too much or too little (depending on the individuals susceptibility) can cause the blood vessel spasm which leads to migraines. Some women develop migraines, others experience total relief on HRT. Progestogens can be implicated as well and a change of dose and type of HRT is indicated.

Oestrogen-dependent conditions such as fibroids and endometriosis can be aggravated by HRT, and this may require cessation of treatment.

Women on HRT who develop bleeding between periods, after sex, or when not normally expected should immediately visit their doctor. A hysteroscopy and biopsy of the endometrium is warranted to rule out endometrial cancer.

Reasons to avoid HRT

According to the *Australian Prescription Products Guide*, the contraindications for HRT include:

- Known or suspected pregnancy.
- Known or suspected cancer of the breast.
- Known or suspected oestrogen-dependent cancer.
- Undiagnosed abnormal vaginal bleeding.
- Active thrombophlebitis (inflammation of a vein with clot formation), or diseases associated with blood clotting abnormalities including recent heart attack or stroke.
- Liver, kidney, or pancreatic disease, and diabetes. Women with these problems may experience a worsening of their condition or additional side effects from HRT. These occur because of the diverse effects of oestrogen on the metabolism of sugars, the workings of the liver and pancreas, and the excretion of minerals in the urine.

Drugs with a hormone-blocking effect

GnRH agonists

GnRH is secreted by the hypothalamus to initiate the release of luteinising and follicle-stimulating hormone from the pituitary gland. Drugs with a similar chemical structure to GnRH are called GnRH analogues. GnRH analogues either mimic the action or stop the secretion of an individual's GnRH, depending on the chemical structure of the drug and the way it is administered. Given continuously, they stop ovulation and are called GnRH agonists. They are primarily used to treat endometriosis and fibroids.

The GnRH agonists are used increasingly to reduce the fibroid size and the amount of blood vessels which surround it prior to a myomectomy because of the reduced rate of bleeding and the relative ease in removing a smaller fibroid. There is also the advantage of reducing excess menstruation pre-operatively which allows time for anaemia to be corrected prior to surgery. They are not used unless surgery is to follow because once these drugs are stopped, the fibroid invariably grows again.

GnRH agonists can be used to treat endometriosis by inducing a temporary menopausal state. Compared to danazol, the GnRH agonists are equally effective in reducing the symptoms and the size of endometrial growths, but obvious side effects are less severe.[39] (Bone density loss causes no symptoms until late in life, but should be considered in the decision to use GnRH agonists.) On average, endometriomas (endometrial cysts) have returned to their initial size four months after stopping the treatment,[40] making some sort of additional treatment necessary. GnRH agonists have no additional benefits in improving fertility.[41]

GnRH agonists have also been trialled in combination with the Pill as 'add back therapy' for premenstrual symptoms including premenstrual breast pain.[42] These sorts of treatments are controversial and are reserved for severe and intractable cases of PMS. They are very occasionally used for abnormal bleeding which has failed to respond adequately to other methods.

GnRH agonists cannot be used as oral preparations because of their chemical make-up. Instead, they are either given as an injection (Zoladex), usually once per month in a long-acting form; or as a nasal spray (Synarel). They cause a pseudo-menopause and a temporary cessation of the period, but ovulation returns within about four weeks of stopping the drugs.[43] Menopausal symptoms such as hot flushes, dry vagina and headaches are common, and some women have difficulty with sexual intercourse because of vaginal dryness and lowered libido.

There is an early and significant bone density loss after commencing GnRH agonists.[44] Radial bone density (in the wrist) is not affected, but the bone density of the spine shows significant changes.[45] For some women, this may not be reversible and should be considered as part of their decision to use GnRH agonists. Oestrogen and progesterone given at the same time (add back therapy) might prevent bone density loss (but aggravate the condition the GnRH were prescribed for) and this regime is currently under review.

Occasionally, women will develop ovarian cysts in the first two months of treatment with GnRH agonists, especially if they have a previous history of polycystic ovarian disease. These cysts will often resolve as the treatment progresses, but can grow large enough to require surgery or cessation of the drug.

Women who take GnRH agonists should ensure that their calcium and magnesium intake is adequate. Information on calcium is included on pages 150–1 and on magnesium on pages 272–3.

Bromocriptine

Bromocriptine (Parlodel) reduces elevated prolactin, stops lactation and re-instates ovulation, cyclic regularity and fertility when women have hyperprolactinaemia. Prolactin-secreting tumours can decrease in size with continued use and because bromocriptine also improves oestrogen levels, it is always considered when there is a risk of low bone density.

Bromocriptine has also been used to treat PMS and breast pain,[46] but the validity of this treatment has been questioned. Breast soreness is the only symptom to consistently respond and the drug often causes unacceptable side effects.[47] These include nausea, vomiting, dizziness, headaches and a blocked nose. These are usually only transitory and can be reduced if the drug is taken at night or given as a suppository.

Women on bromocriptine continue or start to ovulate. If they do not want to become pregnant they will need to use a barrier contraceptive such as a diaphragm or condoms. The inhibitory (dopamine-like) effect on the hypothalamus is only temporary and most women with hyperprolactinaemia who discontinue the drug stop menstruating again.

Tamoxifen, Tamoxifen citrate (Genox, Nolvadex)

Tamoxifen is a synthetic anti-oestrogen compound that competes with endogenous oestradiol for oestrogen receptors and, in addition, lowers prolactin levels. It is prescribed as an oestrogen-blocking agent, at doses between 20–40 mg, when women have oestrogen-dependent cancers. It has also been used for severe premenstrual breast symptoms at doses of 10 mg, however the long-term safety of tamoxifen for pre-menopausal women without malignancy has not been determined and it is usually only recommended for premenstrual complaints when other drugs fail.

Side effects include hot flushes, vaginal bleeding, vaginal dryness and irritation, menstrual irregularity, and an increased risk of endometrial hyperplasia, polyps and cancer.

Other drugs used for gynaecological complaints

Prostaglandins inhibitors

More correctly called the prostaglandins synthetase inhibitors, these drugs prevent the production of the series 2 prostaglandins (by inhibiting the enzyme synthetase) which cause increased uterine muscle spasm and heavier periods. These drugs are also known as 'non-steroidal anti-inflammatory drugs (NSAIDs). They can be bought without a prescription from a chemist. Aspirin is a well-known prostaglandins inhibitor, but is not very effective for period pain. The newer and more effective drugs in this class include Ponstan, Naprogesic, ACT 3, and Nurofen.

Prostaglandins inhibitors are rapidly absorbed and can reduce pain in about half an hour. They can be used for the relief of primary or secondary dysmenorrhoea, or to relieve moderate to severe period pain associated with endometriosis.[48] Some women use them only when they have pain, others prefer to start to take them before the expected onset of the period. There seems to be no difference in effectiveness if the drugs are taken before the start of the period,[49] but it is wise to commence treatment early if vomiting accompanies pain. Otherwise, keeping the dose in the lowest effective range is always sound advice.

These drugs reduce menstrual blood loss by blocking the conversion of prostaglandins into prostacyclin 2.[50] Prostacyclin 2 stops platelets from clumping together, and dilates blood vessels: the net result being an increase in bleeding. Women who have heavy periods, and who continue to ovulate seem to respond better to these drugs than women who are not ovulating. They also seem to work better in combination with the Pill or progesterone tablets, and some doctors recommend these treatments be combined.[51]

Ponstan (mefenamic acid) has also been used to treat mood swings, fatigue, headache, breast pain and the general aches and pains which accompany PMS.[52] The series 2 prostaglandins cause vasodilation in the breast which leads to engorgement and pain. Prostaglandins inhibitors improve cyclic breast pain by reducing these effects. These drugs should be restricted to a seven day interval,[53] making them unsuitable for the many women who experience breast pain or PMS for more than seven days before their period.

Prostaglandins inhibitors do not reverse the prostaglandins imbalance which causes excessive menstruation, pain or PMS and will have to be used indefinitely until the cause/s of the imbalance are identified and rectified. This prospect is not appealing to many women, especially since these drugs have many side effects.

About 25 per cent of people using prostaglandins inhibitors experience side effects associated with the gastrointestinal system. Symptoms can include nausea, vomiting, stomach pain, indigestion, diarrhoea, heartburn, abdominal cramps, constipation, abdominal bloating and flatulence.[54] These drugs should always be taken with food to try to minimise the risk of gastric ulceration and should be avoided by women with a history of gastrointestinal disease.

A number of other complaints can be aggravated by the use of prostaglandins inhibitors and they may cause problems for those who have poor liver function, asthma, clotting disorders, lupus, and heart disease. Women with any of these disorders should seek medical advice before using these drugs. Prostaglandins inhibitors can mask the signs of infection and should not be taken when period pain is known or suspected to be caused by pelvic inflammatory disease.

Prostaglandins inhibitors are given to control symptoms and are only necessary while the complaint occurs. Slippery elm can help to prevent gastric ulceration associated with these drugs. One teaspoon mixed into apple juice, or equal quantities of apple juice mixed with yoghurt, and taken at the same time helps to protect the stomach lining.

Diuretics

Diuretics have been one of the most commonly prescribed drugs for bloating and breast tenderness associated with PMS, based on the assumption that increased levels of aldosterone in the premenstrual phase causes fluid retention. The results of trials using different types of diuretics has been conflicting, and due to a tendency for some women to take more tablets than recommended, their use has diminished.[55]

Some diuretics deplete potassium levels and supplements may be required, but ask the prescribing doctor first before self-prescribing. Herbal diuretics such as dandelion leaf, one or two teaspoons per cup, twice daily, is a suitable alternative. Dandelion leaf has high levels of potassium and additional supplements are not required.

Anti-depressants and anxiolytics

A variety of anti-depressants and anxiolytics (anti-anxiety drugs) are sometimes used for mood disorders associated with menstrual complaints, particularly PMS and around menopause. These symptomatic treatments are unacceptable to many women and are often not useful.

The minor tranquillisers, such as the benzodiazapines (Valium) may add to the fatigue and lethargy often associated with hormonal changes;[56] and when tri-cyclic anti-depressants or other major tranquillisers are prescribed for mood disorders, they must be taken continually and not just when symptoms worsen with hormonal fluctuations.

The herbal alternatives to reduce tension and the effects of stress are the nervines. These are milder in action than drugs and tend to have fewer side effects. They are described on page 199.

SURGERY

Hysteroscopy

A hysteroscope is a small pencil-sized instrument which is inserted into the cervix to view the inner cavity of the uterus. A general anaesthetic is recommended by most doctors because, unless the woman has given birth to at least one child, her cervix will be too small to pass the instrument through without considerable discomfort. Sometimes, however, a hysteroscopy is performed with a local anaesthetic in the specialist's rooms.

This procedure has the diagnostic advantage of being able to see which parts of the endometrium appear to be diseased. Prior to hysteroscopies, any procedures, such as a curette, were performed 'blind' which resulted in up to one quarter of pathologies being missed.

A diagnostic hysteroscopy is used before *any* treatment to exclude serious conditions when abnormal bleeding or other worrying symptoms are present, especially when women are over 40. It is performed by inflating the uterine cavity with gas so that a good view is possible. If hysteroscopic treatment is possible, for example, for the removal of uterine polyps, sub-mucous fibroids or abnormal tissue changes in the endometrium, the uterine cavity is distended with a viscous fluid to enable the doctor to successfully perform the operation.

The procedure is very short and only takes about half an hour. If a general anaesthetic has been used, a four-hour recovery time in hospital is necessary to observe for complications associated with the anaesthetic. Most women go home on the same day and feel completely well the next day following a hysteroscopy.

Laparoscopy

A laparoscopy is performed, either as a diagnostic or therapeutic procedure, with a laparoscope. This thin, pencil-like instrument has fibre-optics through which the operator can view the inner organs. The procedure requires a general anaesthetic, and a number of small incisions are made, usually one under the navel and another just above the pubic bone, to insert the laparoscope, so that a good view of all of the pelvic organs is possible.

Frequently, the abdomen is filled with gas so that the abdominal wall does not interfere with the surgeon's view of the pelvic contents. After the procedure, the gas is allowed to escape, but some may remain in the abdominal cavity and cause pain until it eventually dissipates after a few days. (Gas which is trapped under the diaphragm causes irritation of nerves and referred shoulder-tip pain.)

Laparoscopy has a number of advantages. An accurate diagnosis can be made because the gynaecologist can view the entire pelvic cavity. Additionally, minor surgical procedures can be performed during a laparoscopy such as laser or diathermy to burn patches of endometriosis, and the removal of small ovarian cysts or adhesions. These surgical procedures generally only involve a day in hospital; and pain and post-operative complications are minimal because major abdominal incisions are not required.

Recovery time is usually a few days depending on the extent of the additional surgery and the type of complaint treated. Even though the external wounds can be quite small, the internal organs might take a while to recover. Pain is a good indicator of how much to do and when rest is needed.

Laparotomy

A laparotomy involves an abdominal incision, usually just above the pubic bone and below 'the bikini line' and is indicated when extensive surgery is needed. This can include removal of extensive and inaccessible adhesions, removal of larger ovarian cysts (cysts larger than 3 mm are usually removed at laparotomy), diathermy or laser of extensive and difficult to reach endometriosis, or for reconstruction and microsurgery to improve fertility.

A laparotomy can take from between half an hour to several hours, depending on the type of surgery to be performed. Recovery time is longer than after a laparoscopy because the abdominal wounds are larger and the surgery is usually more extensive. The advice on pre- and post-operative care will be useful to improve recovery.

Endometrial ablation

An endometrial ablation is destruction of the lining of the uterus (endometrium) either with a laser or by cauterisation. It is usually performed for heavy bleeding and the preferred outcome is that only a little or no endometrium is left behind, and menstruation ceases.

There are many critics of this procedure, and disadvantages include a high failure rate. Menstruation often continues, especially when women have adenomyosis. For some though, when all other treatments have failed, this procedure offers a possible alternative to the conventional hysterectomy.

Myomectomy

A myomectomy is the surgical removal of a fibroid. It is usually performed through a laparotomy incision and can be a difficult operation to perform. A myomectomy is suggested when the woman wants to conserve her uterus, but the fibroid needs to be removed because of the following circumstances:

- the fibroid is larger than a 12–14 week pregnancy
- the fibroid is growing
- the fibroid is associated with heavy bleeding
- the fibroid is pedunculated (attached to a stem)
- the fibroid interferes with fertility

Surgery or not?
Size is often quoted as a reason for removing a fibroid, whether it is causing symptoms or not. In direct opposition to this recommendation, a recent comment in the *American Journal of Obstetrics and Gynecology* suggested that regardless of size, the presence and severity of significant symptoms 'should be the most important considerations in the individualisation of treatment strategies'.[57] In other words, if it's not causing problems, leave it alone.

Fibroids are also blamed for problems with fertility and removal is sometimes suggested before a woman tries to become pregnant, just in case. It is unlikely, however, that the fibroids will affect fertility and conception rates. The same study showed that there was an increased rate of Caesarean section when a woman has fibroids, particularly if they are situated in the lower portion of the uterus, but no change in fertility rate.[58] Women with fibroids have an increased risk of severe bleeding following childbirth, however, caused by the fibroid interfering with uterine contractions. The risks associated with pregnancy when women have fibroids need careful evaluation and the need for surgery should be discussed with all of these points in mind.

Myomectomy or hysterectomy?
For women past their child-bearing years or those not wishing to become pregnant a hysterectomy is usually recommended, but for others, a myomectomy (removal of the fibroid, but leaving the uterus in place) may be suggested. A myomectomy or hysterectomy may be performed as an abdominal operation or using laser surgery during a laparoscopy.

Some doctors are reluctant to perform a myomectomy, especially for women who do not want to have (more) children and may suggest a hysterectomy instead. It is difficult for even the most experienced gynaecologist to predict how easily a fibroid can be removed. Severe bleeding can occur and may mean that a hysterectomy will have to be performed anyway, and under less than optimum conditions. Sometimes the exact location of the fibroid will only be discovered during the surgery. It may be in a position where it is difficult to reach, or surrounded by delicate structures. It may be fed by more blood vessels than usual.

Other reasons for not wanting to perform a myomectomy are that the fibroids may grow back or the heavy menstrual bleeding associated with the fibroid prior to its removal may not stop. An unspoken reason for suggesting hysterectomy is the common medical opinion that women who do not intend to have a child have no need for a uterus. This, combined with the unpredictability of a myomectomy, means that a hysterectomy may be offered first and a myomectomy discussed only when the women requests the information.

This decision is often difficult for many women. When a hysterectomy has been advised, but is not a suitable option, a second opinion from a gynaecologist experienced in the technique of myomectomy is advisable. Removal of fibroids using laser is reported to decrease adhesion formation, reduce bleeding at the time of surgery and improve the fertility rate of women wanting to conceive.[59]

Sometimes a hysterectomy may be the only option. A myomectomy might just be too risky, complicated or unpredictable. There may be too many fibroids (although I do know of a 45-year-old woman whose gynaecologist removed 42 fibroids rather than perform a hysterectomy!) or there may be other gynaecological reasons why a hysterectomy is a better option.

Good pre-operative preparation is essential before major surgery and can greatly influence the recovery time (see page 404). Both hysterectomy and myomectomy are elective procedures and so it is possible to arrange an auto-transfusion (where a women gives her own blood some days before the operation and then is transfused with this blood during the procedure if bleeding occurs). A woman giving blood for an auto-transfusion should take iron supplements and increase her daily intake of iron-containing foods (see the information on iron on page 189).

Hysterectomy

A hysterectomy is the removal of the uterus and can be performed through an abdominal incision—an abdominal hysterectomy; or through the vagina—a vaginal hysterectomy. The decision to perform one over the other depends somewhat on the preference of the surgeon and on the type of condition present. A hysterectomy for endometriosis, for example, is often performed abdominally if there are multiple adhesions which make vaginal removal too difficult.

A hysterectomy is the removal of the uterus. When the uterus, tubes and ovaries are removed, the procedure is called a hysterectomy and bilateral salpingo-oopherectomy. A hysterectomy where the ovaries are left *in situ* is used for conditions like excessive menstrual loss, fibroids, prolapses, and when women have severe pain and bleeding associated with adenomyosis.

For conditions which are oestrogen-dependent, such as severe and non-responsive endometriosis and some types of cancer, a hysterectomy and uni/bilateral salpingo-oopherectomy is frequently recommended. Removing the ovaries can prevent or slow the growth of these oestrogen-sensitive tissues.

PREPARING FOR AN OPERATION

Recovery from any abdominal surgery, including a hysterectomy, myomectomy, laser surgery, laparotomy or Caesarean section can be improved by following a few pre-operative strategies to improve wound healing and reduce wound infections; assist with early post-operative mobility; and reduce the discomfort caused by bowel problems.

Vitamin C promotes collagen formation and has been shown to improve wound-healing time.[60] Zinc supplements also have a beneficial effect on wound healing and zinc as a topical lotion is one of the oldest wound-healing agents known. It was used as far back as 100 BC by the Egyptians in the form of calamine lotion to promote the healing of wounds. More than half of all Australian women consume less than the recommended daily intake for zinc and many vegetarians are zinc deficient. Surgery increases zinc requirements because zinc is needed to enhance cell proliferation during wound healing.[61] Pre-operative zinc supplements can be recommended for most women. Information on zinc is included in Chapter 7 'Adolescence'.

Vitamin A plays an important role in wound healing by increasing cellular activity required for repair. A post-operation supplement of vitamin A can also increase collagen synthesis, and improve the bursting strength of the scar. Vitamin A applied topically improves healing and the appearance of scars. A vitamin A deficiency usually occurs without symptoms. Dietary sources of vitamin A are full-cream dairy products, egg yolk, yellow and green vegetables, and yellow or orange fruit.[62]

Vitamin E, which prevents internal scar tissue formation (adhesions), is very beneficial when fertility must be conserved following surgery. Small doses of around 100–250 IU should be taken pre-operatively because of the (very slight) risk of increased bleeding during surgery. Once food is commenced following surgery doses of around 400–500 IU can be taken. Vitamin E can also be rubbed into the wound to hasten healing and reduce scarring. Oral vitamin E reduces the risk of post-operative blood clots.

Echinacea, a herb commonly used to improve resistance to infection, also seems to increase the formation of keloid scar tissue (thick, raised scars), and should be taken cautiously.

Poor muscle strength and agility can hamper recovery time post-operatively because getting out of bed and walking around is much more difficult. Weak leg and abdominal muscles can be improved pre-operatively by specific exercises such as yoga exercises, squats, walking, sit-ups and gym work. Being physically active post-operatively improves recovery time and stamina, and reduces the risk of blood clots and respiratory infections. About a month is usually needed to dramatically improve muscle strength, but even a few days is better than nothing.

Post-operative recovery can be hampered by the abdominal discomfort caused by the handling of the bowel during surgery. Fortunately, a few dietary changes in the *weeks prior to surgery* can often help to prevent or reduce the symptoms.

- The seed breakfast (page 230) should be started about one week before the operation and continued as soon as solid foods can be eaten after surgery.
- Daily salads of grated raw carrot and beetroot or a medium sized cooked beetroot to help prevent post-operative constipation.
- Yoghurt or cultured milk drinks colonise the bowel with healthy bacterial colonies and minimise flatulence. Drink or eat about one cup per day. Check that the yoghurt has live cultures and no sugar.
- Avoid refined sugars which tend to increase fermentation and flatulence.
- Avoid foods known to cause flatulence, constipation or diarrhoea.
- Pre- and post-operatively, three to six cups daily (two teaspoons of mixture per cup) of the herbal tea combination of equal parts of *Melissa officinalis*, *Matricaria recutita* and *Mentha piperita*. Make up a jar to take to hospital.
- Post-operative nausea is relieved by ginger root. Two studies which compared the degree of nausea experienced after a laparoscopy[63]

and major gynaecological surgery,[64] with and without ginger root, found that the women who were given ginger root had much less nausea than those given a placebo. The usual dose is between 0.5–1g every four hours in tablet form, or between 10–20 drops as a fluid extract, but check with the medical staff first.

CONVALESCENCE, OR MEETING THE DEMANDS OF STRESS

People have forgotten how to convalesce. With the increase in laser surgery, and shorter hospital stays, many women start housework or return to work within days of surgical procedures and then wonder why they spend the rest of the year feeling dreadful. The financial strains on the average household also mean a shortened convalescent period for many people.

Many women recovering from operations are astonished by their doctors' predictions of 'you'll be back at the gym in a week' or 'you'll be up and walking by tomorrow' when they feel nothing like going to the gym (or anything else for that matter). It may be worth pointing out that recovery times vary considerably and are influenced by factors such as smoking, lack of previous fitness, an inability to take it easy and let the body heal, or more surgery than was originally planned. It is better to be guided by pain and stamina and to do a little more every day than to resume former levels of work and exercise too quickly.

When the body is under stress or recovering from an illness, the nutrient requirements increase dramatically. Unfortunately, this often occurs at a time when the appetite is diminished and when there is little interest in food. Any stress, whether it be from surgery, burns, difficult times, a car accident, or excessive working, has a similar effect on the body.

Some general guidelines

- Requirements for all nutrients increase dramatically, but especially for protein, the B vitamins generally and particularly vitamin B_5 (pantothenic acid), vitamin C, and the minerals potassium, magnesium and zinc. A vitamin B complex tablet which has 50 mg of B_5 and B_6, with a multi-mineral supplement and 1–2 g of vitamin C can be used to supplement the diet.
- Rapid energy fluctuations can be reduced by eating small, but frequent meals of complex carbohydrate (potato, rice, bread, oat-

meal and pasta), combined with *small* amounts of protein such as yoghurt, cheese, tofu, hoummos, tuna or egg.

- Any food which acts as a 'body stressor', such as the stimulant caffeine and refined sugars should be avoided.
- Some exercise is vital. Exercise every second day allows for one day of recovery after energy expenditure. As strength improves, exercise every day will increase stamina and a sense of well-being.
  Exercise should be taken at a much slower pace. People tend to over-estimate their capabilities so a good rule of thumb is to start at *half* the level you imagine you could comfortably manage *now*; if it is too little, no harm will be done. Long slow distance exercise is best (see page 169).
- Simple, easily digested soups and 'energy drinks' provide concentrated nutrients.
- Have one serve of a cooked green *leafy* vegetable every day while in the recovery period such as spinach, Chinese cabbage or silverbeet.
- Never skip breakfast and have a cooked breakfast (oatmeal, egg on toast, cooked rice cereal, vegetable soup) at least every second day.
- Use the 'suggested menus' given for the hypoglycaemic diet (pages 129–30) as a basis for the diet with the additional recipes provided.

Suggested convalescent recipes

Soups

Soups are useful recovery foods. The best types are those based on grains, especially barley and rice; beans, such as tofu, orange lentils, fresh soya beans and red kidney beans; or root vegetables like potato, carrot and sweet potato.

Chicken broth
Many societies use chicken broth as a convalescent food. Use free-range chicken carcasses. The broth can be prepared with a particular flavour, for example, Thai (lemon grass, lime leaves, galangal, chilli), or Western (celery, bay leaves, onion, carrot and peppercorns).

High protein drinks

High protein drinks are useful meal substitutes or for between meals, particularly when digestion and appetite are poor.

Almond Smoothie
    1 tablespoon of almond meal
    1 teaspoon rice bran
    1 teaspoon wheatgerm
    1 cup soya milk (Bonsoy™, Aussie Soy™, Vitasoy™)
    1 teaspoon of malt extract

Blend all ingredients until smooth.

Variation
Substitute $\frac{1}{2}$ cup of yoghurt and $\frac{1}{2}$ cup fruit juice for the soya milk and malt extract.

Berry Drink
$\frac{1}{2}$ punnet blueberries, strawberries, raspberries or other berry fruit in season
$\frac{1}{2}$–$\frac{3}{4}$ cup yoghurt or soya milk (yoghurt and berries tends to be fairly tangy and may not be to everyone's liking)
2 teaspoons almond meal, ground cashews, or seeds (the 'seed mix' for irritable syndrome is suitable)

Blend all ingredients together until smooth.

Tofu Drink I
50 g soft tofu
6 dried apricots soaked overnight in 1 cup water
1 tablespoon almond meal
1 teaspoon slippery elm powder

Blend all ingredients together until smooth.

Tofu Drink II
50 g soft tofu
1 banana
1 teaspoon slippery elm powder (or 1 teaspoon rice bran)
2 teaspoons almond meal
1 cup fruit juice

Blend all ingredients together until smooth.

Tofu Drink III
50 g soft tofu
1 cup freshly squeezed orange juice
2–4 teaspoons almond meal
2–4 teaspoons ground cashew nuts or seed mix
1 teaspoon slippery elm powder

Blend all ingredients together until smooth.

Appendix

Patterns of disharmony

The qualities

Heat

Heat, like all of the qualities, is vital to life. In balanced degree, Heat is necessary for good health and the normal functioning of the organs.

Excess heat
The state of imbalance associated with excesses of Heat is caused by inappropriate diet, lack of fluids, constipation, exposure to the elements, or extreme emotions. Heat which has been introduced into the body due to Hot foods, exposure to too much sun, or hot weather is common and easily recognised. Internal Heat, caused by pent-up emotions, failure to eliminate toxins (constipation) or excess activity are more complex presentations of disharmony which are often referred to as 'Hot blood' or 'Heat in the blood'. People with a temperament related to excess Heat are usually called 'hot-blooded', referring to their impulsiveness, to their sexual appetite or their bad temper.

Abnormal bleeding, pelvic inflammatory disease (PID), and some cervical and vaginal infections are examples of conditions women might experience that are associated with excess Heat. Other symptoms are described below.

Visible signs
- The body and face are hot to the touch, and the face is red
- Perspiration is increased
- A tendency to develop red and inflamed skin eruptions
- Respiratory tract infections are accompanied by fevers, inflamed mucous membranes and may either be Moist or Dry
- Discharges are likely to be thick and yellow, often with a foul odour
- The urine is dark, scant and strong smelling

- There is a tendency to Heat signs in the upper body (heat rises)
- Hot disorders may either be associated with Heat alone, Heat with Moistness, or Heat with Dryness
- The tongue is red and often dry, rough or coated with yellow fur
- The pulse is rapid. It may be full or thready depending on the strength of the individual

Symptoms
- Sensation of being uncomfortably hot
- Symptoms aggravated by heat
- Fatigue similar to the tiredness felt on a very hot day, feeling drained, depleted and too tired to move about (physical activity generates more heat and aggravates the symptoms)
- Thirst, especially for cold drinks
- Burning and irritation which can affect any of the mucous membranes, or organs. Examples might be burning stomach pain, burning and dry nose or eyes, burning and discomfort on passing urine, hot and burning passage of stool, hot and painful throat
- Coughs tend to be dry and irritating, perhaps with some expectoration of blood
- Constipation
- Headaches which are relieved by cool applications
- Increased libido
- Pain described as burning and/or throbbing
- Bitter taste in the mouth; bad breath

Preferences
- A liking for cold foods or drink, cold applications, cool weather; dislike of spicy and hot (temperature) foods, drinks, applications
- Dislike of summer and hot weather

Temperament
- Heat is an aspect of the Sanguine and the Choleric temperaments An abundance of Heat will tend to contribute to the enthusiasm, impulsiveness and ardour of the Sanguine individual, and make the Choleric type more irascible and quick-tempered
- A Hot person is likely to overreact to emotional experiences, have difficulty with relaxing and sleeping, or dream vividly

In gynaecology
- Heat is frequently associated with abnormal bleeding or infections
- Menstrual bleeding is usually heavier, and brighter, and may contain many small clots
- Infections are associated with symptoms of burning, throbbing or itching
- Vaginal discharges are usually yellowish, irritating and may have an offensive odour

Outcome
- Excess Heat will eventually cause Dryness as the body fluids dissipate
- An extreme form of Heat, caused by exposure to the elements or an external heat source, can cause high fever, red and dry skin, restlessness or lassitude, and eventually loss of consciousness. This is common in heat stroke
- In extreme and prolonged cases of Heat, the disharmony will eventually become Cold due to diminishing stores of vitality caused by the frantic activity of the Heat

Common problems with diagnosis
Although it is common to associate infections with Heat, many people with quite severe infections will not have any of the symptoms outlined above. This is true of conditions like PID which, although caused by an infection, may not be accompanied by any of the signs or symptoms of Heat. PID of this type is likely to be associated with other types of disharmony and the treatment will need to reflect the rectification of the appropriate imbalance.

The symptoms of abnormal sweating and hot flushes encountered during times of debility, anxiety, and at menopause, at first glance, would appear to be caused by Heat. More often, however, they are the body's reaction to an abnormal situation, and cannot be seen to represent a condition in and of themselves. If all of the other symptoms point to other qualities predominating in the symptom picture, for example, when a woman with hot flushes talks of Cold symptoms, these are likely to represent the true picture for that individual. (Also discussed in the sections on adrenal exhaustion, neurasthenia and menopause.)

Cold

Cold provides balance to Heat. Cold generally reduces activity of the organs and the mind, thereby allowing rest, recuperation and harmony in the body's activities.

Excess Cold
Problems occur when Cold is either introduced into the body or develops as a result of lack of Heat and vitality. Introduced Cold is frequently associated with exposure to the cold weather, sudden temperature changes from hot to cold, drinking too many iced drinks, or eating cold foods such as ice-cream, cucumber and watermelon. It is easier for a person to suffer from a disharmony associated with Cold if they are already depleted in vitality or Heat.

Introduced Cold will affect the part of the body which has been most exposed to its influence: the stomach and bowel if Cold foods have been eaten, the limbs and lungs if a person was exposed to cold weather. 'Internal' Cold conditions associated with a lack of vitality and

Heat (in other words, those not introduced by an external factor) will tend to sink and cause disharmony in the lower body.

As one of the causes of disharmony in gynaecology, Cold can present in one of two ways. It can be seen as an indication of the lack of Heat, often associated with poor vitality; or as an externally introduced factor which has the potential to aggravate a condition, or in some cases, cause one. Historically, the problem of Cold for women was acknowledged by recommending that menstruating women should not swim, get cold, sit on cold ground or eat cold food. Of course, many of these recommendations became confused with social mores, and many of them have been abandoned today as 'old wives tales'. However, for women who lack vital energy, and for whom the spectre of Cold as an externally introduced aggravating factor is real, these early prescriptions are still useful.

Visible signs
- The face is blanched or pale
- There is evidence of poor circulation with cold limbs and extremities, purple nail beds, diminished mental ability
- The skin is mottled, purplish or white, and cold to the touch
- Respiratory tract infections tend to become 'catarrhal'
- Chills are more frequent than fevers
- Discharges tend to be clear or white and copious
- There are frequent urges to pass urine, without pain or discomfort
- Large volumes of pale urine are passed
- Complaints associated with part of body exposed to cold, or predominantly to the lower portions of the body
- Disorders caused by Cold may either be associated with Cold alone, Cold and Moistness, or Cold and Dryness
- The tongue is pale and sometimes large, with a white coat
- The pulse tends to be slow, deep and thin

Symptoms
- There is an unusual dislike of cold either in the form of food, drink, weather, draughts, or changes in weather from hot to cold
- The person tends to feel chilled, and wears more clothes than others. There is difficulty getting warm even with increased clothing
- All complaints are aggravated by cold
- There is a tendency to be fatigued, especially where the Cold is caused by a diminution of the vitality and Heat
- There is a diminished desire for fluids, or a desire only for warm drinks
- Pain is strong, and tends to remain in one position (fixed). It is either colicky or stabbing
- Digestion is poor and the appetite diminished. Bloating is common
- Poor libido
- Joints are stiff and painful to move, especially in cold weather

Preferences
- A tendency to want hot or spicy foods, with an aversion to salads and cold foods generally
- Likes baths and hot applications
- Suffers more in winter

Temperament
- Cold is an aspect of the Melancholic and Phlegmatic temperaments. Excess Cold will tend to cause the Phlegmatic individual to become fixed in their opinions and pragmatic; or even to become mentally dull and slow. The Melancholic is liable to slip into deep depression or to exhibit signs of catatonic and withdrawn behaviour
- There is the inclination to brood, withdraw, become pensive and to have a poor memory. Sleep is often taken in excess and there is difficulty waking or remaining alert

In gynaecology
- Menstrual pain which tends to be intense and relieved by heat
- Bleeding which is characterised by dark or clotted blood which flows slowly and is accompanied by pain
- Periods are inclined to be late, or cycles too long
- Vaginal discharges are usually copious, white and non-irritating

Outcome
- Response to illness tends to be slow, 'chronic' and be characterised by underactivity of the body
- Cold conditions may become Cold and Moist over time. The reduction in bodily functions, particularly the weakening of digestion and elimination, lead to an accumulation of 'toxins' in the gut and eventually, catarrhal complaints
- Similarly Cold conditions may become Cold and Dry over time
- The cycle of transmutation may continue, and a Cold and Moist disorder might become eventually Moist and Hot; a Cold and Dry disorder might change to Dry and Hot

Common problems with diagnosis
The most difficult interpretation of Cold disorders is whether they are predominantly introduced or related to an internal weakness of vitality and Heat. In reality, the two conditions intermingle, since introduced Cold will affect an individual who is already depleted much more easily. Cold associated with a lack of Heat and vitality will require tonics to improve vitality, restore Heat, and replenish the Blood (which is Hot and Moist), as well as warming herbs and foods.

Moist

Moistness is an essential quality to lubricate the tissues and organs and to facilitate elimination from the body.

Excess Moistness

('Moist' is the term favoured by Culpeper and other writers of the humoral theory, and will be used here instead of Damp which is used in Traditional Chinese Medicine. Related terms are 'catarrh' and 'lymphatic congestion' which are descriptions of conditions rather than qualities.)

Excesses of Moisture are associated with any condition which is characterised by too much fluid, with puffiness, fluid retention and deranged digestion with a tendency to diarrhoea. There is a tendency to discharges; poor resistance to infections; poor elimination accompanied by foul body odours; flatulence; bad breath and fluid retention.

Excessive Moistness causes swelling and heaviness, makes movement difficult and results in sluggishness of the mental faculties as well as the body. It can be caused by over-eating; eating rich, fatty or sweet food; humid weather; prolonged immersion in water; working or living in a damp environment; sedentary lifestyle; or emotional turmoil.

As with the other qualities, excess Moistness can be externally acquired or can result from disharmony within the body. The dietary excesses and environmental factors described above are examples of introduced Moisture; while physical underactivity, emotional lability, poor vitality, lack of Heat, and faulty elimination are both the causes and effects of 'internal' Moisture.

Women who suffer from an excess of the Moist quality will have vaginal discharges, obvious mucus in their menstrual blood, and will often suffer greatly if they develop PMT. Their fluid retention will be pronounced; they will become tired, muddled-headed, clumsy; and they will often suffer from thick, heavy headaches with nausea and vomiting (migraines).

Moistness is a passive quality and will usually combine with one of the active qualities, Heat or Cold. (The additional quality will be included, where relevant, in brackets.)

Visible signs
- The complexion is greasy, oily and sallow
- Skin diseases are characterised by watery blisters, ulcers and abscesses with oozing discharge
- Complaints tend to be accompanied by thick coloured mucus (Heat) or clear, or white mucus (Cold)
- Discharges and bodily excretions are often offensive (Heat)
- Moisture settles and is often found in the lower body (especially if associated with Cold)
- The urine is cloudy with mucus and a strong smell (Heat)
- The pulse slippery and rapid (Heat) or slow and deep (Cold)
- The tongue is wet with a thick mucous-like white coat (Cold) or a greasy yellow coat (Heat)

Symptoms
- The preference is for dry and hot weather and there is an unusual dislike of wet or cold places and weather (Cold)

  Or
- There is an unusual aversion to hot and humid weather, hot baths, and steam rooms, and attraction to dry and cool environments (Heat)
- Fatigue and debility is accompanied by heaviness of the limbs. This is often described as a sensation of walking through glue or treacle
- The joints are sore and stiff
- Tiredness and stiffness worsens with rest, and gradually improves with movement (especially with Cold)
- The head is heavy and thick, sometimes with a sense of the head being tightly bound
- The appetite is diminished with nausea and indigestion, particularly from eating rich or fatty foods or alcohol (Heat)
- Any pain is dull, persistent and congestive. Moisture combined with Cold causes sharper and crampy pain; if mingled with Heat, the pain will tend to have the characteristics of burning and stabbing
- There is fullness and bloating in the chest, stomach and abdomen
- Diarrhoea will be either copious, possibly containing mucous (Cold); or burning and offensive (Heat)
- Resistance to, and recovery from infections tends to be poor
- Eliminative processes are often faulty resulting in constipation and fluid retention or oedema
- Diseases of the liver and gall bladder are often associated with Moist and Hot disorders
- Excessive amounts of sleep are needed but this does not refresh or improve fatigue
- The eyelids are puffy on waking

Preferences
- Wants sour, salty and hot foods (Cold and Moist)

  Or
- Craves sour, cold and bitter foods (Hot and Moist)

Temperaments
- Moisture affects the Phlegmatic (Cold and Moist) and Sanguine (Hot and Moist) temperaments. Because an increase in Moisture slows and calms mental faculties, the Sanguine temperament will be less optimistic, ardent and courageous; while the Phlegmatic type will become more inclined to dullness of thought and more set in their ways

In gynaecology
- Vaginal discharges can be of the Hot and Moist type: thick, yellow, corrosive and offensive; or of the Cold and Moist type: bland, white or clear leucorrhoea

- Fungal infections, especially thrush or Candida will be very irritating if associated with Heat, and have a copious, less irritant discharge if associated with Cold
- PMT symptoms are associated with heaviness, clumsiness fluid retention, bloating, headaches, skin eruptions and fatigue

Outcome
- Symptoms tend to linger and are difficult to eradicate
- Excess Moisture gives rise to conditions that are turbid and foul in nature. It arises from sluggish bodily functions, as well as making the bodily functions slow down

Dry

Dryness is the counterbalance to Moisture in the body. It regulates the fluid balance and allows for dispersion and lightness.

Excess Dryness
The quality of Dryness may be introduced into the body as a result of excessively Dry and often windy weather, Drying foods, inappropriate fasting, or lack of nutritious food. In other circumstances, a lack of fluids bought about by excessive Heat, by excessive physical activity (causing a loss of body fluids), or extreme emotions, may cause Dryness to appear.

Gynaecological conditions associated with Dryness are usually associated with excesses of both the Cold and Dry qualities, brought about because of an absence of Heat and Moisture (Blood). This can cause late and scanty periods, while excessive menstrual loss may be one of the causes of a relative preponderance of Cold and Dry.

Dry is a passive quality and will combine with Heat or Cold. Where appropriate, these are indicated in brackets.

Visible signs
- The skin is dry, rough and chapped and readily absorbs oils, ointments or creams
- The mouth, mucus membranes, nose and lips are dry, cracked and chaffed
- The eyes are often dry and red (Heat)
- Inflamed, dry and itchy skin or mucus membranes; or tissues which crack and bleed indicate Dryness with Heat
- If Cold is a factor, the skin is dry, pale, scaly and cold. This is particularly apparent on the lower extremities
- Respiratory tract infections are characterised by difficulty in breathing in dry environments, wheezing, shortness of breath, dry throat, dry cough with little phlegm. The presence of blood indicates Heat
- The tongue is dry and red (Heat) or pale (Cold)
- The pulse is indistinct and either rapid (Heat) or slow (Cold)

Symptoms
- Dislikes dry, windy weather
- Conditions will tend to worsen in autumn
- There is a preference for humid and wet weather rather than hot and dry or cold and dry seasons
- The thirst cannot be easily satisfied
- Conditions may be accompanied by muscle-wasting and weakness
- The bones are often weak and fragile as is seen in osteoporosis
- Allergic conditions such as allergic rhinitis, conjunctivitis and dry eczema predominate, and the symptoms tend to worsen in autumn
- Insomnia associated with Heat is caused by a lack of the quietening and relaxing qualities of Cold and Moist
- The stools are dry
- There is poor resistance to infections of the skin, mucus membranes and respiratory tract due to breaches in the continuity of the tissues caused by Dryness

Preferences
- Unusual dislike of dry foods
- Unusual and insatiable thirst
- Often takes baths, goes swimming
- Likes to be near water and in moist environments

Temperaments
- Dryness is associated with the Choleric and Melancholic temperaments. Excess of Dryness will diminish the creativity of the Melancholic type and increase the irritability of the Choleric type.

In gynaecology
- The Blood Humour is both Hot and Moist, and excess loss of Blood will cause a relative excess of the Cold and Dry qualities. This is likely to mean that women will have fewer periods, lower libido and have a heavy and cold sensation in the lower abdomen
- Alternatively, excess of the Cold and Dry qualities from other causes outlined above can be a cause of infrequent or absent menstruation
- Excess of Hot and Dry qualities may be associated with small, sticky and dark clots in the menstrual blood, and with burning, smarting or stitch-like pains

Outcome
- Dryness is most likely to transform into Heat because of the drying of the body fluids
- However, when the Dryness is associated with loss of the Blood Humour, Coldness and Dryness will predominate and this may eventually transform into a Cold and Moist disharmony, particularly if the Blood loss is pronounced and the vitality is diminished.

Rules governing the qualities

The qualities Hot, Cold, Dry and Moist are governed by a number of rules:

- One quality cannot form an element: elements consist of two qualities combined in various proportions
- Hot and Cold are the active qualities, while Dry and Moist are passive
- Hot and Cold are opposites as are Dry and Moist
- An active quality will combine with a passive one, but not with its opposite quality. That is Hot cannot combine directly with Cold; Dry cannot combine directly with Moist
- It is not possible for more than two qualities to combine in one element since opposites will come together and cancel each other out
- Adjacent qualities intermingle to create the elements: Hot and Dry produce Fire; Cold and Moist produce Water; Hot and Moist produce Air; Cold and Dry produce Earth

The elements

Of the elements, Air and Fire are light and tend to move upwards. They are the positive and active elements. Earth and Water are heavy; they tend to move downwards and are the negative, passive elements. In a diagnostic sense, this means that Air and Fire tend to be related to conditions that are quick to develop, that affect the upper body and that are associated with overactivity, inflammation, fever and infection. Water and Earth tend to be related to conditions that are associated with slow-moving complaints of a more chronic nature, with constriction, slowing down and signs of underactivity.

Fire

Fire is described as the most rarefied and light of the elements. It is composed of the Hot and Dry qualities and is always represented as being above the other elements. It prevails over Cold and permeates Air, with which it has much in common. Its active, positive and dispersive attributes lessen solidity and encourage the intermingling of the humours. Fire refines the mind and bestows drive, energy, passion and wakefulness. It is related to Yellow Bile and the Choleric temperament.

Air

Air is seen to be Hot and Moist and is related to Blood and the Sanguine temperament. Its natural tendency is to float and to dissipate, ensuring lightness and ease of movement. The Moistness of Air dispels the Dryness of Fire, and it overcomes the Dry and Cold attributes of its opposite, Earth. With Water it shares the Moist quality, but its Heat counterbalances the tendency of Water to become Cold and stagnant. Air confers the characteristics of quickness, passion and courage to the temperament. It is depicted as being above Earth and Water, but below Fire.

Water

Water is comprised of the Cold and Moist qualities and has the tendency to flow, change in shape and disperse. It is found between Air and Earth in nature and is related to the Phlegmatic temperament and the Phlegm humour. Its passive and Cold qualities impart an inclination to moderate bodily processes, to soothe and to reduce inflammation. Water adds Moistness to Earth and gives it form; dampens the Heat and Dryness of Fire; and calms the Heat of Air. Water imparts calm, peaceful and passive attributes to the character.

Earth

Although Earth is said to be below all of the other elements, it is central to life. Earth gives the body form and solidity. It is passive, Cold and Dry; and by far, the heaviest of the elements. Because of its solidity, it attracts all of the other elements to it: Earth modifies the Heat of the Fire element; the Moistness of the Water element; and counterbalances the light, floating and insubstantial qualities of the Air element. Although inclined to changeability, Earth imparts insight, vision and intellectual brilliance to the mental capacities.

Rules governing the elements

Like the qualities, the elements Fire, Earth, Air and Water are governed by a number of rules:
- All earthly things consist of the four elements combined in various proportions
- Fire and Water are opposites, as are Earth and Air; and both pairs are mutually exclusive
- The elements adjacent to one another share one quality; Fire and Earth share Dry; Earth and Water share Cold; Water and Air share Moist; and Air and Fire share Hot
- Hot dominates dry in the Fire element; Moist dominates Heat in the Air element; Cold is dominant over Moist in the Water element; and Dry dominates over Cold in the Earth element
- Each of the elements endeavours to behave naturally: Fire tries to rise, Water wants to flow, Air to float, and Earth to fall
- The relative preponderance of one quality in relation to another may alter allowing one element to transform into another and eventually even into its opposite element
- Irrespective of the transformation of one element into another, the

worldwide quantity of any given element will remain the same. (This is similar to the first law of thermodynamics.)

- Elemental opposites are kept apart by the force of repulsion, which causes disease and degeneration; and are brought together by the force of attraction bringing health and regeneration
- Attraction and repulsion wax and wane over the seasons and the throughout the life cycle, creating an oscillation like that between Yin and Yang
- Elemental opposites are connected by the intermediate element and the qualities they share: Fire is connected to Air and Earth by the qualities of Heat and Dryness; Earth to Fire and Water because it shares Cold and Dry; Water is connected to Earth and Air because of the qualities Coldness and Moisture; and Air is connected to Water and Fire because of the qualities Moistness and Heat

The humours

The 'body fluids' known as the humours are Blood, Phlegm, Yellow Bile, and Black Bile. They are believed to arise from the liver, and from the ingestion, digestion and evacuation of food and medicine. When any of the aspects of life become unbalanced; if for example, there is not enough rest, the diet is inappropriate, or evacuation is impaired, there is a corresponding imbalance in the humours and disease occurs. The inherent strength of the body determines whether the person succumbs to the disease, and the relative strength of the organs determines its type and location.

Identifying and correcting humoral imbalance continues to be an important aspect of diagnosis and treatment in the Unani Tibb system of medicine.

Blood

According to the humoral theory, Blood is made from the best quality, thoroughly digested foods (Culpeper says 'blood is made of meat perfectly concocted'). It is then transmuted into flesh, and the normal bodily secretions, including sperm, menstrual blood and breast milk (which was believed to be blood with the redness taken out). Blood humour improves the judgement and fortifies the digestion. It is carried by the blood vessels and through them, is dispersed throughout the body. It is Hot and Moist.

Phlegm

Phlegm humour is described as being made from the not so perfectly digested and next-best quality food. It makes the sweat, saliva, mucus and digestive juices and it is normally found in the lungs. Phlegm is believed to stabilise the emotions and the mind, and to prevent the irritability associated with Yellow Bile because of its Cooling and Moistening effect. Phlegm humour assists with elimination of wastes by allowing the bowels to function normally and mucus to be cleared from the respiratory passages. It is Cold and Moist.

Yellow bile

This humour is thought to be made from the coarser and less refined nutrients. It makes the bile, is stored in the gall bladder and strengthens the body's ability to assimilate nutrients. Yellow bile dispels apprehension and provides the necessary qualities for continued activity. Through these attributes, it is believed to give courage and passion. It warms the body and is Hot and Dry.

Black bile

Black Bile is composed of the least digestible and least nutritious part of food. It is stored in the spleen and strengthens the body's ability to retain food until it can be properly digested. It is seen to affect the temperament by fortifying the memory and improving the ability to concentrate and study. It calms lust and conveys a solid and steady quality to the personality. It is Cold and Dry.

The temperaments

The temperament is the personality expressed according to the humoral prevalence and provides a theoretical basis for interpreting the intellect and the emotions. Much of the following is adapted from the writings of Hildegard of Bingen who gave a detailed account of how the four temperaments specifically influence a woman's personality, her sexual behaviour and her reproductive capacity.

Sanguine

The sanguine type is described as being optimistic, courageous, hopeful, and amorous. This temperament is associated with Blood, the element Air and comprised of the Hot and Moist qualities. Women of this temperament were often described as being well-mannered and serene. They were seen to have few gynaecological complaints, normal periods and few difficulties with fertility.

Choleric

A choleric person is described as impatient, passionate, quick to anger, bilious and irritable. They are inclined to a sallow complexion, and are physically inclined to be well-built but slender. Both Hildegard and the unknown author of the *Medieval Woman's Guide to Health* describe choleric women as being subject to heavy periods with hot, red and fiery blood.

Phlegmatic

The phlegmatic temperament is represented in the even-tempered, serene individual. They are governed by the phlegmatic humour, the Water element and the Cold and Moist qualities. Their periods are not excessively troublesome, flowing neither too much or too lightly, and they are usually of an average build.

Melancholic

Melancholic individuals are ruled by Black Bile, the element Earth and the Cold and Dry qualities. They are often described as being intellectually gifted, creative and inclined to be spiritual. Of all of the temperaments, the melancholic is inclined to have more difficulty with heavy periods and infertility. They are physically weaker too, and often succumb to illness especially when depressed.

Physiology according to the humoral theory

The humoral theory, like other traditional medicines, describes a system of 'forces' which govern the overall functioning of the body and maintain a state of equilibrium. The three physiological forces, the vital spirit, the *anima*, and the natural spirit, are known variously as 'the forces of conservation' (Culpepper), the 'three natural faculties' (Unani Tibb), or the three treasures, *san bao* (Chinese medicine). These three physiological forces are inseparable and interdependent; an absence of one or more is incompatible with life.

Pneuma is the primary generative energy, usually described as being of cosmic origin, which both creates and governs the physiological forces. (See Figure A:1)

In the humoral theory, the vital spirit is housed in the heart, circulated throughout the body by the arteries, where it oversees the 'administering qualities of attraction, digestion, retention and expulsion. It gives rise to consciousness of self and the emotions.

The *anima* or soul spirit (called the animal spirit by Culpeper), resides in the brain and governs consciousness and the five senses. It is conveyed via the nervous system.

The natural spirit, housed in the liver, controls the production of the four humours and is the basis for vitality, growth and reproduction. The humours were believed to be conveyed throughout the body by the veins.

The concept of some form of vital force has informed the practice of natural medicine worldwide: in many traditions it has been associated with a deity, the sun or some other cosmic force. Whatever the origin

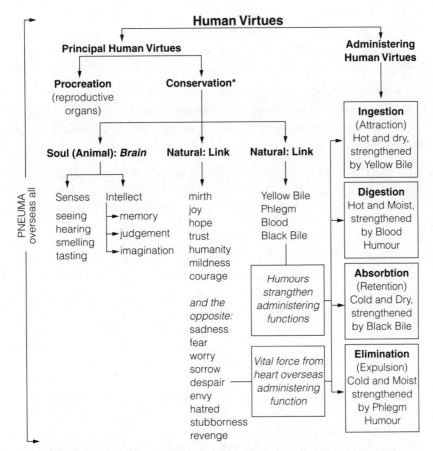

Figure A.I Physiology according to the humoral theory

* Conservation refers to the doctrine of preservation of energy such that the total energy of any system of bodies can be neither increased nor diminished.

Figure A.I Physiology according to the humoral theory

of this energy, its very existence has stimulated spirited debate for centuries. The contemporary argument revolves around what has been referred to as the mechanistic theory and the vitalistic theory.

Mechanism believes that life is dependent on the complexity of the arrangement of the organism: the more complex the organism the more complicated the arrangement of parts. Vitalism takes this theory one step further with the belief that a 'vital force' is necessary for this complex arrangement of parts to function.

At a very fundamental level, the vitalism of an organism is seen to be that factor which defines the difference between life and death; the force that allows a particular collection of organs, cells and structures to continue to grow and organise itself in a coherent and coordinated manner. For natural therapists, it is the vital force, and not the complexity of the arrangement of the organs and cells which governs an individual's unique complexity. The vital force is also inherently corrective, and throughout life it seeks to achieve a state of homeostasis through repair and reorganisation. Its ability to do this is dependent upon its quality and strength, which are themselves reliant on a number of factors:

- the amount of vitality inherited from one's forebears
- the amount generated from the digestion and assimilation of food
- the amount remaining after the demands of daily living, stress or disease processes.

The vital energy determines the way in which an individual will react to disease: will they recover quickly and completely as would a vital and healthy person, or will disease or vague ill-health linger interminably?

An individual with poor vitality might be easily fatigued, unusually weak or always unwell. Any or all of the body's recuperative, defensive, digestive or reproductive functions may be underactive. They may have complaints which come on after physical exertion or any expenditure of energy. Their mental capacity and memory is often diminished; their eyes are dull and lack the sparkle of the healthy person. They may have a large moist tongue. Their vitality, stamina and physical strength is poor and they usually feel the cold easily since vitality generates heat.

Over the normal lifetime the vitality or pneuma is gradually whittled away. This process is accelerated by poor eating, an unhealthy lifestyle, illness and the normal wear and tear on the body; and slowed down by reducing stress, eating well, exercise, and freedom from ill-health.

All traditional medicine, which is based on a belief in vitalistic concepts, strives to maintain and support the individuals inherent vital energy, qi or prana. Central to this theme is that medicines should do no harm, and that correctly administered, they will assist with the conservation of, or the return to, a state of health.

Glossary

abortifacient an agent which is used to terminate a pregnancy.

adaptogen a non-toxic substance that increases resistance to physical, environmental, emotional or biological stressors; a substance which can help to re-establish normal physiological function.

adenoma a benign tumour in which the cells form recognisable glandular structures.

adenomyoma a well-defined and benign tumour-like mass which forms in the uterine muscle.

adenomyosis the growth of abnormally-situated endometrium between the muscle fibres of the uterus.

adhesions scar tissue which forms internally after trauma, infection or blood loss.

aldosterone a hormone secreted by the adrenal gland which regulates water and electrolyte balance.

alpha-linolenic acid first omega-3 fatty acid found in linseeds, canola, walnut and soya bean oils.

amenorrhoea the absence of the period for six months during the menstrual years or the failure to commence menstruation.

anabolic constructive metabolism; growth-promoting.

androgen hormone produced by both men and women with masculinising effects when present in large quantities. Women secrete androgens from their ovaries and adrenal glands.

androgenic alopecia male pattern baldness, usually an inherited trait.

androgenising drug a drug which produces masculinising effects such as hirsutism, deepening of the voice, clitoral enlargement, atrophy of the breasts, weight gain and acne.

androstenedione androgen, weaker than testosterone, secreted by the ovary and adrenal gland (and testes in men).

anodyne an agent with pain-relieving properties.

anorexia nervosa an eating disorder characterised by extreme weight loss.

anovulatory not associated with the release of an ovum.

anti-haemorrhagic a agent which can stop bleeding.

anti-oestrogen an agent that blocks the action of oestrogen by competing for receptor binding sites. Examples are the phyto-oestrogens and the drug tamoxiphen.

anti-oxidant food or herbal component which protects against oxidation and free radical damage.

antispasmodic an agent that relieves or prevents smooth or skeletal muscle spasm.

anxiety depression a depressive state accompanied by anxiety.

arachidonic acid an omega-6 fatty acid found in cell membranes of animals.

aromatase an enzyme which converts androgens to oestrogens.

aromatisation an enzymatic process which occurs in adipose tissue, muscle and in the ovary, leading to the conversion of androgens to oestrogens.

astringent (herbal medicine) a herb which stops bleeding or discharge from tissues via a tissue 'tightening' effect.

atherosclerosis a condition involving the deposition of cholesterol-containing plaques in arteries.

auto-immune disease a condition characterised by the immune system reacting against the body's tissues.

basal body temperature the temperature of the body at complete rest; taken first thing in the morning after sleep.

beta-carotene a provitamin that is converted to vitamin A in the liver and intestines. Found in many green leafy and yellow vegetables.

beta-glucuronidase an enzyme produced by intestinal bacteria that converts oestrogen into the (deconjugated) form that can be absorbed from the bowel.

beta-hydrogenase an enzyme vital to the production of oestrogen in the ovary.

beta-sitosterol a steroid-like substance of plant origin.

biochanin A one of the isoflavone phyto-oestrogens found in soya products and a number of other plants.

bioflavonoid a group of compounds, widely distributed in plants, that maintain the health of small blood vessel walls.

biopsy a procedure where a small sample of tissue is taken for examination and identification.

bitters herbs or foods that has a bitter taste; Liver herbs.

body mass index (BMI) a value obtained by dividing the weight in kilograms by the height in metres squared. Used as a means of assessing the relative health risks of being above or below average weight for body height.

bone density ratio of bone mass to bone volume.

bulimia nervosa an eating disorder characterised by intermittent feasting, vomiting and fasting.

caffeine a stimulating and diuretic substance found in a number of plants, including tea and coffee.

carcinogen any cancer-producing substance.

cardiovascular disease a disease process affecting the heart and blood vessels.

carminative a medicine that relieves flatulence, and assuages gastric and abdominal discomfort.

cellulose a type of plant fibre.

chloasma well-defined, patchy area of increased pigmentation, usually distributed over the cheeks and forehead, and sometimes on the upper lip and neck. Frequently associated with pregnancy, menopause and the Pill. Also called the 'mask of pregnancy'.

chromium one of the trace minerals necessary for health.

climacteric medical term for the peri-menopause.

Cold (humoral theory) one of the four qualities.

competitive inhibition the process whereby one substance prevents another from occupying receptor binding sites and where the receptor is unable to respond in the same way, resulting in an inhibition of some process.

congestive dysmenorrhoea period pain described as aching, heavy and/or dragging.

conjugated oestrogen oestrogen excreted by pregnant mares in their urine. Administered orally as hormone replacement therapy, e.g. Premarin.

corpus albicans literally, the 'white body'. This is the scar left on the ovary after ovulation.

corpus luteum the 'yellow body' which is the structure left after ovulation has occurred and which is responsible for the secretion of oestrogen and progesterone.

cortisol The major glucocorticoid hormone secreted by the adrenal cortex; the body's own cortisone. During periods of stress, cortisol levels increase dramatically, primarily affecting carbohydrate metabolism, muscle tone, circulation, reaction to injury and the immune response.

coumestan plant compound, structurally similar to isoflavones, which possesses oestrogenic activity. The important coumestan is coumestrol.

coumestrol a phyto-oestrogen found in legumes; the amount increases when the legume is sprouting.

cystadenoma a cystic tumour composed of glandular tissue that can occur in the ovary.

D&C a surgical procedure performed under a general anaesthetic where the lining of the uterus is removed and/or biopsied.

daidzein one of the isoflavone phyto-oestrogens which is converted by intestinal bacteria to equol.

danazol (Danocrine) a progestogen which can cause pronounced androgenic effects.

deconjugated oestrogen the form of oestrogen produced by the action of enzymes present in intestinal bacteria, which can be reabsorbed from the bowel.

dehydroepiandrosterone an androgen.

diagnostic D&C see D&C.

diethylstilboestrol (DES) a synthetic oestrogen.

dihydrotestosterone a powerful androgenic hormone.

dihydroxytestosterone an androgen.

docosahexaenoic acid (DHA) the fatty acid which is the last step in the omega-3 pathway; found in fish.

dopamine a central nervous system neurotransmitter, also known as prolactin-inhibiting factor.

Dry (humoral theory) one of the four qualities.

dydrogesterone a progestogen which has mild androgenic effects, e.g. Duphaston.

dysmenorrhoea painful menstruation, usually associated with colicky pain.

eicosanoids a class of biologically active hormone-like compounds which include the prostaglandins, leukotrienes and thromboxanes.

eicosapentaenoic acid (EPA) an omega-3 fatty acid found in fish, which has many therapeutic properties.

elements (humoral theory) the basic building blocks of the universe: Earth, Air, Fire and Water.

embryo a fertilised ovum is called an embryo between two weeks and seven or eight weeks.

emmenagogue a herb which increases the strength and frequency of uterine contractions.

endogenous oestrogen oestrogen which is produced within the body.

endometrial hyperplasia abnormal increase in the growth of the lining of the uterus.

endometrioma a non-cancerous collection of endometrium which often forms in scar tissue or on the ovaries. Associated with endometriosis.

endometriosis a collection of endometrial cells growing on the outside of the uterus, usually in the pelvic cavity.

endometrium the lining of the uterus which is shed at each period.

endorphin a morphine-like substance found in the brain.

enterodiol a mammalian lignan with oestrogenic activity, formed from the activity of intestinal bacteria on plant lignans.

enterolactone a mammalian lignan with oestrogenic activity, formed from the activity of intestinal bacteria on plant lignans.

epinephrine a hormone secreted by the adrenal gland. It increases both metabolic activities and blood pressure.

equol an oestrogenic substance formed by the activity of intestinal bacteria on the phyto-oestrogen, daidzein.

essential fatty acids alpha-linoleic acid, an omega-3 and linoleic acid, an omega-6 fatty acid. They are necessary for growth and development and cannot be made by the body.

ethinyl oestradiol a relatively potent synthetic oestrogen often used in the Pill, e.g. Estigyn.

fatty acid the basic unit found in fats and oils, made from chains of carbon atoms.

feed-back loop the hormonal communication between the hypothalamus, the pituitary gland and the ovaries.

fertilised ovum an ovum which has been fertilised by sperm and which is less than two weeks old.

fibroadenoma an adenoma containing fibrous tissue.

fibroma a tumour consisting mainly of fibrous tissue; a fibroid.

fimbria a fringed border or edge; the finger-like end of the Fallopian tube which encircles the ovary.

flavonoids a group of compounds widely distributed in plants which have a number of actions including the strengthening of tissues and oestrogen-like effects.

foetus an embryo becomes a foetus from about seven to eight weeks until birth.

follicle the structure in the ovary which can contain the ovum if development proceeds to ovulation.

follicle-stimulating hormone (FSH) a pituitary gland hormone which stimulates the growth of follicles.

follicular atresia the degeneration and reabsorption of a secondary ovarian follicle before it reaches maturity and ruptures.

follicular cyst a closed cavity or sac produced by the enlargement of the developing follicle.

follicular phase the time in the menstrual cycle between the end of the period and ovulation when the follicle develops.

formononetin a phyto-oestrogen; one of the isoflavones converted to daidzein by the plant.

fornix (vaginal) the recess formed between the vaginal wall and the vaginal part of the cervix.

functional hypoglycaemia a syndrome characterised by fluctuating blood sugar levels, usually related to the over-consumption of refined carbohydrates and prolonged stress.

galactorrhoea an excessive or spontaneous flow of breast milk.

gamma-linolenic acid the fatty acid found in some seed oils including evening primrose oil and star flower oil.

genistein one of the phyto-oestrogenic isoflavones, produced by the conversion of biochanin A.

genitalia the external and internal organs concerned with reproduction.

glucocorticoids the corticosteroids produced by the adrenal gland.

glucose tolerance test a blood test to measure the rate of clearance of glucose from the blood following the ingestion of a standard dose of glucose.

GnRH agonist a drug which, when given continuously, inhibits ovulation and creates a menopausal state.

gonadotrophin-releasing hormone (GnRH) a hormone secreted by the hypothalamus which initiates the release of luteinising and follicle-stimulating hormones (the gonadotrophins) from the pituitary gland.

haemostasis cessation of blood flow.

haemostatic an agent which can arrest blood loss.

HDL cholesterol high density lipoprotein—the fat and protein carrier molecule that transports cholesterol to the liver for storage or conversion; known as 'good cholesterol'.

hirsutism abnormal hairiness in women especially with male pattern distribution.

hormone replacement therapy (HRT) oestrogens and progestogens given after the menopause to treat effects of low oestrogen.

Hot (humoral theory) one of the four qualities.

HRT see hormone replacement therapy.

humoral theory an early system for understanding the workings of the body which proposed that all bodily processes are due to the actions of one or more of the four humours: Black Bile, Yellow Bile, Blood and Phlegm.

humour (humoral theory) one of the 'body fluids': Blood, Phlegm, Yellow Bile or Black Bile.

hydrogenated fat the process of adding hydrogen to an unsaturated fat. This can occur naturally, but is also a commercial process used to protect oils from rancidity, or to solidify oils when making margarine.

2–hydroxyoestrone a metabolite of oestradiol which is believed to protect against the development of breast cancer.

16–hydroxyoestrone a metabolite of oestradiol which is elevated when women have breast cancer.

hyperplasia an abnormal increase in the number of cells in an organ or structure.

hyperprolactinaemia increased levels of prolactin in the blood.

hyperthecosis a cystic condition of the ovaries associated with abnormal hormone levels, and sometimes with hirsutism and amenorrhoea.

hypothalamic–pituitary–ovarian axis the hormonal axis; the interplay between the major endocrine glands which regulates all of the events of the menstrual cycle.

hypothalamus the gland situated in the base of the brain which secretes, amongst other hormones, gonadotrophin-releasing hormone (GnRH) and dopamine.

hysterectomy surgical removal of the uterus.

hysteroscopy examination of the interior of the uterus.

IBS see irritable bowel syndrome.

imperforate hymen complete closure of the vaginal orifice by the hymen.

inco-ordinate uterine activity frequent, irregular, ineffectual and very painful contractions which fail to dilate the cervix. A common cause of 'failure to progress' in a woman delivering her first child.

insulin resistance a syndrome where insulin levels and hepatic glucose output increase because insulin is incapable of transporting glucose into the cell. Commonly associated with obesity.

in vitro fertilisation union of ovum and sperm that takes place out of the body; *in vitro*—in glass.

irritable bowel syndrome a syndrome characterised by abdominal discomfort, flatulence and alternating constipation and diarrhoea brought about by abnormal activity of the musculature of the bowel.

ischaemia lack of blood supply to an organ or part of the body.

isoflavonoid a group of substances, ubiquitous in the plant world, which has a variety of physiological effects.

IVF see *in vitro* fertilisation.

lactose intolerance an inability to digest the milk sugar, lactose.

laparoscopy examination of the interior of the abdomen or pelvic cavity using a laparoscope.

laparotomy a surgical excision into the abdomen to gain access to the abdominal or pelvic cavity.

latent hyperprolactinaemia a syndrome believed to be related to decreased progesterone which results in an increased sensitivity to normal or mildly elevated prolactin levels.

LDL cholesterol low density lipoprotein—the fat and protein carrier molecule that transports cholesterol into the blood vessel walls: known as 'bad cholesterol'.

leucorrhoea a whitish vaginal discharge.

leukotrienes eicosanoids which regulate allergic and inflammatory responses.

LH see luteinising hormone.

lignans mammalian lignans are phyto-oestrogens which are formed in the body from fibre called lignins.

linoleic acid an omega-6 fatty acid found in many seed and vegetable oils, nuts, organ meats and human milk.

luteal cyst a cyst occurring in the corpus luteum of the ovary.

luteal phase the time between ovulation and the commencement of the period.

luteal phase defect a hormonal defect that occurs after ovulation.

luteinising hormone (LH) the hormone produced by the pituitary gland which sustains the corpus luteum.

mastalgia breast pain.

medroxyprogesterone a progestogen that tends not to affect blood lipids or have strong androgenic effects.

melasma see chloasma.

menarche the time in a woman's life when she first starts to menstruate.

menopause the cessation of menstruation for more than a year; characterised by low oestrogen and elevated FSH; usually around 50 years.

menorrhagia excessively heavy menstrual flow at the time of the period.

methionine a naturally-occurring amino acid.

mittelschmerz intermenstrual pain.

Moist (humoral theory) one of the four qualities.

monounsaturated fat a major component of olive and canola oil.

myometrium the uterine muscle.

nervine (herbal medicine) a herb that has an effect on the nervous system.

neurotransmitter a substance released from the ends of nerves which can transmit messages to a target cell.

norepinephrine (noradrenaline) a neurohormone secreted by the adrenal gland in response to stress.

norethisterone a progesterone which has mild androgenic effects and adversely alters blood lipids with prolonged administration, e.g. Primolut N.

oestradiol the most potent endogenous oestrogen.

oestriol a weak endogenous oestrogen excreted in large amounts in the urine.

oestrogen receptor a structure in or on specific cells that responds to the stimulus of oestrogen.

oestrone an endogenous oestrogen formed from oestradiol and by peripheral conversion of androgens, with a potency between that of oestradiol and oestriol.

oligomenorrhoea infrequent or scanty menstrual flow.

omega-3 fatty acids the fatty acids in the omega-3 pathway, principally alpha-linolenic acid, eicosapentaenoic acid and docosahexaenoic acid.

omega-6 fatty acids the fatty acids in the omega-6 pathway, principally linoleic acid, gamma-linolenic acid and arachidonic acid.

omega-3 pathway metabolic process describing the conversion of alpha-linolenic acid to docosahexaenoic acid.

omega-6 pathway metabolic process describing the conversion of linoleic acid to arachidonic acid.

ovum the egg produced by the ovary each menstrual cycle.

partus praeparator (herbal medicine) a plant or combination of plants given to improve labour.

pathology disease; evidence of localised tissue change indicating a disease process.

pedicle the stalk or stem which attaches a structure to the body.

pedunculated a structure growing on a short stalk, often a cyst or fibroid.

pelvic inflammatory disease inflammation of one or more of the pelvic organs usually in response to infection.

peri-menopause the years both before and after the menopause when a woman experiences symptoms associated with changing hormone levels.

perineum the muscular floor of the pelvis; the area between the vagina and anus.

peripheral conversion the conversion of androgens to oestrone, which largely occurs in the fat and muscle.

peritoneal fluid free fluid in the peritoneal (abdominal or pelvic) cavity.

peritoneum the membrane which lines the abdominal and pelvic cavities, and the organs therein.

phenomenology the study of phenomena. Hence, a phenomenological approach seeks to explain the world on the basis of those events that are already understood. For example, heat dries wood, therefore dry skin must be caused by excess inner Heat.

photosensitivity the development of an abnormally high reactivity of the skin to sunlight.

phyto-oestrogen a substance produced by a plant which can exert oestrogen-like effects.

phytosterol steroid-like compounds found in plants; can have mild oestrogen-like effects.

PID see pelvic inflammatory disease.

pilo-sebaceous unit the hair follicle and its sebaceous gland.

pituitary adenoma (micro/macro) a tumour of the glandular tissue of the pituitary gland. A microadenoma is less than 10 millimetres in diameter—if larger it is classed as a macroadenoma.

pituitary gland the gland situated at the base of the brain, and in close communication with the hypothalamus, which secretes a number of hormones including LH and FSH.

PMS and PMT see premenstrual syndrome.

pneuma (humoral theory) vital energy, life force.

polycystic ovarian disease a condition which is characterised by multiple ovarian cysts, an abnormal hormone profile and irregular cycles or amenorrhoea.

polysaccharide a carbohydrate containing many (poly) simple sugars.

polyunsaturated fat a fat found in oils and margarine, seeds, nuts, fish and some vegetables, which is less stable than saturated fat.

post-menopause all of the years following the last menstrual period.

pouch of Douglas a pocket-like space between the rectum and the uterus which is lined with peritoneum.

prana (Ayurvedic medicine) vital energy, life force.

pregnenolone a precursor to endogenous progesterone.

pre-menopause technically all of the years between the commencement of the period in the teens and the menopause, but often used specifically in reference to the decade between 40 and 50.

premenstrual the time before the onset of the period, usually the week before.

premenstrual syndrome (PMS) also known as premenstrual tension (PMT); the symptoms which recur each month before the beginning of the period, and which include irritability, headaches, bloating, breast soreness and tearfulness.

primary amenorrhoea failure of menstruation to become established by age seventeen.

primary follicle the follicle which will develop and produce the ovum.

proanthocyanidins flavonoids with strong anti-oxidant and collagen-stabilising abilities.

progestogen the term used to describe a synthetic progesterone.

prolactin one of the hormones secreted by the pituitary gland that stimulate lactation.

prostacyclin an eicosanoid which reduces blood clotting and dilates blood vessels.

prostaglandin a hormone-like substance involved in a variety of inflammatory, vascular and muscle-related activities throughout the body.

pycnogenol a compound found in various plants with powerful anti-oxidant and collagen-stabilising abilities.

qi vital energy, life force.

qualities (humoral theory) Dry, Hot, Moist and Cold.

receptor site the site on or in the cell where hormones and other substances can 'dock' and interact with cellular structures.

relative hormone imbalance when the absolute levels of a hormone are within 'normal' range, but when compared to another hormone, the ratio is sufficiently changed to cause symptoms.

resorcylic acid lactone a type of phyto-oestrogen.

sapogenin the compound absorbed into the blood stream after intestinal bacteria cleave a glucose molecule from a saponin.

saponin a soapy substance in plants which can have hormone-like effects.

sarcoma a tumour of connective tissue, often highly malignant.

saturated fat a fat abundant in animal products and tropical oils; often solid at room temperature.

scoliosis a lateral curvature of the spine.

secondary amenorrhoea absence of menstruation for more than 6 months after it has been established at puberty.

secretory phase the phase in the menstrual cycle between ovulation and menstruation when the breast and the endometrium undergo secretory changes because of progesterone.

serum ferritin the iron found in the serum.

sex hormone-binding globulin (SHBG) a protein that carries sex hormones (androgens and oestradiol) in the bloodstream.

spasmodic dysmenorrhoea period pain that is sharp and colicky due to uterine spasm.

spasmolytic a substance which can relax muscle; often used to describe herbs with this quality.

spiral arterioles vascular structures supplying the endometrium, which contract during the period to reduce blood loss.

steroid hormone any of the hormones which have a central structural component based on cholesterol, including the corticosteroids, androgens, oestrogens, and progesterone.

steroidal saponins compounds found in plants with the ability to interact with steroid hormone regulation and metabolism.

temperament (humoral theory) character or personality, of which there are four types—Sanguine, Choleric, Phlegmatic or Melancholic.

teratoma a tumour that originates from germ cells in either the testis or the ovary and which may contain hair, teeth, bone, cartilage, nervous and endocrine tissue and epithelium.

terminal phenolic group relating to phyto-oestrogens; the chemical structure that imparts the oestrogen-like ability.

testosterone an androgen, produced in the testes of the male and also produced by females at low levels.

theophylline one of the xanthines found in tea leaves (and also produced synthetically) which has central nervous system-stimulating, smooth muscle-relaxing and diuretic effects.

therapeutic diet a diet given to achieve a therapeutic outcome.

thromboembolism a blood clot.

thromboxanes eicosanoids which are primarily involved with blood clotting and blood vessel activity.

torsion the twisting of a structure about an axis, as in the twisting of a pedunculated fibroid or cyst.

trans-cortin a carrier protein that binds to cortisol and progesterone; also called cortisol-binding globulin.

trans-**fatty acids** fatty acids which are produced by hydrogenation and which tend to behave like saturated fats.

triglyceride a compound consisting of three molecules of fatty acid joined to a glycerol molecule.

trimester a time period of three months.

triterpenoid saponin saponins found in plants with diverse physiological effects. Some have weak oestrogen-like actions.

ultrasound high frequency sound waves used for diagnostic or therapeutic purposes.

uterine tone the normal degree of tension in the uterine muscle.

uterine tonic a group of herbs that re-establish normal function of the uterine muscle.

vaginal septum a congenital malformation where a bridge of tissue divides the vagina.

virilisation the development of male secondary sexual characteristics due to the presence of excessive amounts of androgenic hormones, including the development of facial hair, male pattern fat distribution, enlarged clitoris and deepening of the voice.

vital force subtle force which permeates the universe and organises and animates all living things. The energy which makes growth, healing and repair possible in the face of entropy and disease.

xanthine compounds found in tea, coffee and cocoa: caffeine, theobromine and theophylline.

xeno-oestrogen any oestrogen-like substance, not of plant origin, which has been introduced into the body.

zearalenone a phyto-oestrogenic mould which contaminates cereal crops.

Notes

Chapter I

1 Griggs, B. 1981. *Green Pharmacy*, Hale, London. p. 5.

2 Riddle, J.M. 1991. 'Oral Contraceptives and early-term abortifacients during classical antiquity and the Middle Ages', *Past and Present* **132**, pp. 3–32.

3 ibid. pp. 3–32.

4 Weiss, R.F. 1988. *Herbal Medicine*, AB Arcanum, Gothenburg, p. 320.

5 Dharmananda, S. 1986. *Your Nature, Your Health*, Institute for Traditional Medicine & Preventative Health Care, Portland, p. 1.

6 Griggs, B. 1981. *Green Pharmacy*, Hale, London. p. 89.

7 Markham, G. 1638. 'The English House-wife', *A Way to Get Wealth*.

8 Author unknown. Publication early 1800s, *The Family Doctor: An Encyclopaedia of Domestic Medicine and Household Surgery, Vol. I & II*, Houlston and Wright, London.

9 Broadbent, J. 1887. *The Australian Botanic Guide*, self-published.

10 Warren, Ira. 1870. The Household Physician, Guy McLellan, Melbourne; Beard, G.M. 1883. *The New Cyclopaedia of Family Medicine*, E.B. Treat, Sydney; Miller, John A. 1891. *Home Treatment for Diseases of Women and Some Favorite Prescriptions*, John Miller Publication(s), San Francisco; No author. Published early 1900s, *The Dictionary of Daily Wants*, Houlston and Sons, London; Muskett, Philip E. 1892. *The Art of Living in Australia*, Eyre and Spottiswoode, London; Muskett, Philip E. 1903. *The Illustrated Australian Guide*, William Brooks and Co. Ltd, Sydney; McArthur, A. 1940s, *The Encyclopaedia of Health and Wealth*. No publisher recorded.

11 Rawson, Mrs Lance, 1910. *Australian Enquiry Book of Household and General Information*, E.W. Cole, Melbourne.

12 Richards, Eulalia S. 1939. *Ladies Handbook of Home Treatment*, Signs Publishing Company, Warbuton, Australia.

13 Ferguson, M. 1980.*The Aquarian Conspiracy*, Paladin, London, p. 270.

14 ibid. pp. 270–1.

15 Porkert, M. 1982. *Chinese Medicine*, William Morrow and Company Inc., New York, p. 16.

16 Kaptchuk, T. 1983. *The Web that has no Weaver*, Congdon and Weed, New York.

Chapter 3

1   Crawford, P. 1981. 'Attitudes to menstruation in seventeenth-century England', *Past and Present* **91**, pp. 47–73.

2   Bennett, J. 1991. *Lilies of the Hearth*, Camden House, Ontario, Canada. p. 26.

3   Rowland, B. 1981. *Medieval woman's guide to health: the first English gynecological handbook*, Kent State University Press, Kent, Ohio.

4   Bullough, V. and Voght, M. 1973. 'Women, menstruation and nineteenth-century medicine', *Bull Hist Med.* **47**, pp. 66–82.

5   Toufexis, A. 1993. *A woman's best defense?* Time, Oct 4, pp. 60–1.

6   Grimwade, J. 1995. *The Body of Knowledge* William Heinemann Australia, Melbourne, p. 18.

7   Sharp, Jane, 1671. republished 1985. *The Midwives Book*, Garland Publishing Inc., New York, p. 312.

Chapter 4

1   Bradlow, H.L., Hershcopf, R.E. and Fishman, J.F. 1986. 'Oestradiol 16 α = hydroxylase: a risk marker for breast cancer', *Cancer Surv 5*, pp. 573–83.

2   Davis, D.L. and Bradlow, H.L. 1995. 'Can environmental estrogens cause breast cancer?' *Sci Am*, Oct: pp. 144–9.

3   Soto, A.M. Chung, K.L. and Sonnerschein, C. 1994. 'The pesticides endosulphan, toxaphene, and dieldrin have estrogenic effects on human estrogen-sensitive cells', *Environ Health Perspect* **102**(4), pp. 380–3.

4   Truelove, J.F. Tanner, J.R. Langlois, I.A. et al., 1990. 'Effect of polychlorinated biphenyls on several endocrine reproductive parameters in the female rhesus monkey', *Arch Environ Contam Toxicol* **19**(6), pp. 939–43.

5   Robinson, A.K. Schmidt, W.A. and Stancel, G.M. 1985. 'Estrogenic activity of DDT: estrogen-receptor profiles and the responses of individual uterine cell types following o,p'-DDT administration', *J Toxicol Environ Health*, **16**(3–4), pp. 493–508.

6   Soto, A.M. Justicia, H. Wray, J.W. et al., 1991. 'p-Nonyl-phenol: an estrogenic xenobiotic released from "modified" polystyrene', *Environ Health Perspect* **92**, pp. 167–73.

7   Brotons, J.A. Olea-Serrano, M.F. Villalobos, M. et al., 1995. 'Xenoestrogens released from lacquer coatings in food cans', *Environ Health Perspect* **103**(6), pp. 608–12.

8   Saxena, S.P. Khare, C. Farooq, A. et al., 1987. 'DDT and its metabolites in leiomyomatous and normal human uterine tissue', *Arch Toxicol* **59**(6) pp. 453–5

9   Sharpe, R.M. and Skakkebaek, N.E. 1993. 'Are oestrogens involved in falling sperm counts and disorders of the male reproductive tract?' *Lancet* **341**(8857), pp. 1392–5.

10 Adami, H.O. Lipworth, L. Titus-Ernstoff, L. et al., 1995. 'Organochlorine compounds and estrogen-related cancers in women', *Cancer Causes Control* **6**(6) pp. 551–66; Krieger, N. Wolff, M.S. Hiatt, R.A. et al., 1994. 'Breast cancer and serum organochlorines: a prospective study among white, black, and Asian women', *J Natl Cancer Inst* **86**(8) pp. 589–99.

11 Arnold, S.F. Klotz, D.M., Collins, B.M., et al., 1996. 'Synergistic activation of estrogen receptor with combinations of environmental chemicals', *Science*, **272**, pp. 1489–92.

Chapter 5

1   Goldin, B.R. and Gorbach, S.L. 1976. 'The relationship between diet and rat fecal bacterial enzymes implicated in colon cancer', *J Natl Cancer Instit* **57**, pp. 371–75.

2   Goldin, B.R. Adlercreutz, H. Gorbach, S.L. et al., 1986. 'The relationship between estrogen levels and diets of Caucasian American and Oriental immigrant women', *Am J Clin Nutr* **44**(6) pp. 945–53.

3   Longcope, C. Gorbach, S. Goldin, B. et al., 1987. 'Effect of low fat diet on oestrogen metabolism', *J Clin Endocrinol Metab* **64**(6), pp. 1246–9.

4   Chu, S.Y. Lee, N.C. Wingo, P.A. et al., 1991. 'The relationship between body mass and breast cancer among women enrolled in the Cancer and Steroid Hormone Study', *J Clin Epidemiol* **44**(11), pp. 1197–206; Austin, H. Austin, J.M. Partridge, E.E. et al., 1991. 'Endometrial cancer, obesity and body fat distribution', *Cancer Res* **51**(2), pp. 568–72.

5   Colditz, G.A. 1993. 'Epidemiology of breast cancer. Findings from the nurses' health study', *Cancer* **71**(4 Suppl), pp. 1480–9.

6   Ross, R.K. Pike, M.C. Vessey, M.P. et al., 1986. 'Risk factors for uterine fibroids: reduced risk associated with oral contraceptives', *Br Med J Clin Res Ed* **293**(6543), pp. 359–62.

7   McCann, S.E. Freudenheim, J.L. Darrow S.L. et al., 1993. 'Endometriosis and body fat distribution', *Obstet Gynecol* **82**(4 Pt 1), pp. 545–9.

8   Brodsky, I.G. and Devlin, J.T. 1994. 'Hormone and nutrient interactions', *Modern Nutrition in Health and Disease*, 8th Edition, eds M.E. Shils, J.A. Olson, and M. Shike, Lea & Febiger, Philadelphia, p. 617.

9   Goldin, B.R. Woods, M.N. Spiegelman, D.L. et al., 1994. 'The effect of dietary fat and fiber on serum estrogen concentrations in premenopausal women under controlled dietary conditions', *Cancer* **74**(3 Suppl), pp. 1125–31; Rose, D.P. Goldman, M. Connolly, J.M. et al., 1991. 'High-fiber diet reduces serum estrogen concentrations in premenopausal women', *Am J Clin Nutr* **54**(3), pp. 520–5; Woods, M.N. Gorbach, S.L. Longcope, C. et al., 1989. 'Low-fat, high-fiber diet and serum estrone sulfate in premenopausal women', *Am J Clin Nutr* **49**(6), pp. 1179–83.

10   Goldin, B.R. and Gorbach, S.L. 1984. 'The effect of milk and lactobacillus feeding on human intestinal bacterial enzyme activity', *Am J Clin Nutr* **39**, pp. 756–61.

11   Gorbach, S.L. 1984. 'Estrogens, breast cancer and intestinal flora', *Rev Inf Dis* **6**(S 1), pp. S85-S90.

12   van't Veer, P. Dekker, J.M. Lamers, J.W.J. et al., 1989. 'Consumption of fermented milk products and breast cancer: a case-control study in the Netherlands', *Cancer Res.* **49**, pp. 4020–23.

13   Adlercreutz, H. Bannwart, C. Wahala, K. et al., 1993. 'Inhibition of human aromatase by mammalian lignans and isoflavonoid phytoestrogens', *J Steroid Biochem Mol Biol* **44**(2), pp. 147–53.

14   Setchell, K.D.R. and Adlercreutz, H. 1988. 'Mammalian lignans and phyto-oestrogens. Recent studies on their formation, metabolism and biological role in health and disease', *Role of the Gut Flora in Toxicity and Cancer*, ed I. Rowland, Academic Press Limited, London. pp. 315–45; Adlercreutz, H. Hockerstedt, K. Bannwart, C. et al., 1987. 'Effect of dietary components, including lignans and phytoestrogens, on enterohepatic circulation and liver metabolism of estrogens and on sex hormone binding globulin (SHBG)', *J Steroid Biochem* **27**(4–6), pp. 1135–44.

15   Michnovicz, J.J. and Bradlow, H.L. 1990. 'Induction of estradiol metabolism by dietary indole–3-carbinol in humans', *J Natl Cancer Inst* **82**(11), pp. 947–9; Jellinck, P.H. Forkett, P.G. Riddick, D.S. et al., 1993. 'Ah receptor binding properties of indole carbinols and induction of hepatic estradiol hydroxylation',

Biochem Pharmacol 45(5), pp. 1129–36; Bradlow, H.L. Michnovicz, J.J. Halper, M. et al., 1994. 'Long-term responses of women to indole–3-carbinol or a high fiber diet', *Cancer Epidemiol Biomarkers Prev* 3(7), pp. 591–5.

16 Lui, H. Wormke, M. Safe, S.H. et al., 1994. 'Indolo[3,2-b]carbazole: a dietary-derived factor that exhibits both antiestrogenic and estrogenic activity', *J Natl Cancer Inst* 86(23), pp. 1758–65.

17 Tiwari, R.K. Guo, L. and Bradlow, H.L. 1994. 'Selective responsiveness of human breast cancer cells to indole–3-carbinol, a chemopreventive agent', *J Natl Cancer Inst* 86(2), pp. 126–31.

18 Anderson, K.E. Kappas, A. Conney, A.H. et al., 1984. 'The influence of dietary protein on the principal oxidative biotransformations of estradiol in normal subjects', *J Clin Endocrinol Metab* 59(1), pp. 103–7.

19 Bell, E. 1980. 'The excretion of a vitamin B6 metabolite and the probability of recurrence of early breast cancer', *Eur J Cancer* 16, pp. 297–8.

20 Bender, D.A. 1987. 'Oestrogen and vitamin B6—actions and interactions, *Wld Rev Nutr Diet* 51, pp. 140–88.

21 Webster, L.A. and Weiss, N.S. 1989. 'Alcoholic beverage consumption and the risk of endometrial cancer. Cancer and Steroid Hormone Study Group', *Int J Epidemiol* 18(4), pp. 786–91.

22 Byers, T. 1994. 'Nutritional risk factors for breast cancer', *Cancer* Suppl, 74(1), pp. 288–95.

23 Harlow, S.D. and Campbell, B.C. 1994. 'Host factors that influence the duration of menstrual bleeding', *Epidemiology* 5(3), pp. 352–5.

24 Mishell, D.R. and Davajan, V. 1994. 'Differential diagnosis of secondary amenor-rhea', *Management of Common Problems in Obstetrics and Gynecology*, eds D.R. Mishell and P.F. Brenner, Blackwell Scientific Publications, Boston. p. 607.

25 Feng, W. Marshall, R. Lewis-Barned, N.J. et al., 1993. 'Low follicular oestrogen levels in New Zealand women consuming high fibre diets: a risk factor for osteopenia?' *NZ Med J* 106(965), pp. 419–22.

26 Snow-Harter, C.M. 1994. 'Bone health and prevention of osteoporosis in active and athletic women', *Clin Sports Med* 13(2), pp. 389–404.

27 Baron, J.A. La Vecchia, C. and Levi, F. 1990. 'The antiestrogenic effect of cigarette smoking in women', *Am J Obstet Gynecol* 162(2), pp. 502–14.

28 Shen L. Du J.Y. and Yang J.Y. 1994. 'Preliminary study on prevention of bone loss in post-menopausal women with kidney invigoration', *Chung Kuo Chung Hsi I Chieh Ho Tsa Chih* 14(9), pp. 515–8; Ding, G.Z. Zhang, Z.L. and Zhou, Y. 1995. 'Clinical study on effect of bushen jiangu capsule on postmenopausal osteoporosis', *Chung Kuo Chung Hsi I Chieh Ho Tsa Chih* 15(7), pp. 392–4.

29 Arjmandi, B.H. Alekel, L. Hollis, B.W. et al., 1996. 'Dietary soybean protein prevents bone loss in an ovariectomised rat model of osteroporosis', *J Nutr* 126(2), pp. 161–7.

30 Tsutsumi, N. 1995. 'Effect of coumesterol on bone metabolism in organ culture', *Biol Pharm Bull* 18(7), pp. 1012–5.

31 Johnson, I.T. Gee, J.M. and Price, K.R. 1986. 'Influence of saponins on gut permeability and active nutritive transport in vitro', *J Nutr* 116, pp. 2270–7.

32 Manilow, M.R. 1984. 'Saponins and cholesterol metabolism', *Athersclerosis* 50, pp. 117–8.

33 Bopp, B. and Shoupe, D. 1993. 'Luteal phase defects', *J Reprod Med* May, 38(5), pp. 348–56.

34 Shoupe, D. Mishell, D.R. and LaCarra, M. 1989. 'Correlation of endometrial maturation with 4 methods of estimating day of ovulation', *Obstet Gynecol* 73, pp. 88–92.

35 Filicori, M. Butler, J.P. and Crowley, W.R. 1984. 'Neuroendocrine regulation of the corpus luteum in the human', *J Clin Invest* 73, pp. 1638.

Chapter 6

1 Behrman, H.R. Rahway, N.J. and Anderson, G.G. 1974. 'Prostaglandins in reproduction', *Arch Intern Med* **133**, pp. 77–84.

2 Kelly, R.W. Lumsden, M.A. Abel, M.H. et al., 1984. 'The relationship between
   menstrual blood loss and prostaglandin production in the human: evidence for
   increased availability of arachidonic acid in women suffering from menorrhagia',
   Prost Leuk Med **16**, pp. 69–77.

3 Kelly, R.W. Lumsden, M.A. et al., 1984. 'The relationship between menstrual blood
   loss and prostaglandin production in the human: evidence for increased availability
   of arachidonic acid in women suffering from menorrhagia', *Prost Leuk Med* **16**,
   pp. 69–77.

4 Horrobin, D.F. 1979. 'Cellular basis of prolactin action', *Med Hypothesis* **5**,
   pp. 599–620.

5 Nigam, S. Benedetto, C. and Zonca, M. 1991. 'Increased concentrations of
   eicosanoids and platelet-activating factor in menstrual blood from women with
   primary dysmenorrhoea', *Eicosanoids* **4**(3), pp. 137–41.

6 Pungetti, D. Lenzi, M. and Travisani, D. 1987. 'Prostanoids in peritoneal fluid
   of infertile women with pelvic endometriosis and PID', *Acta Eur Fertil* **18**(3),
   pp. 189–92.

7 Abou-el-Ela, S.H. Prasse, K.W. Farrell, K.W. et al., 1989. 'Effects of D.L-2-dif-
   luoromethylornitnine and indomethacin on mammary tumour promotion in rats
   fed high n–3 and/or n–6 fat diets', *Cancer Res* **49**(6), pp. 1434–40.

8 Linscheer, W.G. and Vergroesen, A.J. 1994. 'Lipids', *Modern Nutrition in Health
   and Disease*, eds M.E. Shils, J.A. Olsen and M Shike, Lea & Febiger, Philadelphia,
   pp. 47–88.

9 Horrobin, D.F. 1983. 'Regulation of prostaglandin biosynthesis by the manipulation of essential fatty acid metabolism', *Rev Pure and Appl Pharmacol Sci* **4**(4),
   pp. 339–83.

10 Erasmus, U. 1993. 'Fats that Heal, Fats that Kill', Alive Books, Burnaby, BC,
    Canada, pp. 258–65.

11 Mantzioris, E. James, M.J. Gibson, RA. et al., 1994. 'Dietary substitution with an
    alpha-linolenic acid-rich vegetable oil increases eicosapentaenoic acid concentra-
    tions in tissues', *Am J* Clin Nutr **59**, pp. 1304–9.

12 Emken, E.A., Adlof, R.O., Rhowedder, W.K. et al., 1992. 'Comparison of dietary
    linolenic acid and linoleic metabolism in man: influence of dietary linoleic acid,'
    *Essential Fatty Acids and Eicosanoids. Invited Papers from the Third International
    Congress*, eds A. Sinclair and R. Gibson, American Oil Chemists Society, Illinois,
    pp. 23–5.

13 Dryberg, J. Jorgensen, K.A. 1982. 'Marine oils and thrombogenesis' *Prog Lipid
    Res* **21**, pp. 255–69.

14 Linscheer, W.G. and Vergroesen, A.J. 1994. 'Lipids', *Modern Nutrition in Health
    and Disease*, eds M.E. Shils, J.A. Olsen and M Shike, Lea & Febiger, Philadelphia,
    pp. 47–88.

15 Kelly, R.W. Lumsden, M.A. et al., 1984. 'The relationship between menstrual blood
    loss and prostaglandin production in the human: evidence for increased availability
    of arachidonic acid in women suffering from menorrhagia', *Prost Leuk Med* **16**,
    pp. 69–77.

16 Smith, S.K. Abel, M.H. Kelly, R.W. et al., 1981. 'A role for prostacyclin (PGI2)
    in excessive menstrual bleeding', *Lancet* **1**, pp. 522–25.

17 Fraser, I.S. Shearman, R.P. McIlveen, J. et al., 1981. 'Efficacy of mefenamic acid
    in patients with a complaint of menorrhagia', *Obstet Gynecol* **58**(5), pp. 543–551.

18 Covens, A.L. Christopher, P. and Casper, R.F. 1988. 'The effect of dietary

supplementation with fish oil fatty acids on surgically induced endometriosis in the rabbit', *Fertil Steril* **49**(4), pp. 698–703.

19 Pullman-Mooar, S. Laposata, M. Lem, D. et al., 1990. 'Alteration of the cellular fatty acid profile and the production of eicosanoids in human monocytes by gamma-linoleic acid', *Arthritis Rheum* **33**(10), pp. 1526–33.

20 Goldin, B.R. Adlercreutz, H. Gorbach, S.L. et al., 1986. 'The relationship between estrogen levels and diets of Caucasian American and Oriental immigrant women', *Am J Clin Nutr* **44**(6), pp. 945–53.

21 Rees, M.C.P. 1990. 'Human menstruation and Eicosanoids', *Reprod Fertil Dev* **2**, pp. 467–76.

22 Nigam, S. Benedetto, C. Zonca, M. et al., 1991. 'Increased concentrations of eicosanoids and platelet-activating factor in menstrual blood from women with primary dysmenorrhoea', *Eicosanoids* **4**(3), pp. 137–41.

23 Nigam, S. 1992. 'Evidence for relief from severe menstrual cramps by fish diet in patients with primary dysmenorrhoea', *Program and Abstracts*, eds R. Gibson and A. Sinclair, Third International Congress on Essential Fatty Acids and Eicosanoids, Adelaide, p. 20.

24 Puolakka J. Makarainen L. Vinikka, L. et al., 1985. 'Biochemical and clinical effects of treating the premenstrual syndrome with prostaglandin synthesis precursors', *J Reprod Med* **30**(3), pp. 149–153; Mira, M. McNell, D. Fransen, I.S. et al., 1986. 'Mefenamic acid in the treatment of premenstrual syndrome', *Obstet Gynecol* **68**, pp. 395–8

25 Brush, M.G. 1983. 'Evening primrose oil in the treatment of premenstrual syndrome', *Clinical Uses of Essential Fatty Acids*, ed D.F. Horrobin, Eden Press, Montreal.

26 Horrobin, D.F. 1983. 'The role of essential fatty acids and prostaglandins in premenstrual syndrome, *J Reprod Med* **28**(7), pp. 465–8.

27 Collins, A. Cerin, A. Coleman, G. et al., 1993. 'Essential fatty acids in the treatment of premenstrual syndrome', *Obstet Gynecol* **81**(1), pp. 93–8; Khoo, S.K. Munro, C. and Battistutta, D. 1990. 'Evening primrose oil and treatment of premenstrual syndrome', *Med J Aust* **153**, pp. 189–92.

28 Koike, H. Egawa, H. Ohtsuka, T. et al., 1992. 'Correlation between dysmenorrheic severity and prostaglandin production in women with endometriosis', *Prost Leukot EFAs* **46**(2), pp. 133–7.

29 Sharma, SC. Barry-Kinsella, C. Cottell, E. et al., 1994. 'A mid-luteal phase comparison of peritoneal fluid volume and its contents of PGF2 alpha and PGE2 in women with minimal stage endometriosis and a normal pelvis', *Prostaglandins* **47**(1), pp. 9–16.

30 Pungetti, D. Lenzi, M. Travisani, D. et al., 1987. 'Prostanoids in peritoneal fluid of infertile women with pelvic endometriosis and PID', *Acta Eur Fertil* **18**(3), pp. 189–92

31 Dunselman, G.A. Hendrix, M.G. Bouckaert, P.X. et al., 1988. 'Functional aspects of peritoneal macrophages in endometriosis of women', *J Reprod Fertil* **82**(2), pp. 707–10.

32 Yano, Y. 1992. 'Effect of dietary supplementation with eicosapentaenoic acid on surgically induced endometriosis in the rabbit', *Nippon Sanka Fujinka Gakkai Zasshi* **44**(3), pp. 282–8; Covens, A.L. Christopher, P. and Casper, R.F. 1988. 'The effect of dietary supplementation with fish oil fatty acids on surgically induced endometriosis in the rabbit', *Fertil Steril* **49**(4), pp. 698–703.

33 Ziboh, V.A. and Fletcher, M.P. 1992. 'Dose-response effects of dietary gamma-linolenic acid-enriched oils on human polymorphonuclear-neutrophil biosynthesis of leukotriene B4', *Am J Clin Nutr* **55**(1), pp. 39–45.

34 Fletcher, M.P. and Ziboh, V.A. 1990. 'Effects of dietary supplementation with

eicosapentanoic acid and gamma-linolenic acid on neutrophil phospholipid fatty acid composition and activation responses', *Inflammation* **14**(5), pp. 585–97.

35 Fan Y.Y. and Chapkin, R.S. 1992. 'Mouse peritoneal macrophage prostaglandin E1 synthesis is altered by dietary gamma-linolenic acid', *J Nutr* **122**(8), pp. 1600–6.

36 Abou-el-Ela, S.H. Prasse, K.W. Farrell, K.W. et al., 1989. 'Effects of D.L–2-difluoromethylornithine and indomethacin on mammary tumour promotion in rats fed high n–3 and/or n–6 fat diets', *Cancer Res* **49**(6), pp. 1434–40.

37 Fritsche, K.L. and Johnston P.V. 1990. 'Effect of dietary alpha-linolenic acid on growth, metastasis, fatty acid profile and prostaglandin production of two murine mammary adenocarcinomas', *J Nutr* **120**(12), pp. 1601–9; Takata, T. Minoura, T. Takada, H. et al., 1990.'Specific inhibitory effect of dietary eicosapentaenoic acid on N-nitroso-N-methylurea-induced mammary carcinogenesis in female Sprague-Dawley rats', *Carcinogenesis* **11**(11), pp. 2015–9.

38 Horrobin, D.F. 1979. 'Cellular basis of prolactin action', *Med Hypothesis* 5, pp. 599–620.

Chapter 7

1 Frisch, R.E. 1990. 'The right weight: body fat, menarche and ovulation', *Baillieres Clin Obstet Gynaecol* **4**(3), pp. 419–39.

2 Baghurst, K.I. Dreosti, I.E. Syrette, J.A. et al., 1991. 'Zinc and magnesium status of Australian adults', *Nutr Res* **11**, pp. 23–32.

3 Vivoli, G. Fantuzzi, G. Bergomi, M. et al., 1990. 'Relationship between zinc in serum and hair and some hormones during sexual maturation in humans', *Sci Total Env* (Netherlands) **95**, pp. 29–40.

4 Baghurst, K.I. Dreosti, I.E. Syrette, J.A. et al., 1991. 'Zinc and magnesium status of Australian adults', *Nutr Res* **11**, pp. 23–32.

5 Baghurst, K. Record, S. Powis, G. et al., 1993. *What are Australians Eating? 1985 & 1990 Victorian Nutrition Surveys*, CSIRO Division of Human Nutrition, Adelaide, pp. 46–7.

6 Carr-Gregg, M. 1995. Fact Sheet 5: 'Young People and Depression', Centre for Adolescent Health in association with VicHealth, Royal Children's Hospital, Melbourne.

7 Carr-Gregg, M. 1995. Fact Sheet 16: 'Young People and Panic Disorders', Centre for Adolescent Health in association with VicHealth, Royal Children's Hospital, Melbourne.

8 Carr-Gregg, M. 1995. Fact Sheet 2: 'Youth Suicide', Centre for Adolescent Health in association with VicHealth, Royal Children's Hospital, Melbourne.

9 Vivoli, G. Fantuzzi, G. Bergomi, M. et al., 1990. 'Relationship between zinc in serum and hair and some hormones during sexual maturation in humans', *Sci Total Env* (Netherlands) **95**, pp. 29–40.

10 Werbach, M.R. 1989. *Nutritional Influences on Illness*, Thorsons Publishing Group, England, p. 8.

Chapter 8

1 Abraham, G. 1983. 'Nutritional factors in the etiology of the premenstrual tension syndromes', *J Reprod Med* **28**(7), pp. 446–64.

2 Janiger, O. Riffenburgh, R. and Kersh, R. 1972. 'Cross cultural study of premenstrual symptoms', *Psychosomatics* **13**, pp. 226–35.

3   Dennerstein, L. 1994. 'Psychiatry of women', *Foundations of Clinical Psychiatry*, eds S. Bloch and B.S. Singh, Melbourne University Press, Melbourne, pp. 289–99.

4   Hammarback, S. Damer, J.E. and Backstrom, T. 1989. 'Relationship between symptom severity and hormone changes in women with premenstrual syndrome', *J Clin Endocr Metab* **68**, pp. 125–30.

5   Backstrom, T. and Carstensen, H. 1974. 'Estrogen and progesterone in plasma in relation to premenstrual tension', *J Ster Biochem* **5**, pp. 257–60.

6   Munday, M.R. Brush, M.G. and Taylor, R.W. 1981. 'Correlations between progesterone, estradiol, and aldosterone levels in the premenstrual syndrome', *Clin Endocrinol* **14**, pp. 1–9.

7   Rubinow, D.R. Hoban, M.C. and Grover, G.N. 1988. 'Changes in plasma hormones across the menstrual cycle in patients with menstrually related mood disorder and in control subjects', *Am J Obstet Gynecol* **158**, pp. 5–11.

8   Merraim, G.R. Brody, S.A. and Almedia, O.F. 1983. 'Endocrinology of the menstrual cycle, Implication for premenstrual syndrome', *Proceedings of the National Institute of Mental Health Premenstrual Syndrome Workshop*, National Institute of Mental Health, Bethesda, MD.

9   Dalton, K. 1990. 'The aetiology of premenstrual syndrome is with the progesterone receptors', *Med Hypotheses* **31**, pp. 323–27.

10 Nock, B. 1986. 'Noradrenergic regulation of progestin receptors, New findings', *Reproduction: A Behavioural and Neuroendocrine Perspective*, eds B.R. Komusaruk et al., *Annals New York Acad Sci* New York, pp. 415–22.

11 Dalton, K. 1990. 'The aetiology of premenstrual syndrome is with the progesterone receptors', *Med Hypotheses* **31**, pp. 323–27.

12 Rabin, D.S. Schmidt, P.J. Campbell, G. et al., 1990. 'Hypothalamic-pituitary-adrenal function in patients with premenstrual syndrome', *J Clin Endocrinol Metab* **71**(5), pp. 1158–62.

13 Reid, R.L. and Yen, S.S.C. 1981. 'Premenstrual syndrome', *Am J Obstet Gynecol* **139**, pp. 85–104.

14 Reid, R.L. and Yen, S.S.C. 1981. 'Premenstrual syndrome', *Am J Obstet Gynecol* **139**, pp. 85–104; Lurie, S. and Borenstein, R. 1990. 'The premenstrual syndrome', *Obst. Gyn Surv* **45**(4), pp. 220–228; O'Brien, P.M.S. and Symonds, E.M. 1982. 'Prolactin levels in the premenstrual syndrome', *Br J Obstet Gyn* **89**, pp. 306–308.

15 Chuong, C.J. Coulam, C.B. Kao, P.C. et al., 1985. 'Neuropeptide levels in premenstrual syndrome', *Fertil Steril* **44**, pp. 760–5.

16 Reid, R.L. and Yen, S.S.C. 1981. 'Premenstrual syndrome', *Am J Obstet Gynecol* **139**, pp. 85–104.

17 Quigley, M.E. and Yen, S.S.C. 1980. 'The role of endogenous opiates on LH secretion during the menstrual cycle', *J Clin Endocrinol Metab* **51**, pp. 179.

18 Bosches, B. and Arbit, J. 1970. 'A controlled study of the effect of L-dopa on selected cognitive and behavioural functions', *Trans Am Neurol Assoc* **55**, pp. 59–62.

19 Abraham, G.E. 1980. 'Premenstrual tension', *Curr Probs Obstet Gynecol* **3**(12), pp. 1–39.

20 Briggs, M. 1972. 'Relationship between monoamine oxidase activity and sex hormone concentration in human blood plasma', *J Reprod Fertil* **29**, pp. 447–9.

21 Lurie, S. and Borenstein, R. 1990. 'The premenstrual syndrome', *Obst Gyn Surv* **45**(4), pp. 220–228.

22 Puolakka, J. Makarainen, L. Viinikka, L. et al., 1985. 'Biochemical and clinical effects of treating the premenstrual syndrome with prostaglandin synthesis precursors', *J Reprod Med* **30**(3), pp. 149–53.

23 Mira, M. McNell, D. Fransen, I.S. et al., 1986. 'Mefenamic acid in the treatment of premenstrual syndrome', *Obstet Gynecol* **68**, pp. 395–8.

24 van den Berg, H. Louwerse, E.S. Bruinse, H.W. et al., 1986. 'Vitamin B6 status

of women suffering from premenstrual syndrome', *Hum Nutr Clin Nutr* **40C**, pp. 441–50.

25 Chuong, J.C. Dawson, E.B. Smith, E.R. et al., 1990. 'Vitamin E levels in premenstrual syndrome', *Am J Obstet Gynecol* **163**, pp. 1591–5.

26 Chuong, J.C. Dawson, E.B. and Smith E.R. 1990. 'Vitamin A levels in premenstrual syndrome', *Fertil Steril* **54**(4), pp. 643–7.

27 Rose, D.P. and Braidman, I.P. 1971. 'Oral contraceptives and tryptophan metabolism: effects of oestrogen in low dose combined with progestogen and of a progestogen (megestrol acetate) given alone', *J Clin Path* **25**, pp. 252–8.

28 Kleijnen, J. Ter Riet, G. and Knipschild, P. 1990. 'Vitamin B6 in the treatment of the premenstrual syndrome—a review', *Brit J Obstet Gyn* **97**, pp. 847–52.

29 Axelrod, J. 1977. 'Regulation of the synthesis, release and actions of catecholamine neurotransmitters', 'First European Symposium on Hormones and Cell Regulation', eds J. Dumont and J. Nunez, North Holland Biomedical Press, pp. 137–55.

30 Abraham, G.E. Schwartz, U.D. and Lubran, M.M. 1981. 'Effect of vitamin B6 on serum and red cell magnesium levels in premenopausal women', *Ann Clin Lab Sci* **11**(4), pp. 333–6.

31 Bender, D.A. 1987. 'Oestrogens and B6—actions and interactions', *Wld Rev Nutr Diet* **51**, pp. 140–88.

32 Parry, G.J. and Bredesen, D.E. 1985. 'Sensory neuropathy with low-dose pyridoxine', *Neurology* **35**, pp. 1466–8.

33 Williams, M.J. Harris, R.I. and Dean, B.C. 1985. 'Controlled trial of pyridoxine in the premenstrual syndrome', *J Int Med Res* **13**, pp. 174–9; Brush, M.G. Bennet, T. and Hansen, K. 1988. 'Pyridoxine in the treatment of premenstrual syndrome: a retrospective survey of 630 patients', *Br J Clin Prac* **42**(11), pp. 448–52.

34 Fuchs, N. Hakim, M. and Abraham, G.E. 1985. 'The effect of a nutritional supplement, Optivite for women, on pre-menstrual tension syndromes: 1. Effect on blood chemistry and serum steroid levels during the mid luteal phase', *J Appl Nutr* **37**, pp. 1–11.

35 Parry, G.J. and Bredesen, D.E. 1985. 'Sensory neuropathy with low-dose pyridoxine', *Neurology* **35**, pp. 1466–8.

36 Frizel, D. Coppen, A. and Marks, V. 1969. 'Plasma magnesium and calcium in depression', *Brit J Psychiat* **115**, pp. 1375–77.

37 Poenaru, S. Rouhani, S. Durlach, J. et al., 1989. 'Magnesium and monoaminergic neurotransmitters: Elements of human and experimental pathophysiology', *Magnesium in Health and Disease*, eds Y. Itakawa and J. Durlach, J. Libby, London, pp. 291–7.

38 Ishizuka, J. Bold, R.J. Townsend, C.M. et al., 1994. 'In vitro relationship between magnesium and insulin secretion', *Mag Res.* **7**(1), pp. 17–22.

39 Goei, G.S. Ralston, J.L. and Abraham, G.E. 1982. 'Dietary patterns of patients with premenstrual tension', *J Applied Nutrition* **34**(1), pp. 4–11.

40 Abraham, G.E. and Lubran, M.M. 1981. 'Serum and red cell magnesium levels in patients with PMT', *Am J Clin Nut* **34**, pp. 2364–6; Sherwood, R.A. Rocks, B.F. Stewart, A. et al., 1986. 'Magnesium and the premenstrual syndrome', *Ann Clin Biochem* **23**, pp. 667–70; Facchinetti, F. Borella, P. Valentini, M. et al., 1988. 'Premenstrual increase of intracellular magnesium levels in women with ovulatory, asymptomatic menstrual cycles', *Gynecol Endocrinol* **2**, pp. 249–56.

41 Facchinetti, F. Borella, P. Sances, G. et al., 1991. 'Oral magnesium successfully relieves premenstrual mood changes', *Obstet Gynecol* **78**, pp. 177–81.

42 Elin, R.J. 1987. 'Assessment of magnesium status', *Clin Chem* **33**, pp. 1965–70.

43 London, R.S. Sundaram G.S. and Murphy, L. 1983. 'Evaluation and treatment of breast symptoms in patients with the premenstrual syndrome', *J Reprod Med* **28**, pp. 503–8.

44 London, R.S. Sundaram, G.S. and Murphy, L. et al., 1982. 'The effect of alpha-tocopherol

on premenstrual symptomatology: a double-blind trial', *J Am Coll Nutr* **2**, pp. 115–22; London, R.S. Murphy, L. Kitlowski, K. et al., 1987. 'Efficacy of alpha-tocopherol in the treatment of premenstrual syndrome', *J Reprod Med* **32**, pp. 400–4.

45 London, R.S. Sundaram, G.S. Schultz, M. et al., 1981. 'Endocrine parameters and alpha-tocopherol therapy of patients with mammary dysplasia', *Cancer Res* **41**, pp. 3811–13.

46 Fasold, H. 1937. 'Uber die Wirkung des Vitamin A auf das Ovar des PubertŠtsalters', *Klin Wchnschr* **16**, pp. 90; Argonz, J. Abinzano, C. 1950. 'Premenstrual tension treated with vitamin A', *J Clin Endocrinol* **10**, pp. 1579–1590.

47 Block, E. 1960. 'The use of vitamin A in pre-menstrual tension', *Acta Obst Gynec Scand* **39**, pp. 587–92.

48 Stewart, A.C. Tooley, S. and Stewart, M. 1991. 'Effect of a nutritional programme on PMS: A retrospective analysis', *Comp Med Res* **5**(1), pp. 8–11; Goei, G.S. Abraham, G.E. 1983. 'Effect of nutritional supplement, Optivite, on symptoms of premenstrual tension', *J Reprod Med* **28**, pp. 528–31.

49 Horrobin, D.F. 1983. 'The role of essential fatty acids and prostaglandins in the premenstrual syndrome', *J Reprod Med* **28**(7), pp. 465–8.

50 Graham, J. 1984. *Evening Primrose Oil*, Thorson's, London, pp. 37–8.

51 Roy, S.K. Ghosh, B.P. and Bhattacharjee, S.K. 1971. 'Changes in oral glucose tolerance during normal menstrual cycle', *J Ind Med Assoc* **57**(6), pp. 201–4.

52 Price, W.A. Dimarzio, M.S. and Gardner, P.R. 1986. 'Biopsychosocial approach to premenstrual syndrome', *AFP* **33**(6), pp. 117–22; Engel, G.I. 1977. 'The need for a new medical model: A challenge for biomedicine', *Science* **196**, pp. 129–36.

53 Dennerstein, L. 1994. 'Psychiatry of women', *Foundations of Clinical Psychiatry*, eds S Bloch and B.S. Singh, Melbourne University Press, Melbourne, pp. 289–99.

54 Price, W.A. Dimarzio, M.S. and Gardner, P.R. 1986. 'Biopsychosocial approach to premenstrual syndrome', *AFP* **33**(6), pp. 117–22.

55 Puolakka, J. Makarainen, L. Viinikka, L. et al., 1985. 'Biochemical and clinical effects of treating the promenstrual syndrome with prostaglandin synthesis precursors', *J Reprod Med* **30**(3), pp. 149–53.

56 Abraham, G. 1983. 'Nutritional factors in the etiology of the premenstrual tension syndromes', *J Reprod Med* **28**(7), pp. 446–64.

57 Dalton, K. 1994. *PMS: The Essential Guide to Treatment Options*, Thorsons, London, p. 69.

58 Janiger, O. Riffenburgh, R. and Kersh, R. 1972. 'Cross cultural study of premenstrual symptoms', *Psychosomatics* **13**, pp. 226–35.

59 Love, S.M. Gelman, R.S. and Silen, W. 1982. 'Fibrocystic "disease" of the breast—A non-disease', *N Engl J Med* **307**(16), pp. 1010–14; McGinn, K.A. 1992. *The Informed Woman's Guide to Breast Health*, Bull Publishing Company, Palo Alto, California, pp. 19–21.

60 Vorherr, H. 1986. 'Fibrocystic breast disease: pathophysiology, pathomorphology, clinical picture, and managment', *Am J Obstet Gynecol* **154**(1), pp. 161–79.

61 Wise Budoff, P., 1983. 'The use of prostaglandins inhibitors for premenstrual syndrome', *J Reprod Med* **28**(7), pp. 469–78.

62 Vorherr, H., 1986. 'Fibrocystic breast disease: Pathophysiology, pathomorphology, clinical picture and management', *Am J Obstet Gynecol*, **154**, pp. 161–79.

63 Horrobin, D.F., 1983. 'The role of essential fatty acids and prostaglandins in the pre-menstrual syndrome', *J Reprod Med*, **28**(7), pp. 465–8.

64 Wetzig, N.R. 1994. 'Mastalgia: A 3 year Australian study', *Aust NZ J Surg* **64**, pp. 329–331.

65 Consumers' Association, 1992. 'Cyclical breast pain—What works and what doesn't', *Drug Th Bull* **30**(1), pp. 1–3.

66 Boyle, C.A. Berkowitz, G.S. Livolsi, V.A. et al., 1984. 'Caffeine consumption and

fibrocystic breast disease: a case-control epidemiological study', *J Natl Cancer Inst* 72(5), pp. 1015–9.

67 Boyd, N.F. McGuire, V. Shannon, P. et al., 1988 'Effect of a low-fat high-carbohydrate diet on symptoms of cyclical mastopathy', *Lancet* 2, pp. 128–32.

68 London, R.S. Sundaram, G.S. and Goldstein, P.J. 1982. 'Medical management of mammary dysplasia', *Obstet Gynecol* 59(4), pp. 519–23.

69 ibid. pp. 519–23.

70 Consumers' Association, 1992. 'Cyclical breast pain—what works and what doesn't', *Drug Th Bull*, 30(1), pp. 1–3.

71 Copeland, M.M. 1963. 'The treatment of mammary dysplasia with special reference to microcystic and macrosystic disease of the breast', *Am J Surg*, 106, pp. 382–4; McFadyn, I.J. Raab, G.M. Macintyre C.C.A. et al., 1989. 'Progesterone cream for cyclic breast pain', *BMJ* 298, p. 231.

72 London, R.S. Sundaram, G.S. Schultz, M. et al., 1981. 'Endocrine parameters and alpha-tocopherol therapy of patients with mammary dysplasia', *Cancer Res*, 41, pp. 3811–13.

73 Pyke, J.K. Mansel, R.E. and Hughes L.E. 1985. 'Clinical experience of drug treatments for mastalgia', *Lancet* 2(8451), pp. 373–7.

74 Mansel, R.E. Pye, J.K. and Hughes, L.E. 1990. 'Effects of essential fatty acids on cyclical mastalgia and non-cyclical breast disorders', *Omega-6 Essential Fatty Acids. Pathophysiology and Roles in Clinical Medicine*, ed. D Horrobin, Niley-Liss, New York, pp. 557–66.

75 Tamborini, A. and Taurelle, R. 1993. '[Value of standardised Gingko biloba extract (EGB 761) in the management of congestive symptoms of premenstrual syndrome]' *Rev Fr Gynecol Obstet* 88(7–9), pp. 447–57.

76 Rose, D.P. Boyar, A.P. Cohen, C. et al., 1987. 'Effect of a low-fat diet on hormone levels in women with cystic breast disease. I. Serum steroids and gonadotropins', *J Natl Cancer Inst* 78(4), pp. 623–6; Boyd, N.F. McGuire, V. Shannon, P. et al., 1988. 'Effect of a low-fat high-carbohydrate diet on symptoms of cyclical mastopathy', *Lancet* 2, pp. 128–32.

77 Sanders, L.R. Hofeldt, F.D. Kirk, MC. et al., 1982. 'Refined carbohydrate as a contributing factor in reactive hypoglycemia', *South Med J* 75(9), pp. 1072–5.

78 O'Keefe, S. and Marks, V. 1977. 'Lunchtime gin and tonic as a cause of reactive hypoglycemia', *Lancet* 1(8025), pp. 1286–8.

79 Marsoobian, V. Grosvenor, M. Jacob, M. et al., 1995. "Very-low-energy diets alter the counterregulatory response to falling plasma glucose concentrations', *Am J Clin Nutr* Feb; 61(2), pp. 373–8.

80 Anderson, R.A. Polansky, M.M. Bryden, NA. et al., 1987. 'Effects of supplemental chromium on patients with symptoms of reactive hypoglycemia', *Metabolism* Apr; 36(4), pp. 351–5.

81 Shansky, A. 1981. 'Vitamin B3 in the alleviation of hypoglycemia', Drug and Cosmetic Industry 129 (4), p. 68.

82 Werbach, M.R. 1989. *Nutritional Influences on Illness*, Thorsons Publishing Group, England, p. 241.

Chapter 9

1 Mei, Q.B. Tao, J.Y. and Cui, B. 1991. 'Advances in the pharmacological studies of radix Angelica sinensis (Oliv) Diels (Chinese Dang gui)', *Ch Med J* 104(9), pp. 776–81.

2 Thomas, J. ed. 1995. *Australian Prescription Products Guide*, Australian Pharmaceutical Publishing Company Limited, Melbourne, pp. 1097–8.

3   Coney, S. 1991. *The Menopause Industry. A Guide to Medicine's 'Discovery' of the Mid-Life Woman*, Penguin Books, Auckland, New Zealand, p. 132.

4   Siddle, N. Sarrel, P. and Whitehead, M. 1987. 'The effect of hysterectomy on the age of ovarian failure: Indentification of a subgroup of women with premature loss of ovarian function and literature review', *Fert Sterility* 47(1), pp. 94–100.

5   Turney, L. 1993. 'Risk and contraception. What women are not told about tubal ligation', *Women's Studies Int Forum* 16(5), pp. 471–86.

6   Stoppard, M. 1994. *Menopause*, Penguin, Melbourne, p. 32.

7   Dennerstein, L. Smith, A.M.A. and Morse, C. 1993. 'Menopausal symptoms in Australian women', *Med J Aust* 159, pp. 232–6.

8   Adleurcreutz, H. Hamalainen, E. and Gorbach, S. 1992. 'Dietary phyto-oestrogens and the menopause in Japan', *Lancet* 339, p. 1233; Ramoso-Jalbuena, J. 1994. 'Climacteric Filipino women: a preliminary survey in the Philippines', *Maturitas* 19(3), pp. 183–90; Haines, C.J. Chung, T.K. and Leung, D.H. 1994. 'A prospective study of the frequency of acute menopausal symptoms in Hong Kong Chinese women', *Maturitas* 18(3), pp. 175–81.

9   Wilcox, G. Wahlqvist, M.L. Burger, H.G. et al., 1990. 'Oestrogenic effect of plant foods in postmenopausal women', *BMJ* 301, pp. 905–6; Murkies, A.L. Lombard, C. Strauss, B.J.G. et al., 1995. 'Dietary flour supplementation decreases post-menopausal hot flushes: effect of soy and wheat flour', *Maturitas* 21, pp. 189–95.

10 Armstrong, B.K. Brown, JB. Clarke, H.T. et al., 1981. 'Diet and reproductive hormones: a study of vegetarian and nonvegetarian postmenopausal women', *J Natl Cancer Inst* 67, pp. 761–7.

11 Mousavi, Y. and Adleurcreutz, H. 1993. 'Genistein is an effective stimulator of sex hormone-binding globulin production in hepatocarcinoma human liver cells and suppresses proliferation of these cells in culture', *Steroids* 58, pp. 301–4.

12 Khan, S.A. Pace, J.E. Cox, M.L. et al., 1994. 'Climacteric symptoms in healthy middle-aged women', *Br J Clin Pract* 48(5), 240–2.

13 Dennerstein, L. Smith, A.M.A. Morse, C. et al., 1993. 'Menopausal symptoms in Australian women', *Med J Aust* 159, pp. 232–6.

14 Wilcox, G. Wahlqvist, M.L. Burger, H.G. et al., 1990. 'Oestrogenic effects of plant foods in postmenopausal women', *BMJ* 301, pp. 905–6.

15 Bradbury, R.B. and White, D.E. 1954. 'Estrogens and related substances in plants', *Vitams Horm* 12, pp. 207–33; Cheng, E.W. et al., 1954. 'Estrogenic activity of some isoflavone derivatives', *Science* 120, pp. 575.

16 Werbach, M.R. 1988. 'Nutritional Influences on Illness', Thorsons, London, p. 297.

17 ibid. p. 297.

18 Chenoy, R. Hussain, S. Tayob, Y. et al., 1994. 'Effect of oral gamolenic acid from evening primrose oil on menopausal flushing', *BMJ* 308(6927), pp. 501–3.

19 Castelo-Branco, C. Pons, F. Gratacos, E. et al., 1994. 'Relationship between skin collagen and bone changes during aging', *Maturitas* 18(3), pp. 199–206.

20 Willard, T. 1991. *The Wild Rose Scientific Herbal*, Wild Rose College of Natural Healing, Canada, p. 123.

21 Stoll, W. 1987. 'Phytopharmacon influences atrophic vaginal epithelium. Double blind study—*Cimicifuga* vs oestrogenic substances', *Therapeutikon* 1, p. 23.

22 Khan, S.A. Pace, J.E. Cox, M.L. et al., 1994. 'Climacteric symptoms in healthy middle-aged women', *Br J Clin Pract* 48(5), pp. 240–2.

23 Chenoy, R. Hussain, S. Tayob, Y. et al., 1994. 'Effect of oral gamolenic acid from evening primrose oil on menopausal flushing', *BMJ* 308(6927), pp. 501–3.

24 Morse, C.A. 1989. 'Menopausal mood disorders', *Comprehensive Therapy* 15(3), pp. 22–7.

25 Dennerstein, L. Smith, A.M.A. and Morse, C. 1994. 'Psychological well-being, mid-life and the menopause', *Maturitas* 20, pp. 1–11; Morse, C.A. 1989. 'Menopausal mood disorders', *Comprehensive Therapy* 15(3), pp. 22–7.

26 Ballinger, S. 1990.'Stress as a factor in lowered oestrogen levels in early postmenopause', *Ann N Y Acad Sci* **592**, pp. 95–113. Discussion pp. 123–33.

27 Ballinger, S. Cobbin, D. Krivanek, J. et al., 1979. 'Life stresses and depression in the menopause', *Maturitas* **1**(3), pp. 191–9.

28 Hunter, M.S. 1990. 'Emotional well-being, sexual behaviour and hormone replacement therapy', *Maturitas* **12**(3), pp. 299–314.

Chapter 10

1   Dramusic, V. Marjanovic, B. and Erceg, J. 1974. 'Dysmenorrhea in adolescence caused by disturbed family relations', *The Family. Fourth International Congress of Psychosomatic Obstetrics and Gynecology*, ed S.L. Smith, Tel Aviv, pp. 503–6.

2   Tiu, C. 1953. 'The fundamentals of clinical proteinology', *J Clin Nutr* **1**, pp. 232–49.

3   McClain, C.J. Humphries, L.L. and Hill, K.K. 1993. 'Gastrointestinal and nutritional aspects of eating disorders', *J Am Coll Nutr* **12**(4), pp. 466–74.

4   Schauss, A.G. and Bryce-Smith, D. 1987. 'Evidence of zinc deficiency in anorexia nervosa and bulimia nervosa', *'Nutrients and Brain Function'*, ed W.B. Essman, Karger, Basel, pp. 151–62.

5   Taymor M.L. et al., 1964. 'The etiological role of chronic iron deficiency in production of menorrhagia', *JAMA* **187**, pp. 323–7.

6   Harlow, S.D. and Campbell, B.C. 1994. 'Host factors that influence the duration of menstrual bleeding', *Epidemiology* May; **5**(3), pp. 352–5.

7   Barbieri, R.L. 1990. 'Etiology and epidemiology of endometriosis', *Am J Obstet Gynecol* Feb; **162**(2), pp. 565–7.

8   Wetzig, N.R. 1994. 'Mastalgia: A 3 year Australian study', *Aust NZ J Surg* **64**, pp. 329–331.

9   Law, M.R. Wald, N.J. and Meade, T.W. 1991. 'Strategies for prevention of osteoporosis and hip fracture', *BMJ* **303**, pp. 453–9.

10 Krolner, B. Toft, B. Nielson, S. et al., 1983. 'Physical exercise as prophylaxis against involutional vertebral bone loss: A controlled trial', *Clin Sci* **64**, pp. 541–6; Chow, R.K. Harrison, J.E. and Notarius, C. 1987. 'Effect of two randomised exercise programmes on bone mass of healthy postmenopausal women', *Br Med J* **292**, pp. 607–10.

11 Flintoff-King, D. 1995. *Instant Vitality*, Anne O'Donovan, Melbourne.

12 Han, M. Pan, L. Wu, B. et al., 1994. 'A case-control epidemiologic study of endometriosis', *Chin Med Sci J* Jun; **9**(2), pp. 114–8; Pan, L.Y. 1993. 'Menstrual status as risk factors of endometriosis: a case controlled study', *Chung Hua Fa Chan Ko Tsa Chih* Mar; **28**(3), pp. 147–9, 188.

13 Mira, M. and Abraham, S. 1985. 'Amenorrhoea in female runners. What are the problems?" *Patient Management* Sept; pp. 25–31.

14 Constantini, N.W. and Warren, M.P. 1994. 'Special problems of the female athlete', *Baillieres Clin Rheumatol* **8**(1), pp. 199–219.

15 Elias, A.N. and Wilson, A.F. 1993. 'Exercise and gonadal function', *Hum Reprod* **8**(10), pp. 1747–61.

16 Beals, K.A. and Manore, M.M. 1994. 'The prevalence and consequences of subclinical eating disorders in female athletes', *Int J Sport Nutr* Jun; **4**(2), pp. 175–95.

17 Hetland, M.L. Haarbo, J. Christiansen, C. et al., 1994. 'Bone metabolism in female runners. Menstruation disorders are frequent among long-distance runners, but the bone mass is not influenced, with the exception of runners with amenorrhea', *Ugeskr-Laeger* Nov 28; **156**(48), pp. 7219–23.

18 Grodstein, F. Goldman, M.B. and Ryan, L. 1993. 'Relation of female infertility to consumption of caffeinated beverages', *Am J Epidemiol* Jun; 137(12), pp. 1353–60.

19 Grodstein, F. Goldman, M.B. and Cramer, D.W. 1994. 'Infertility in women and moderate alcohol use', *Am J Public Health* Sep, 84(9), pp. 1429–32.

20 ibid. pp. 1429–32.

21 Alfonso, M. Marco, J. and Balvis, I.A. 1991. 'Direct action of ethanol on pituitary prolactin secretion in vitro', *Rev Esp Fisiol* Sep, 47(3), pp. 133–40.

22 Kranzler, H.R. and Wallington, D.J. 1992. 'Serum prolactin level, craving, and early discharge from treatment in cocaine-dependent patients', *Am J Drug Alcohol Abuse* 18(2), pp. 187–95.

23 Goodman and Gilman's 1992. *The Pharmacological Basis of Therapeutics*, eds A. Goodman Gilman, T.W. Rall, A.S. Nies and P. Taylor, 8th Edition, McGraw Hill, Singapore, p. 533.

24 Baron, J.A. La Vecchia C. and Levi, F. 1990. 'The antiestrogenic effect of cigarette smoking in women', *Am J Obstet Gynecol* 162, pp. 502–14.

Chapter 11

1 Smith, S.K. Abel, M.H. Kelly, R.W. et al., 1981. 'A role for prostacyclin (PGI2) in excessive menstrual bleeding', *Lancet* 1, pp. 522–5.

2 Fraser, I.S. Shearman, R.P. McIlveen, J. et al., 1981. 'Efficacy of mefenamic acid in patients with a complaint of menorrhagia', *Obstet Gynecol* 58(5), pp. 543–51.

3 Mezrow, G. 1994. 'Treatment of dysfunctional uterine bleeding', *Management of Common Problems in Obstetrics and Gynecology*, eds D.R. Mishell, and P.F. Brenner, Blackwell Scientific Publishing, USA, p. 444.

4 Taymor, M.L. Sturgis, S.H. and Yahia, C. 1964. 'The role of chronic iron deficiency in production of menorrhagia', *JAMA* 187(5), pp. 323–7.

5 Brabin, L. and Brabin, B.J. 1992. 'The cost of successful adolescent growth and development in relation to iron and vitamin A status', *Am J Clin Nutr* 55(5), pp. 955–8.

6 Siddiqui, N.A. Loughney, A. Thomas, E.J. et al., 1994. 'Cellular retinoid binding proteins and nuclear retinoic acid receptors in endometrial cells', *Hum Reprod* 9(8), pp. 1410–16.

7 Lithgow, D.M. and Politzer, W.M. 1977. 'Vitamin A in the treatment of menorrhagia', *S Afr Med J* 51(7), pp. 191–3.

8 Szarka, C.E. Grana, G. and Engstrom, P.F. 1994. 'Chemoprevention of cancer', *Curr Probl Cancer* XVII(1), pp. 3–78.

9 Pizzorno, J.E. and Murray, M.T. 1985. 'Menorrhagia', *A Textbook of Natural Medicine*, John Bastyr College Publications, Seattle Washington, pp. VI: Menorr, 1–4.

10 Gubner, R. and Ungerleider, H.E. 1944. 'Vitamin K therapy in menorrhagia', *South Med J* 36(10), pp. 556–8.

11 Cohen, H. Scott, S.D. Mackie, I.J. et al., 1988. 'The development of hypoprothrombinaemia following antibiotic therapy in malnourished patients with low serum vitamin K1 levels', *Br J Haematol* Jan, 68(1), pp. 63–6; Schentag, J.J. Welage, L.S. Grasela T.H. et al., 1987. 'Determinants of antibiotic-associated hypoprothombinemia', *Pharmacotherapy* 7(3), pp. 80–6.

12 Havsteen, B. 1983. 'Flavonoids, a class of natural products of high pharmacological potency', *Bioch Pharm* 32(7), pp. 1141–8.

13 Markaverich, B.M. Roberts, R.R. Aleindro, MA. et al., 1988. 'Bioflavonoid interaction with rat uterine type II binding sites and cell growth inhibition', *J Steroid Biochem* 30(1–6), pp. 71–8.

14 Ibrahim, A.R. and Abul-Hajj, Y.J. 1990. 'Aromatase inhibition by flavonoids', *J Steroid Biochem Mol Biol* **37**(2), pp. 257–60.

15 Cohen, J.D. and Rubin, H.W. 1960. 'Functional menorrhagia: treatment with bioflavonoids and vitamin C', *Curr Ther Res* **2**(11), pp. 539–42.

16 Cassidy, A. Bingham, S. and Setchell, K.D.R. 1994. 'Biological effects of a diet of soy protein rich in isoflavones on the menstrual cycle of premenopausal women', *Am J Clin Nutr* **60**, pp. 333–40.

17 Rowland, Beryl, 1981. *Medieval Woman's Guide to Health: The First English Gynecological Handbook*, Kent State University Press, Kent, Ohio.

18 March, C.M. 1994. 'Uterine leiomyomas', *Management of Common Problems in Obstetrics and Gynecology*, eds D.R. Mishell and P.F. Brenner, Blackwell Scientific Publications, Boston, p. 467.

19 Christiansen, J.K. 1993. 'The facts about fibroids', *Postgrad Med* **94**(3), pp. 129–37.

20 Saxena, S.P. Khare, C. Farooq, A. et al., 1987. 'DDT and its metabolites in leiomyomatous and normal human uterine tissue', *Arch Toxicol* **59**(6), pp. 453–5.

21 Ross, R.K. Pike, MC. Vessey, M.P. et al., 1986. 'Risk factors for uterine fibroids: reduced risk associated with oral contraceptives', *Br Med J Clin Res Ed* **293**(6543), pp. 359–62.

22 Stalder, R. Bexter, A. Wurzner, H.P. et al., 1990. 'A carcinogenicity study of instant coffee in Swiss mice', *Food Chem Toxicol* **28**(12), pp. 829–37.

23 Drife, J. 1990. 'Benefits and risks of oral contraceptives', *Adv Contracept* **6** Suppl, pp. 15–25.

24 Parazzini, F. La-Vecchia, C. Negri, E. et al., 1988. 'Epidemiologic characteristics of women with uterine fibroids: a case-control study', *Obstet Gynecol* **72**(6), pp. 853–7.

25 Parrazini, F. Negri, E. La-Vecchia, C. et al., 1992. 'Oral contraceptive use and risk of uterine fibroids', *Obstet Gynecol* **79**(3), 430–3; Schesselman, J.J. 1991. 'Oral contraceptives and neoplasia of the uterine corpus', *Contraception* **43**(6), pp. 557–79.

26 Baron, J.A. La-Vecchia, C. and Levi, F. 1990. 'The antioestrogenic effect of cigarette smoking in women', *Am J Obstet Gynecol* **162**(2), pp. 502–14.

27 Parazzini, F. La-Vecchia, C. Negri, E. et al., 1988. 'Epidemiologic characteristics of women with uterine fibroids: a case-control study', *Obstet Gynecol* **72**(6), pp. 853–7.

28 Sakamoto, S. Yoshino, H. Shirahata, Y. et al., 1992. 'Pharmacotherapeutic effects of Kuei-chih-fu-ling-wan (Keishi-bukuryo-gan) on human uterine myomas', *Am J Chin Med* **20**(3–4), pp. 313–7.

29 Mori, T., Sakamoto, S. Singtripop, T. et al., 1993. 'Suppression of spontaneous development of uterine adenomyosis by a Chinese herbal medicine, Keishi-bukuryo-gan, in mice', *Planta Med* **59**, pp. 308–11.

Chapter 12

1 Cahill, D.J. Fox, R. Wardle, P.G. et al., 1994. 'Multiple follicular development associated with herbal medicine', *Hum Reprod* (United Kingdom) **9**(8), pp. 1469–70.

2 Kayser, H.W. and Istanbulluoglu, S. 1954. 'Eine Behandlung von Menstruationsstorungen ohne Hormone', *Hippokrates* **25**, pp. 717–8; Probst, V. and Roth, O.A. 1954. 'Uber einen Pflanzenextrakt mit hormonartiger Wirkung', *Dtsch Med Wschr* **79**, pp. 1271–6.

3 Holman P. 1995. 'Pyridoxine—Vitamin B6', *J Aust Coll Nutr Env Med* **14**(1), pp. 5–16.

4 Rivlin, M.E. 1994. 'Endometrial hyperplasia', *Manual of Clinical Problems in Obstetrics and Gynecology*', eds M.E. Rivlin and R.W. Martin, Little, Brown and Company, Boston, pp. 433–7.

5 Phipps, W.R. Martini, M.C. Lampe, J.W. et al., 1993. 'Effect of flaxseed ingestion on the menstrual cycle', *J Clin Endocrinol Metab*, 77(5), pp. 1215–19.

6 Weiss, R.F. 1988. *Herbal Medicine*, AB Arcanum, England, pp. 316–17.

7 Drozdz, M. Tomala, J. Jendryczko, A. et al., 1989. 'Concentration of selenium and vitamin E in the serum of women with malignant neoplasms and their family members' *Ginekol Pol* 60(6), pp. 301–5.

Chapter 13

1 Lobo R.A. and Kletzky O.A. 1982. 'Normalisation of androgen and sex hormone binding globulin levels after treatment of hyperprolactinaemia', *J Clin Endocrinol Metab* 56, pp. 562–6.

2 Lobo RA. and Kletzky O.A. 1982. 'Normalisation of androgen and sex hormone binding globulin levels after treatment of hyperprolactinaemia', *J Clin Endocrinol Metab* 56, pp. 562–6.

3 Schlechte J.A. Sherman B. and Martin R. 1983. 'Bone density in amenorrheic women with and without hyperprolactinaemia', *J Clin Endocrinol Metab* 56, pp. 1120–3.

4 Usuki, S. and Usuki, Y. 1989. 'Hachimijiogan treatment is effective in the management of infertile women with hyperprolactinaemia or bromocriptine-resistant hyperprolactinaemia', *Am J Chin Med* XVII(3–4), pp. 225–41.

5 Ota, H. Fukushima, M. 1988. 'Stimulation by Kanpo prescriptions of aromatase activity in rat follicle cell cultures', *Recent Advances in the Practice of Kanpo Medicine*', eds E. Hosoya and Y. Yamamura, Exerpta Medica, Amsterdam, pp. 177–82.

6 Sluitz, G. Speiser, P. Schultz, A.M. et al., 1993. 'Agnus castus extracts inhibit prolactin secretion of rat pituitary cells', *Horm Metab Res* 25, pp. 253–5; Milewicz, A. Gejdel, E. Sworen, H. et al., 1993. 'Vitex agnus castus in the treatment of luteal phase defects due to latent hyperprolactinaemia: Results of a randomised placebo-controlled double blind study', *Arzneim Forsch Drug Res* 43(II), pp. 752–6.

7 Thomas, J. ed, 1995. *Australian Prescription Products Guide*, Australian Pharmaceutical Publishing Company Limited, Melbourne.

8 Armstrong, B.K. Brown, J.B. Clarke, H.T. et al., 1981. 'Diet and reproductive hormones: a study of vegetarian and nonvegetarian postmenopausal women', *J Natl Cancer Inst* 67, pp. 761–67.

9 Mousavi, Y. and Adleurcreutz, H. 1993. 'Genistein is an effective stimulator of sex hormone-binding globulin production in hepatocarcinoma human liver cells and suppresses proliferation of these cells in culture', *Steroids* 58(7), pp. 301–4.

10 Sakamoto, K. Watanabe, M. and Aburada, M. 1988. 'Effect of Shakuyaku-kanzo-to (TJ68) and glycyrrhetinic acid on hyperandrogenism', *Recent Advances in the Practice of Kanpo Medicine*, eds E Hosoya and Y. Yamamura, Exerpta Medica, Amsterdam, pp. 163–9.

11 Kellogg, J.H. 1902. *The Home Hand-Book of Domestic Hygiene and Rational Medicine*, Echo Publishing Company, Melbourne.

Chapter 14

1 Srihari Rao T. Basu, N. and Siddiqui, H.H. 1982. 'Anti-inflammatory activity of Curcuma analogues', *Agents and Actions* **18**, pp. 407–12.

2 Backon, J. 1989. 'Negative correlation of cigarette smoking and dysmenorrhoea: reduced prostaglandin synthesis due to beta-endorphin, nicotine, or acrolein antagonism', *Med Hypotheses* **28**(3), pp. 213–4.

3 Merzow, G. 1994. 'Dysmenorrhoea', *'Management of Common Problems in Obstetrics and Gynecology'*, eds D.R. Mishell and P.F. Brenner, Blackwell Scientific Publications, Boston, p. 425.

4 Werbach, M.R. and Murray, M.T. 1994. *Botanical Influences on Illness*, Third Line Press, California, p. 307.

Chapter 15

1 Moen, M.H. and Muus, K.M. 1991. 'Endometriosis in pregnant and non-pregnant women at tubal sterilization', *Hum Reprod* **6**(5), pp. 699–702.

2 Vercellini, P. and Crosignani, P.G. 1993. 'Minimal and mild endometriosis. Is there anything new under the sun'? *J Reprod Med* **38**(1), pp. 49–52.

3 Evers, J.L. 1994. 'Endometriosis does not exist; all women have endometriosis', *Hum Reprod* **9**(12), pp. 2206–9.

4 Wardle, P.G. and Hull, M.G. 1993. 'Is endometriosis a disease'? *Baillieres Clin Obstet Gynaecol* **7**(4), pp. 673–85.

5 Barbieri, R.L. Callery, M. and Perez, S.E. 1992. 'Directionality of menstrual flow: cervical os diameter as a determinant of retrograde menstruation', *Fertil Steril* **57**(4), pp. 727–30.

6 Sanfilippo, J.S. Wakim, N.G. Schikler, K.N. et al., 1986. 'Endometriosis in association with uterine anomaly', *Am J Obstet Gynecol* **154**, pp. 39–43.

7 Ayers, J.W.T. and Friedenstab, A.P. 1985. 'Utero-tubal hypotonia associated with pelvic endometriosis', *Proceedings of 41st Annual Meeting of the American Fertility Society*, American Fertility Society, Birmingham, USA, p. 131.

8 Leiva, M.C. Hasty, L.A. Pfeifer, S. et al., 1993. 'Increased chemotactic activity of peritoneal fluid in patients with endometriosis', *Am J Obstet Gynecol* **168**(2), pp. 592–8.

9 Braun, D.P. Gebel, H. Rotman, C. et al., 1992. 'The development of cytotoxicity in peritoneal macrophages from women with endometriosis', *Fertil Steril* **57**(6), pp. 1203–10.

10 Dunselman, G.A. Hendrix, M.G. and Bouckaert, P.X. 1988. 'Functional aspects of peritoneal macrophages in endometriosis of women', *J Reprod Fertil* **82**(2), pp. 707–10.

11 Halme, J. Becker, S. and Wing, R. 1984. 'Accentuated cyclic activation of peritoneal macrophages in patients with endometriosis', *Am J Obstet Gynecol* **148**(1), pp. 85–90.

12 Haney, A.F. 1993. 'Endometriosis, macrophages, and adhesions', *Prog Clin Biol Res* **381**, pp. 19–44.

13 Dmowski, W.P. Gebel, H.M. and Braun, D.P. 1994. 'The role of cell-mediated immunity in pathogenesis of endometriosis', *Acta Obstet Gnecol Scand Suppl* **159**, pp. 7–14.

14 Ramey, J.W. and Archer, D.F. 1993. 'Peritoneal fluid: its relevance to the development of endometriosis', *Fertil Steril* **60**(1), pp. 1–14.

15 Hill, J.A. Faris, H.M. Schiff, I. et al., 1988. 'Characterisation of leucocyte sub-

populations in the peritoneal fluid of women with endometriosis', *Fertil Steril* 50(2), pp. 216–22.

16 Oosterlynck, D.J. Cornille, F.J. Waer, M. et al., 1991. 'Women with endometriosis show a defect in natural killer activity resulting in a decreased cytotoxicity to autologous endometrium', *Fertil Steril* 56(1), pp. 45–51.

17 Garzetti, G.G. Ciavattini, A. Provinciali, M. et al., 1993. 'Natural killer cell activity in endometriosis: correlation between serum oestradiol levels and cytotoxicity', *Obstet Gynecol* 81(5(Pt 1)), pp. 665–8; Garzetti, G.G. Ciavattini, A. Provinciali, M. et al., 1995. 'Natural killer activity in stage III and IV endometriosis: impaired cyctoxicity and retained lymphokine responsiveness of natural killer cells', *Gynecol Endocrinol* 9(2), pp. 125–30.

18 Hirata, J. Kikuchi, Y. Imaizumi, E. et al., 1994. 'Endometriotic tissues produce immunosuppressive factors', *Gynecol Obstet Invest* 37 (1), pp. 43–7; Oosterlynck, D.J. Meuleman, C. Waer, M. et al., 1993.'Immunosuppressive activity of peritoneal fluid in women with endometriosis', *Obstet Gynecol* 82(2), pp. 206–12.

19 Nakayama, K. Masuzawa, H. Li, S.F. et al., 1994. 'Immunohistochemical analysis of the peritoneum adjacent to endometriotic lesions using antibodies for Ber-EP4 antigen, estrogen receptors, and progesterone receptors: implication of peritoneal metaplasia in the pathogenesis of endometriosis', *Int J Gynecol Pathol* 13(4), pp. 348–58.

20 Han, M. Pan, L. Wu, B. et al., 1994. 'A case-control epidemiologic study of endometriosis', *Chin Med Sci J* 9(2), pp. 114–8; Parazzini, F. Ferraroni, M. Fedele, L. et al., 1995. 'Pelvic endometriosis: reproductive and menstrual risk factors at different stages in Lombardy, northern Italy', *J Epidemiol Community Health* 49(1), pp. 61–4; Pan, L.Y. 1993. 'Menstrual status as risk factors of endometriosis: a case controlled study', *Chung Hua Fa Chan Ko Tsa Chih* 28(3), pp. 147–9, 188; Candiani, G.B. Danesino, V. Gastaldi, A. et al., 1991. 'Reproductive and menstrual factors and risk of peritoneal and ovarian endometriosis', *Fertil Steril* 56(2), pp. 230–4.

21 Moen, M.H. and Magnus, P. 1993. 'The familial risk of endometriosis', *Acta Obstet Gynecol Scand* 72(7), pp. 560–4.

22 Han, M. Pan, L. Wu, B. et al., 1994. 'A case-control epidemiologic study of endometriosis', *Chin Med Sci J* 9(2), pp. 114–8; Pan, L.Y. 1993. 'Menstrual status as risk factors of endometriosis: a case controlled study', *Chung Hua Fa Chan Ko Tsa Chih* 28(3), pp. 147–9, 188.

23 Barbieri, R.L. 1990. 'Etiology and epidemiology of endometriosis', *Am J Obstet Gynecol* 162(2), pp. 565–7.

24 Parazzini, F. Ferraroni, M. Fedele, L. et al., 1995. 'Pelvic endometriosis, reproductive and menstrual risk factors at different stages in Lombardy, northern Italy', *J Epidemiol Community Health* 49(1), pp. 61–4; Candiani, G.B., Danesino, V. Gastaldi, A. et al., 1991. 'Reproductive and menstrual factors and risk of peritoneal and ovarian endometriosis', *Fertil Steril* 56(2), pp. 230–4.

25 Kirshon, B. Poindexter, A.N. et al., 1988. 'Contraception: a risk factor for endometriosis', *Obstet Gynecol* 71(6 (Pt 1)), pp. 829–31.

26 Tang, D.C. and Wu, X.R. 1991. 'Dynamic changes of myometrial activity, levels of PGF2 alpha and E2 in rabbits after insertion of four types of IUDs', *Adv Contracept* 7(1), pp. 29–38.

27 Vercellini, P. Ragni, G. Trespidi, L. et al., 1993. 'Does contraception modify the risk of endometriosis?' *Hum Reprod* 8(4), pp. 547–51.

28 Vessey, M.P. Villard-Mackintosh, L. and Painter, R. 1993. 'Epidemiology of endometriosis in women attending family planning clinics', *BMJ* 306(6871), pp. 182–4.

29 Grodstein, F. Goldman, M.B. and Ryan, L. et al., 1993. 'Relation of female infertility to consumption of caffeinated beverages', *Am J Epidemiol* 137(12), pp. 1353–60.

30 Perper, M.M. Breitkopf, L.J. Breitstein, R. et al., 1993. 'MAST scores, alcohol consumption, and gynecological symptoms in endometriosis patients', *Alcohol Clin Exp Res* 17(2), pp. 272–8.

31 Grodstein, F. Goldman, M.B. and Cramer, D.W. 1994. 'Infertility in women and moderate alcohol use', *Am J Public Health* 84(9), pp. 1429–32.

32 Filer, R.B. and Wu, C.H. 1989. 'Coitus during the menses. Its effect on endometriosis and pelvic inflammatory disease', *J Reprod Med* 34(11), pp. 887–90.

33 Lamb, K. and Berg, N. 1985. 'Tampon use in women with endometriosis', *J Community Health* Winter, 10(4), pp. 215–25.

34 Darrow, S.L. Vena, J.E. Batt, R.E. et al., 1993. 'Menstrual cycle characteristics and risk of endometriosis', *Epidemiology* 4(2), pp. 135–42.

35 Cramer, D.W. Wilson, E. Stillman, R.J. et al., 1986. 'The relationship of endometriosis to menstrual characteristics, smoking, and exercise', *JAMA* 255(14), pp. 1904–8.

36 Sutton, C.J. Ewen, S.P. Whitelaw, N. et al., 1994. 'Prospective, randomised, double-blind, controlled trial of laser laparoscopy in the treatment of pelvic pain associated with minimal, mild, and moderate endometriosis', *Fertil Steril* Oct, 62(4), pp. 696–700.

37 Israel, R. 1994. 'Endometriosis: Treatment', *Management of Common Problems in Obstetrics and Gynecology*, eds D.R. Mishell, and P.F. Brenner, Blackwell Scientific Publications, Boston, USA.

38 Mahmood, T.A. and Templeton, A. 1990. 'Pathophysiology of mild endometriosis: review of literature', *Hum Reprod* 5(7), pp. 765–84; Booker, M.W. 1988. 'Endometriosis', *Br J Hosp Med* 39(5), pp. 440–5.

39 Mio, Y. Toda, T. Harada, T. et al., 1992. 'Luteinized unruptured follicle in the early stages of endometriosis as a cause of unexplained infertility', *Am J Obstet Gynecol* 167(1), pp. 271–3; Holtz, G., Williamson, H.O., Mathur R.S. et al., 1985. 'Luteinized unruptured follicle syndrome in mild endometriosis. Assessment with biochemical parameters', *J Reprod Med* 30(9), pp. 643–5.

40 Cahill, D.J. Fox, R. Wardle, P.G. et al., 1994. 'Multiple follicular development associated with herbal medicine', *Hum Reprod* 9(8), pp. 1469–70.

41 Kalfarentzos, F. Spiliotis, J. Kaklamanis, L. et al., 1987. 'Prevention of peritoneal adhesion formation in mice by vitamin E', *J R Coll Surg Edinb* 32(5), pp. 288–90; Hemadeh, O. Chilukuri, S. Bonet, V. et al., 1993. 'Prevention of adhesions by administration of sodium carboxymethyl cellulose and vitamin E', *Surgery* 114(5), pp. 907–10; Kagoma, P. Burger, S.N. Seifter, E. et al., 1985. 'The effect of vitamin E on experimentally induced peritoneal adhesions in mice', *Arch Surg* 120(8), pp. 949–51.

42 Sakamoto, W. Fujie, K. Nishihira, J. et al., 1991. 'Inhibition of PGE2 production in macrophages from vitamin E-treated rats', *Prostaglandins Leukot Essent Fatty Acids* 44(2), pp. 89–92.

43 Tengerdy, R.P. 1990. 'The role of vitamin E in immune response and disease resistance', *Ann N Y Acad Sci* 587, pp. 24–33.

44 Rowland Beryl, 1981. *Medieval woman's guide to health: A Middle English treatise associated with Trotula*, The Kent State University Press, Kent, Ohio, p. 65.

45 Ross, Jeremy, 1985. *Zang Fu, The Organ Systems of Traditional Chinese Medicine*, Churchill Livingstone, Edinburgh, p. 101.

46 Resnick, C. 1995. *Nutritional Regulation of Detoxification*, American Association of Naturopathic Physicians, Tree Farm Cassettes (audio tape).

Chapter 16

1   Insler, V. and Lunenfeld, B. 1991. 'Pathophysiology of polycystic ovarian disease: new insights', *Hum Reprod* 6(8), pp. 1025–9.
2   Insler, V. Shoman, Z., Barash, A. et al., 1993. 'Polycystic ovaries in non-obese and obese patients: possible pathophysiological mechanisms based on new interpretation of facts and findings', *Hum Reprod* 8(3), pp. 379–84; Anttila, L. Ding, Y.Q. Ruutianen, K. et al., 1991. 'Clinical features and circulating gonadotrophin, insulin, and androgen interactions in women with polycystic ovarian disease', *Fertil Steril* 55(6), pp. 1057–61.
3   Eden, J.A. 1991. *Women's hormone problems*, Booklet published in conjunction with Royal Hospital for Women Paddington, Sydney, pp. 12–13.
4   Amann, W. 1975. 'Akne vulgaris and *Agnus castus* (Agnolyt®)', *Allg Med* 51 (35), pp. 1645–8.
5   Jarry, H. Leonhardt, S., Gorkow, C. et al., 1994. 'In vitro prolactin but not LH and FSH release is inhibited by compounds in extracts of *Agnus castus*: direct evidence for a dopaminergic principle by the dopamine receptor assay', *Exp Clin Endocrinol* 102, pp. 448–54.

Chapter 17

1   Budowski, P. and Crawford, M. 1985. 'Alpa-linolenic acid as a regulator of the metabolism of arachidonic acid: dietary implications of the ratio, n-6: n-3 fatty acids', *Proceedings of the Nutrition Society of Australia*, 44, pp. 221–9.
2   Miettinen, T.A. and Kesaniemi, Y.A. 1989. 'Cholesterol absorption: regulation of cholesterol synthesis and elimination and within-population variations of serum cholesterol levels', *Am J Clin Nutr* 49, pp. 629–635.
3   Muldoon, M.F. Manuck, S.B. and Matthews, K.A. 1990. 'Lowering cholesterol concentrations and mortality; a quantitive review of primary prevention trials', *Br Med J* 301, pp. 309–314.
4   McCully, K.S. 1990. 'Atherosclerosis, serum cholesterol and the homocysteine theory: a study of 194 consecutive autopsies', *Am J Med Sci* 299(4), pp. 217–21.
5   Crouse, J.R. 1989. 'Gender, lipoproteins, diet and cardiovascular risk', *Lancet* 1, pp. 318–20.
6   Mensik, R.P. and Katan, M.B. 1989. 'Effect of a diet enriched with mono-unsaturated or poly-unsaturated fatty acids on levels of low-density lipoprotein cholesterol in healthy women and men', *New Engl J Med* 321(7), pp. 436–41.
7   Reaven, P.D. and Witztum, J.L. 1993. 'Comparison of supplementation of RRR-alpha-tocopherol and racemic alpha-tocopherol in humans. Effects on lipid levels and lipoprotein susceptibility to oxidation', *Arterioscler Thromb* 13(4), pp. 601–8.
8   Werbach, M.R. and Murray, M.J. *Botanical Influences on Illness*, Third Line Press, Tarzana, California, pp. 27–8.
9   Mensik, R.P. and Katan, M.B. 1989. 'Effect of a diet enriched with mono-unsaturated or poly-unsaturated fatty acids on levels of low-density lipoprotein cholesterol in healthy women and men', *New Engl J Med* 321(7), pp. 436–441.
10 Erasmus, U. 1993. '*Fats That Heal, Fats That Kill*', Alive Books, Burnaby, BC. Canada, p. 57.
11 Cobiac, L. 1994. *Lactose: a review of intakes and of importance to health of Australians and New Zealanders*, CSIRO Division of Human Nutrition, Adelaide, SA.
12 ibid. *Lactose: a review of intakes and of importance to health of Australians and New Zealanders*, CSIRO Division of Human Nutrition, Adelaide, SA.

13 Lothe, L. and Lindberg, T. 1989. 'Cow's milk whey protein elicits symptoms of infantile colic in colicky formula-fed infants', *Pediatrics* **83**(2), pp. 262–6.

14 van't Veer, P. Dekker, J.M. Lamers, J.W.J. et al., 1989. 'Consumption of fermented milk products and breast cancer: a case-control study in the Netherlands', *Cancer Res* **49**, pp. 4020–3.

15 Savaiano, D.A. 1990. 'Lactose absorption and tolerance: the role of cultured dairy foods, *Proceedings of the XXIII International Dairy Congress*, Montreal, **2**, pp. 1238–46.

16 Alm, L. 1982. 'Effects of fermentation on curd size and digestibility of milk proteins in vitro of Swedish fermented milk products', *J Dairy Sci* **65**, pp. 509–14.

17 Crim, M.C. and Munro, H.N. 1994. 'Proteins and amino acids', *Modern Nutrition in Health and Disease*, eds M.E. Shils, J.A. Olson, M. Shike, Lea and Febiger, Philadelphia, p. 27.

18 Baghurst, K. Record, S. Powis, G. et al., 1993. *What are Australians Eating?* CSIRO Division of Human Nutrition, Adelaide, SA.

19 ibid. 1993. *What are Australians Eating*'? CSIRO Division of Human Nutrition, Adelaide, SA.

20 Callinan, P. 1991. 'The Pros and Cons of Your Daily Cuppa', *Australian Wellbeing* p. 43.

21 Wilcox, A. Weinberg, C. and Baird, D. 1988. 'Caffeinated beverages and decreased fertility', *Lancet* **2**, pp. 1453–6.

22 Pols, R. and Hawks, D. 1991. *Is there a safe level of daily consumption of alcohol for men and women. Recommendations regarding responsible drinking behaviour*, NH&MRC pamphlet, Canberra.

23 Block, G. Patterson, B. and Subar, A. 1992. 'Fruit, vegetables, and cancer prevention: a review of the epidemiological data', *Nutr Cancer* **18**, pp. 1–29.

24 Katsouyanni, K. Trichopolous, D. Boyle, P. et al., 1986. 'Diet and breast cancer: a case-control study in Greece', *Int J Cancer* **38**(6), pp. 815–20.

25 Szarka, C.E. Grana, G. and Engstrom, P.F. 1994. 'Chemoprevention of cancer', *Curr Probl Cancer* **17**(1), pp. 3–78.

26 Batieha, A.M. Armenian, H.K. Norkus, E.P. et al., 1993. 'Serum micronutrients and the subsequent risk of cervical cancers in a population-based nested case-control study', *Cancer Epidemiol Biomarkers Prev* **2**(4), pp. 335–9.

27 Potischman, N. McCulloch, C.E. Byers, T. et al., 1990. 'Breast cancer and dietary and plasma concentrations of carotenoids and vitamin A', *Am J Clin Nutr* **52**(5), pp. 909–15.

28 Le-Marchand, L. Yoshizawa, C.N. Kolonel, L.N. et al., 1989. 'Vegetable consumption and lung cancer risk: a population-based-control study in Hawaii', *J Natl Cancer Inst* **81**(15), pp. 1158–64; Schiffman, M.H. Pickle, L.W. and Fontham, E. et al., 1988. 'Case-control study of diet and mesothelioma in Louisiana', *Cancer Res* **48**(10), pp. 2911–15.

29 Young, T.B. and Wolf, D.A. 1988. 'Case-control study of proximal and distal colon cancer and diet in Wisconsin', *Int J Cancer* **42**(2), pp. 167–75; Lee, H.P. Gourley, L. Duffy, S.W. et al., 1989. 'Colorectal cancer and diet in an Asian population—a case-control study among Singapore Chinese', *Int J Cancer* **43**(6), pp. 1007–16.

30 Olsen, G.W. Mandel, J.S. Gibson, R.W. et al., 1989. 'A case-control study of pancreatic cancer and cigarettes, alcohol, coffee and diet', *Am J Public Health* **79**(8), pp. 1016–19.

31 Michnovicz, J.J. and Bradlow, H.L. 1991. 'Altered estrogen metabolism and excretion in humans following consumption of indole–3-carbinol', *Nutr Cancer* **16**(1), pp. 59–66; Niwa, T. Swaneck, G. Bradlow, H.L. 1994. 'Alterations in estradiol metabolism in MCF-7 cells induced by treatment with indole-3-carbinol', *Steroids* **59**(9), pp. 523–7.

32 Grubbs, C.J. Steele, V.E. Casebolt, T. et al., 1995. 'Chemoprevention of

chemically-induced mammary carcinogenesis by indole–3-carbinol', *Anticancer Res* **15**(3), pp. 709–16; Kojima, T. Tanaka, T. and Mori, H. 1994. 'Chemoprevention of spontaneous endometrial cancer in female Donryu rats by dietary indole–3-carbinol', *Cancer Res* **54**(6), pp. 1446–9.

33 Steinmetz, K.A. Kushi, L.H. Bostick, R.M. et al., 1994. 'Vegetables, fruit, and colon cancer in the Iowa Women's Health Study', *Am J Epidemiol* **139**(1), pp. 1–15; Han, J. 1993. 'Highlights of the cancer chemoprevention studies in China', *Prev Med* **22**(5), pp. 712–22; Cipriani, F. Buiatti, E. and Palli, D. 1991. 'Gastric cancer in Italy', *Ital J Gastroenterol* **23**(7), pp. 429–35.

34 Ip, C. and Lisk, D.J. 1994. 'Enrichment of selenium in allium vegetables for cancer prevention', *Carcinogenesis* **15**(9), pp. 1881–5; Ip, C. Lisk, D.J. and Scimeca, J.A. 1994. 'Potential of food modification in cancer prevention', *Cancer Res* **54**(7 Suppl), pp. 1957S–1959S.

35 Ip, C. and Lisk, D.J. 1994. 'Characterization of tissue selenium profiles and anticarcinogenic responses in rats fed natural sources of selenium-rich products', *Carcinogenesis* **15**(4), pp. 573–6.

36 Ip, C. Lisk, D.J. and Stoewsand, G.S. 1992. 'Mammary cancer prevention by regular garlic and selenium-enriched garlic', *Nutr Cancer* **17**(3), pp. 279–86.

37 Dorant, E. van den Brandt, P.A. and Goldbohm, R.A. 1995. 'Allium vegetable consumption, garlic supplement intake, and female breast carcinoma incidence', *Breast Cancer Res Treat* **33**(2), pp. 163–70.

38 Zhao, Z.Z. and Huang, M.T. 1992. '[A SOS induction test screening study for vegetables inhibiting mutagenicity caused by antineoplastic drugs'] *Chung Hua Yu Fang I Hsueh Tsa Chih* **26**(2), pp. 92–3.

39 Franceschi, S. Bidoli, E. La Vecchia, C. et al., 1994. 'Tomatoes and risk of digestive tract cancers', *Int J Cancer* **59**(2), pp. 181–4.

40 Morant, R. Jungi, W.F. Koehli, C. et al., 1991. 'Why do cancer patients use alternative medicine'?, *Schweiz Med Wochenschr* **121**(27–28), pp. 1029–34; Obrist, R. von Meiss, M. and Obrecht, J.P. 1986. 'The use of paramedical treatment methods by cancer patients. A inquiry on 101 ambulatory patients', *Dtsch Med Wochenschr* **111**(8), pp. 283–7.

41 Zang, F.A. Barrett, N.O. and Cohen, J.A. 1994. 'Differences in nutritional risk factors for breast cancer among New York City white, Hispanic, and black college students', *Ethn Dis* **4**(1), pp. 28–40.

42 Messina, M. and Barnes, S. 1991. 'The role of soy products in reducing risk of cancer', *J Nat Cancer Inst* **83**(8), pp. 541–6.

43 Messina, M. Persky, V. Setchel, K.D.R. et al., 1994. 'Soy intake and cancer risk: a review of the in vitro and in vivo data', *Nutr Cancer* **21**, pp. 113–31.

44 Gao, Y.T. McLaughlin, J.K. Blot, W.J. et al., 1994. 'Reduced risk of esophageal cancer associated with green tea consumption', *J Natl Cancer Inst* **86**(11), pp. 855–8; Yan, Y.S. 1993. 'The experiment of tumor-inhibiting effect of green tea extract in animal and human body', *Chung Hua Yu Fang I Hsueh Tsa Chih* **27**(3), pp. 129–31; Xu, G.P. Song, P.J. and Reed, P.I. 1993. 'Effects of fruit juices, processed vegetable juice, orange peel and green tea on endogenous formation of N-nitrosoproline in subjects from a high-risk area for gastric cancer in Moping County, China', *Eur J Cancer Prev* **2**(4), pp. 327–35.

45 Klaunig, J.E. 1992. 'Chemopreventive effects of green tea components on hepatic carcinogenesis', *Prev Med* **21**(4), pp. 510–19.

46 Imai, K. and Natachi, K. 1995. 'Cross sectional study of effects of drinking green tea on cardiovascular and liver diseases', *BMJ* **310**(6981), pp. 693–6.

47 Mukhtar, H. Katiyar, S.K. and Agarwal, R. 1994. 'Green tea and skin—anticarcinogenic effects', *J Invest Dermatol* **102**(1), pp. 3–7.

48 Komori, A. Yatsunami, J. Okabe, S. et al., 1993. 'Anticarcinogenic activity of green tea polyphenols', *Jpn J Clin Oncol* **23**(3), pp. 186–90.

49 Imai, K. and Natachi, K. 1995. 'Cross sectional study of effects of drinking green tea on cardiovascular and liver diseases', *BMJ* **310**(6981), pp. 693–6.

50 Mizuno, S. Watanabe, S. Nakamura, K. et al., 1992. 'A multi-institute case-control study on the risk factors of developing pancreatic cancer', *Jpn J Clin Oncol* **22**(4), pp. 286–91.

51 Tewes, F.J. Koo, L.C. Meisgen, T.J. et al., 1990. 'Lung cancer and mutagenicity of tea', *Environ Res* **52**(1), pp. 23–33.

52 Folino, M. McIntyre, A. and Young, G.P. 1995. 'Dietary fibers differ in their effects on large bowel epithelial proliferation and fecal fermentation-dependent events in rats', *J Nutr* June, **125**(6), pp. 1521–8.

53 Slavin, J.L. 1994. 'Epidemiological evidence for the impact of whole grains on health', *Crit Rev Food Sci Nutr* **34**(5–6), pp. 427–34; Thompson, L.U. 1994. 'Antioxidant and hormone-mediated health benefits of whole grains', *Crit Rev Food Sci Nutr* **34**(5–6), pp. 473–97.

54 Alabaster, O. Tang, Z.C. Frost, A. et al., 1993. 'Potential synergism between wheat bran and psyllium: enhanced inhibition of colon cancer', *Cancer Lett* **75**(1), pp. 53–8.

55 van't Veer, P. Dekker, J.M. Lamers, J.W.J. et al., 1989. 'Consumption of fermented milk products and breast cancer: A case-control study in the Netherlands', *Cancer Res* **49**, pp. 4020–3.

56 Lambert, J. 1996. 'Upper gastrointestinal tract disease and probiotics', *Asia Pacific J Clin Nutr* **5**, pp. 31–5.

57 McIntosh, G.H. 1996. 'Probiotics and colon cancer prevention', *Asia Pacific J Clin Nutr* **5**, pp. 48–52.

58 Tanaka, T. Arai, K. and Murota, I. 1985. 'Effects of feeding sour milk in longevity and tumorigenesis in mice and rats', *Bifidobacteria Microflora* **4**, pp. 31–7.

59 van't Veer, P. van Leer, E.M. Rietdijk, A. et al., 1991. 'Combination of dietary factors in relation to breast-cancer occurrence', *Int J Cancer* **47**(5), pp. 649–53.

60 Rosen, M. Nystrom, L. and Wall, S. 1988. '*Diet and cancer mortality in the counties of Sweden*', **127**(1), pp. 42–9.

61 Willett, W.C. Stampfer, M.J. Colditz, G.A. et al., 1987. 'Dietary fat and the risk of breast cancer', *New Eng J Med* **31**, pp. 22–8; Rosen, M. Nystrom, L. Wall, S. 1988. 'Diet and cancer mortality in the counties of Sweden', *Am J Epidemiol* **127**(1), pp. 42–9.

62 Hursting, S.D. Thornquist, M. and Henderson, M.M. 1990. 'Types of dietary fat and the incidence of cancer at five sites', *Prev Med* **19**(3), pp. 242–53.

63 Longnecker, M.P. 1994. 'Alcoholic beverage consumption in relation to risk of breast cancer: meta-analysis and review', *Cancer Causes Control* **5**(1), pp. 73–82; Colditz, G.A. 1993. 'Epidemiology of breast cancer. Findings from the nurses' health study', *Cancer* **71**(4 Suppl), pp. 1480–9.

64 Byers, T. 1994. 'Nutritional risk factors for breast cancer', *Cancer* **74**, pp. 288–95.

65 Kune, G.A. and Vitetta, L. 1992. 'Alcohol consumption and the etiology of colorectal cancer: a review of the scientific evidence from 1957 to 1991', *Nutr Cancer* **18**(2), pp. 97–111.

66 La Vecchia, C. Negri, E. Decarli, A. et al., 1989. 'Dietary factors in the risk of bladder cancer', *Nutr Cancer* **12**(1), pp. 93–101.

67 Benito, E. Obrador, A. Stiggelbout, A. et al., 1990. 'A population-based case-control study of colorectal cancer in Majorca. I. Dietary factors', *Int J Cancer* **45**(1), pp. 69–76.

68 Mesko, T.W. Dunlap, J.N. and Sutherland, C.M. 1990. 'Risk factors for breast cancer', *Compr Ther* **16**(11), pp. 3–9; Ewertz, M. 1993. 'Breast cancer in Denmark. Incidence, risk factors, and characteristics of survival', *Int J Cancer* **32**(6), pp. 595–615; Folsom, A.R. McKenzie, D.R. Bisgard, K.M. et al., 1993. 'No

association between caffeine intake and postmenopausal breast cancer incidence in the Iowa Women's Health Study', *Am J Epidemiol* **138**(6), pp. 380–3.

69 Vatten, L.J. Solvoll, K. and Loken, E.B. 1990. 'Coffee consumption and breast cancer risk. A prospective study of 14,593 Norwegian women', *Br J Cancer* **62**(2), pp. 267–70.

70 Kritchevsky, D. 1990. 'Nutrition and breast cancer', *Cancer* **66**(6 Suppl), pp. 1321–5.

71 English, R. and Lewis, S. 1991. *Food for Health. A Guide to Nutrition with Values for 650 Australian Foods*, Australian Government Publishing Service, Canberra, p. 64; Shils, M. Olson, J.A., Shike M. eds. 1994. *Modern Nutrition in Health and Disease*, Lea & Febiger, USA, pp. A-92–A-98.

Chapter 18

1 Bennets, H.W. Underwood, E.J. and Shier, F.L.A. 1946. 'A specific breeding problem of sheep on subterranean clover pastures in Western Australia', *Aust Vet J* **22**, pp. 2–12.

2 Setchell, K.D.R. and Adlercreutz, H. 1988. 'Mammalian lignans and phyto-oestrogens. Recent studies on their formation, metabolism and biological role in health and disease', *'Role of Gut Flora in Toxicity and Cancer*, Academic Press, London, pp. 315–45.

3 Phipps, W.R. Martini, M.C. Lampe, J.W. et al., 1993. 'Effect of flax seed ingestion on the menstrual cycle', *J Clin Endocrinol Metab* **77**(5), pp. 1215–9; Cassidy, A. Bingham, S. and Setchell, K.D.R. 1994. 'Biological effects of a diet of soy protein rich in isoflavones on the menstrual cycle of premenopausal women', *Am J Clin Nutr* **60**, pp. 333–40.

4 Adlercreutz, H. 1990. 'Western diet and Western diseases: some hormonal and biochemical mechanisms and associations', *Scand J Clin Lab Invest* **50**(S 201), pp. 3–23.

5 Wilcox, G. Wahlqvist, M.L. Burger, H. et al., 1990. 'Oestrogenic effects of foods in postmenopausal women', *BMJ* **301**, pp. 905–6.

6 Goldin, B.R. Adlercreutz, H. and Gorbach, S.L. 1986. 'The relationship between estrogen levels and diets of Caucasian American and Oriental immigrant women', *Am J Clin Nutr* **44**, pp. 945–53.

7 Adlercreutz, H. Hamalainen, E. Gorbach, S. et al., 1992. 'Dietary phyto-oestrogens and the menopause in Japan', *Lancet* **339**, p. 1233.

8 Hughes, C.L. 1988. 'Phyochemical mimicry of reproductive hormones and modulation of herbivore fertility by phyoestrogens', *Environ Health Pers* **78**, pp. 171–5.

9 Shemesh, M. Lindner, H.R. and Ayalon, N. 1972. 'Affinity of rabbit uterine oestradiol receptor for phyto-oestrogens and its use in a competitive protein-binding radioassay for plasma coumestrol', *J Reprod Fert* **29**, pp. 1–9.

10 Verdeal, K. and Ryan, D.S. 1979. 'Naurally-occurring estrogens in plant foodstuffs—a review', *J Food Prot* **42**(7), pp. 577–83.

11 Kielczynski, W. 1996. personal communication.

12 Priest, A.W. and Priest, L.R. 1982. *Herbal Medication*, LR Fowler and Co., London, pp. 94.

13 Grieve, M. 1931. *A Modern Herbal*, Penguin, London, pp. 207–8.

14 Chae, Y.H. Marcus, C.B. Ho, D.K. et al., 1991. 'Effects of synthetic and naturally occurring flavonoids on benzo[a]pyrene metabolism by hepatic microsomes prepared from rats treated with cytochrome P-450 inducers', *Cancer Letters* **60**(1), pp. 15–24.

15 Cassady, J.M. and Zennie, T.M., Chae, Y.H. et al., 1988. 'Use of a mammalian

cell culture benzo[a]pyrene metabolism assay for the detection of potential anti-carcinogens from natural products: inhibition of metabolism by biochanin A, an isoflavone from *Trifolium pratense* L', *Cancer Research* 48(22), pp. 6257–61.

16 Adams, N.R. 1979. 'Altered response of cervical and vaginal epithelia to estradiol benzoate in ewes with clover disease after prolonged exposure to oestrogenic pasture', *J Reprod Fertil* 56(2), pp. 611–13.

17 Shemesh, M. Lindner, H.R. and Ayalon, N. 1972. 'Affinity of rabbit uterine oestradiol receptor for phyo-oestrogens and its use in competitive protein binding radioassay for plasma coumesterol', *J Reprod Fertil* 29, pp. 1–9.

18 Adlercreutz, H. Mousav, Y. Clark, J. et al., 1992. 'Dietary phytoestrogens and cancer: in vitro and in vivo studies', *J Steroid Biochem Molec Biol* 41(3–8), pp. 331–7; Adlercreutz, H. 1988. 'Lignans and phytoestrogens: possible preventive role in cancer', *Progress in Diet and Nutrition*, eds C. Horwitz, and P. Rozen, Karger, Basel; Setchell, K.D.R. Borriello, S.P. Hulme, P. et al., 1984. 'Nonsteroidal estrogens of dietary origin: possible roles in hormone dependant disease', *Am J Clin Nutr* 40, 569–78; Messina, M. and Barnes, S. 1991. 'The role of soy products in reducing risk of cancer', *J Nat Cancer Inst* 83(8), pp. 541–6.

19 Messina, M. and Barnes, S. 'The role of soy products' op. cit, pp. 541–6.

20 Rose, D.P. 1992. 'Dietary fibre, phytoestrogens and breast cancer', *Nutrition* 8(1), pp. 45–51.

21 Horn-Ross, P.L. 1995. 'Phytoestrogens, body composition, and breast cancer', *Cancer Causes Control* 6(6), pp. 567–73.

22 Setchell, K.D.R. and Adlercreutz, H. 1988. 'Mammalian lignans and phyto-oestrogens. Recent studies on their formation, metabolism and biological role in health and disease', *'Role of the Gut Flora in Toxicity and Cancer'*, ed I. Rowland, Academic Press Limited, London, pp. 315–45; Rose, D.P. 1993. 'Diet, hormones, and cancer', *Ann. Rev Publ Health* 14, pp. 1–17; Adlercreutz, H. Hockerstedt, K. Bannwart, C. et al., 1987. 'Effect of dietary components, including lignans and phytoestrogens, on enterohepatic circulation and liver metabolism of estrogens and on sex hormone binding globulin (SHBG)', *J Steroid Biochem* 27(4–6), pp. 1135–44.

23 Adleurcreutz, H. Mousavi, Y., Clark, J. et al., 1992. 'Dietary phytoestrogens and cancer: in vitro and in vivo studies', *J Steroid Biochem Mol Biol* Mar; 41(3–8), pp. 331–7.

24 Adlercreutz, H. Bannwart, C. Wahala, K. et al., 1993. 'Inhibition of human aromatase by mammalian lignans and isoflavonoid phytoestrogens', *J Steroid Biochem Mol Biol* Feb, 44(2), pp. 147–53.

25 Cassidy, A. Bingham, S. and Setchell, K.D.R. 1994. 'Biological effects of a diet of soy protein rich in isoflavones on the menstrual cycle of premenopausal women', *Am J Clin Nutr* 60, pp. 333–40.

26 Phipps, W.R. Martini, M.C. Lampe, J.W. et al., 1993. 'Effect of flax seed ingestion on the menstrual cycle', *J Clin Endocrinol Metab* 77(5), pp. 1215–19.

27 Arjmandi, B.H. Alekel, L. Hollis, B.W. et al., 1996. 'Dietary soya protein prevents bone loss in an oviarectomized rat model of oesteoporosis', *J Nutr* 126(1), pp. 161–7.

28 Tsutsumi, N. 1995. 'Effect of coumestrol on bone metabolism in organ culture', *Biol Pharm Bull* 18(7), pp. 1012–5.

29 Murkies, A.L. Lombard, C. Strauss, B.J.G. et al., 1995. 'Dietary flour supplement decreases post-menopausal hot flushes: Effect of soy and wheat', *Maturitas* 21, pp. 189–95.

30 Werbach, M.R. and Murray, M.T. 1994. *Botanical Influences on Illness*, Third Line Press, Tarzana, California, p. 238.

31 Wilcox, G. Wahlqvist, M.L. and Burger, H.G. 1990. 'Oestrogenic effects of plant foods in menopausal women', *Br Med J* 310, pp. 905–6.

32 Whitten, P.L. Russell, E. and Naftolin, F. 1992. 'Effects of a normal, human-con-
    centration, phytoestrogen diet on rat uterine growth', *Steroids* March; **57**,
    pp. 98–106; Whitten, P.L. and Naftolin, F. 1992. 'Effects of a phytoestrogen diet
    of estrogen-dependant reproductive processes in immature female rats', *Steroids*
    57, pp. 56–61; Cheng, E.W. Yoder, L. Story, C.D. et al., 1954. 'Estrogenic activity
    of some isoflavone derivatives', *Science* **120**, p. 575; Perel, E. and Linder, H.R.
    1970. 'Dissociation of uterotrophic action from implantation-inducing activity in
    two non-steroidal oestrogens (coumesterol and genistein')', *J Reprod Fertil* **21**,
    p. 171.

33 The BHMA Scientific Committee, PR Bradley, ed., 1992. *British Herbal Compen-
    dium*, British Herbal Medicine Association, Dorset, p. 34.

34 Jarry, H. Gorkow, C.H. and Wuttke, W. 1993. 'Treatment of menopausal symptoms
    with extracts of *Cimicifuga racemosa: in vivo* and *in vitro* evidence for estrogenic
    activity; *Phytopharmaka in Forschung und Klinischer Anwendung*, eds D. Loew
    and N. Rietbrock, Steinkopff Darmstadt, pp. 99–112.

35 Duker, E.M. Kopanski, L. Jarry, H. et al., 1991. 'Effects of extracts from
    Cimicifuga racemosa on gonadotrophin release in menopausal women and ovari-
    ectomized rats', *Planta Med* **57**, pp. 420–4.

36 Karzel, K. 1974. 'Pharmacological effects of Ginseng. A review', *Proceedings of
    the International Ginseng Symposium*, The Research Institute, Office of Monopoly,
    Seoul, pp. 49–56.

37 Punnonen, R. and Lukola, A. 1980. 'Oestrogen-like effect of ginseng', *BMJ*
    281(6248), pp. 1110.

38 Greenspan, E.M. 1984. 'Ginseng and vaginal bleeding', [letter], *JAMA* Apr,
    249(15), p. 2018.

39 Palmer, B.V. Montgomery, A.C.V. and Monterio, J.C.M.P. 1978, 'Ginseng and
    mastalgia', *BMJ* (i), p. 1284.

40 Tamaya, T. Sato, S. and Okado, H.H. 1986. 'Possible mechanism of steroid action
    of the plant herb extracts glycyrrhizin, glycyrrhetinic acid, and paeoniflorin:
    Inhibition by plant herb extracts of steroid protein binding in the rabbit', *Am J
    Obstet Gynecol* **155**(5), pp. 1134–9.

41 Kumagai, A., Nishino, K. Shimoyama, A., et al., 1967. 'Effect of glycyrrhizin on
    estrogen action', *Endocrinol Japan* **14**, pp. 34–8.

42 Sakamoto, K. Watanabe, M. Aburada, M. et al., 1988. 'Effect of shakuyaku-kanzo-
    to (TJ-68) and glycyrrhetinic acid on hyperandrogenism', *Recent Advances in the
    Pharmacology of Kanpo (Japanese Herbal) Medicines*, eds E. Hosoya and Y.
    Yamamura, Excerpta Medica, Amsterdam, pp. 163–70.

43 Fukushima, M. and Ota, H. 1988. 'Endocrinological effects of Shakuyaku-kanzo-to
    (TJ-68) and Toki-shakayaku-san (TJ-23) in sulpiride-induced hyperprolactinaemic
    rats', ibid. pp. 155–62.

44 Rao, A., Rao, A.R. and Kale, R.K. 1992. 'Diosgenin—A growth stimulator of
    mammary gland of ovariectomised mouse', *Indian J Exp Biol* **30**, pp. 367–70.

45 Bone, K. 1996. personal communication.

46 Dollbaum, C.M. 1996 'Lab analyses of salivary DHEA and progesterone following
    ingestion of yam-containing products', *Townsend Letters for Doctors and Patients*,
    p. 104.

47 Rao, A., Rao, A.R., and Kale, R.K., 1992. 'Diosgenin—A growth stimulator of
    mammary gland of ovariectomised mouse', *Indian J Exp Biol* **30**, pp. 367–70.

48 Malini, T. and Vanithakumari, G. 1993. 'Effect of beta-sitosterol on uterine
    biochemistry: a comparative study with estradiol and progesterone', *Biochem Mol
    Biol Int* **31**(4), pp. 659–68.

49 Elghamry, M.I. and Shihata, I.M. 1966. 'Biological properties of phytoestrogens',
    Planta Med **14**(3), pp. 352–7.

50 Subbiah, M.T.R. 1973. 'Dietary plant sterols: current status in human and animal metabolism', *Am J Clin Nutr* **26**, pp. 219–25.

51 ibid. pp. 219–25.

52 Rao, A.V. and Janezic, S.A. 1992. 'The role of dietary phytosterols in colon carcinogenesis', *Nutr Cancer* **18**(1), pp. 43–52.

53 Weihrauch, J.L. and Gardner, J.M. 1978. 'Sterol content of foods of plant origin', *J Am Diet Ass* **73**, pp. 39–47.

54 Price, K.R. and Fenwick, G.R. 1985. 'Naturally occurring oestrogens in foods—a review', *Food Addit Cont* **2**(2), pp. 73–106.

55 Setchell, K.D.R. 1985. 'Naturally occurring non-steroidal estrogens of dietary origin', *'Estrogens in the Environment II'*, ed. John A. McLachlan, Elsevier, New York, p. 69; Beckham, N. 1995. 'Phyto-oestrogens and coumpounds that affect oestrogen metabolism—Part 1', *Aust J Med Herbalism* **7**(1), pp. 11–16.

Chapter 19

1   Taylor E.J. ed. 1988. *Dorland's Illustrated Medical Dictionary*, W.B. Saunders Company, Philadelphia.

2   Pedersen, M. 1987. *Nutritional Herbology*, Pedersen Publishing, Utah, pp. 220–1.

3   Bisset, N.G. (ed.), 1994. *Herbal Drugs and Phytopharmaceuticals*, Medpharm Scientific Publishers, Stuggart, (orig. pub.: Wichtl, M. (ed.) CRC Press), pp. 434–6.

4   Mabey, R., 1988. *The Complete New Herbal*, Elm Tree Books, London. p 105.

5   Wren, R.C. 1907. rewritten Williamson, E.M. and Evans, F.J. 1988. *Potters New Cyclopaedia of Botanical Drugs and Preparations*, The C.W. Daniel Co. Ltd, Saffron Waldron, Essex, UK, p. 232.

6   Noble, R.L. 1959. *The Report of the Proceedings, Sixth International Conference on Planned Parenthood*, 14–21 Feb, pp. 243–50.

7   Wren R.C. 1907. rewritten Williamson, E.M., and Evans, F.J. 1988. *Potters New Cyclopaedia of Botanical Drugs and Preparations*, The C.W. Daniel Co. Ltd, Saffron Waldron, Essex, UK, p. 232.

8   Whitehouse, B. 1941. 'Fragarine: an inhibitor of uterine action', *Br Med J* **2**, pp. 370–1.

9   Burn, J.H., Withell, E.R. 1941. 'A principle in raspberry leaves which relaxes uterine muscle', *Lancet* **2**(6149), pp. 1–3.

10 ibid. pp. 1–3.

11 Beckett, A.H., Belthle, F.W., Fell, K.R. et al., 1954. The active constituents of raspberry leaves', *J Pharm Pharmacol* **6**, pp. 785–96.

12 Bamford, D.S., Percival, R.C. and Tothill, A.U. 1970. 'Raspberry leaf tea: a new aspect to an old problem', *Br J Pharmacol* **40**, pp. 161P–162P.

13 ibid. pp. 161P–162P.

14 Willard, T. 1991. *The Wild Rose Scientific Herbal*, Wild Rose College of Natural Healing, Alberta, Canada, pp. 283–5.

15 Bensky, D. and Gamble, A. 1986. *Chinese Herbal Medicine Materia Medica*, Eastland Press, Seattle, p. 474.

16 Wang, H. and Peng, R.X. 1994. 'Sodium ferulate alleviated paracetamol-induced liver toxicity in mice', *Chung Kuo Yao Li Hsueh Pao* **15**(1), pp. 81–3.

17 Yan, R.Q. 1986. 'Effect of bifendati and three Chinese traditional medicinal herbs on aflatoxin B1 (AFB1)-induced hepatocarcinogenesis in rats', *Am J Cancer* **5**(2), p. 141.

18 Mei, Q.B. Tao, J.Y. and Cui, B. 1991. 'Advances in the pharmacological studies of radix *Angelica sinensis* (Oliv) Diels (Chinese Danggui)', *Chin Med J Engl* **104**(9), pp. 776–81.

19 ibid. pp. 776–81.

20 Ozaki, Y. 1992. 'Antiinflammatory effect of tetramethylpyrazine and ferulic acid', *Chem Pharm Bull* **40**(4), pp. 954–6.

21 Wang, S.R. Guo, Z.Q. and Liao, J.Z. 1993. '[Experimental study on the effects of 18 kinds of Chinese herbal medicine for synthesis of thromboxane A2 and PGI2]', *Chung Kuo Chung Hsi I Chieh Ho Tsa Chih* **13**(3), pp. 167–70.

22 Chen, Y.C. and Gao, Y.Q. 1994. '[Research on the mechanism of blood-tonifying effect of danggui buxue decocotion]', *Chung Kuo Chung Yao Tsa Chih*, **19**(1), pp. 43–5, 63.

23 Chang H.M. in Bone, K. 1996. *Clinical Applications of Ayurvedic and Chinese Herbs*, Phytotherapy Press, Qld, p. 5.

24 Yoshihiro, K. 1985. 'The physiological actions of Tang-Kuei and Cnidium', Bull Orient Healing Arts Inst (USA), **10**(7), pp. 269–78.

25 Ma, L.F. 1988. 'The effect of *Angelica sinensis* on mouse marrow haemopoiesis', *Chin J Hemat* **9**(3), p. 148.

26 Bensky, D. and Gamble, A. 1986. *Chinese Herbal Medicine Materia Medica*, Eastland Press, Seattle, p. 474.

27 Tao, J.Y. Ruan, Y.P. Mei, Q.B. et al., 1984. '[Studies on the antiasthmatic action of ligustilide of dang-gui, *Angelica sinensis* (Oliv) Diels]', *Yao Hsueh Hsueh Pao* **19**(8), pp. 561–5.

28 Chiangsu New Medical College, 1978. *Dictionary of Chinese Herbal Drugs*, Shanghai Scientific Technology Press, Shanghai, pp. 876–9.

29 Mei Q.B. Tao J.Y. and Cui B. 1991. 'Advances in the pharmacological studies of radix *Angelica sinensis* (Oliv) Diels (Chinese Danggui)', *Chin Med J Engl* **104**(9), pp. 776–81.

30 Ozaki, Y. and Ma, J.P. 1990. 'Inhibitory effects of tetramethylpyrazine and ferulic acid on spontaneous movement of rat uterus', *Chem Pharm Bull* **38**(6), pp. 1620–3.

31 Yoshiro, K. 1985. 'The physiological actions of Tang-kuei and Cnidium', *Bull Orient Healing Arts* **10**(7), pp. 269–78.

32 Harada, M. Suzuki, M. and Ozaki, Y. 1984. 'Effect of Japanese angelica root and peony root on uterine contraction in the rabbit in situ', *J Pharm Dyn* **7**, pp. 304–11.

33 Ozaki, Y. and Ma, J.P. 1990. 'Inhibitory effects of tetramethylpyrazine and ferulic acid on spontaneous movement of rat uterus', *Chem Pharm Bull* **38**(6), pp. 1620–3.

34 Bensky, D. and Gamble, A. 1986. *Chinese Herbal Medicine Materia Medica*, Eastland Press, Seattle, p. 474.

35 Pilcher, J.D. Burman, G.E. and Delzell, W.R. 1916. 'The action of the so-called female remedies on the excised uterus of the guinea-pig', *Arch Int Med* **18**(5), pp. 557–83; Pilcher, J.D. 1916. 'The action of certain drugs on the excised uterus of the guinea-pig', *J Pharm Exp Ther* **8**, pp. 110–11.

36 Scientific Committee, British Herbal Medicine Association, 1983, *British Herbal Pharmacopoeia*. British Herbal Medicine Association, West Yorks, England, pp. 59–60.

37 Mills, S. 1985. *The Dictionary of Modern Herbalism*, Lothian Publishing Company Pty Ltd, Melbourne.

38 ibid. p. 117.

39 Priest, A.W. and Priest, L.R. 1982. *Herbal Medication*, L.N. Fowler and Co. Ltd, London, p. 104.

40 Weiss, R.F. 1988. *Herbal Medicine*, Beaconsfield Arcanum, Gothenburg, Sweden, p. 316.

41 Rao, A. Rao, A.R. and Kale, R.K. 1992. 'Diosgenin—A growth stimulator of mammary gland of ovariectomised mouse', *Indian J Exp Biol* **30**(5), pp. 367–70.

42 Pilcher, J.D. Burman, G.E. and Delzell, W.R. 1916. 'The action of the so-called female remedies on the excised uterus of the guinea-pig', *Arch Int Med* **18**(5),

pp. 557–83; Butler, C.L. and Costello, C.H. 1944. 'Pharmacological studies', I *Aletris farinosa*, *J Am Pharm Assoc* **33**, pp. 177–83.

43 Wren, R.C. 1907. rewritten Williamson, E.M. and Evans, F.J. 1988. *Potters New Cyclopaedia of Botanical Drugs and Preparations*, The C.W. Daniel Co. Ltd, Saffron Waldron, Essex, UK, p. 272.

44 Pilcher, J.D. Burman, G.E. and Delzell, W.R. 1916. 'The action of the so-called female remedies on the excised uterus of the guinea-pig', *Arch Int Med* **18**(5), pp. 557–83; Pilcher, J.D. 1916. 'The action of certain drugs on the excised uterus of the guinea-pig', *J Pharm Exp Ther* **8**, pp. 110–111.

45 Ferguson, H.C. and Edwards, L.D. 1954. 'A pharmacological study of a crystalline glycoside of *Caulophyllum thalictroides*' *J Am Pharm Ass* **43**(1), pp. 16–21.

46 Scientific Committee, British Herbal Medicine Association, 1983. *British Herbal Pharmacopoeia*. British Herbal Medicine Association, West Yorks, England, p. 245.

47 Nicholson, J.A. Darby, T.D. and Jarboe, C.H. 1972. 'Viopudial, a hypotensive and smooth muscle anti-spasmodic from *Viburnum opulus*', *Proc Soc Exp Biol Med.* **140**(2), pp. 457–61.

48 Youngken, H.W. 1932. 'The pharmacognosy, chemistry and pharmacology of *Viburnum*. III. History, botany and pharmacognosy of *Viburnum opulus* L. var. *americanum* (Miller) Ait'. *J Am Pharm Assoc* **22**, pp. 444–62.

49 Woodbury, R.A. 1951. 'The Viburnums', *Drug Standards* **19**(7–8), pp. 143–152.

50 Youngken, H.W. 1932. 'The pharmacognosy, chemistry and pharmacology of *Viburnum*. III. History, botany and pharmacognosy of *Viburnum opulus* L. var. *americanum* (Miller) Ait', *J Am Pharm Assoc* **22**, pp. 444–462.

51 Woodbury, R.A. 1951. 'The Viburnums, *Drug Standards* **19**(7–8), pp. 143–52.

52 Munch, J.C. 1940. 'The uterine sedative action of Viburnums, VIII', *Pharm Arch* **2**(3), pp. 33–7.

53 Youngken, H.W. 1932. 'The pharmacognosy, chemistry and pharmacology of *Viburnum*. III. History, botany and pharmacognosy of *Viburnum opulus* L. var. *americanum* (Miller) Ait', *J Am Pharm Assoc* **22**, pp. 444–62.

54 Munch, J.C. 1939. 'Viburnum studies. V. Uterine sedative action', *J Am Pharm Assoc* **28**(11), pp. 886–7.

55 Woodbury, R.A. 1951. 'The Viburnums', *Drug Standards* **19**(7–8), pp. 143–52.

56 ibid. pp. 143–52.

57 Munch, J.C. 1939. 'Viburnum studies. V. Uterine sedative action', *J Am Pharm Assoc* **28**(11), pp. 886–7; Munch, J.C. 1940. 'The uterine sedative action of authentic Viburnum. X', *Proc Penna Acad Sci* **14**, pp. 118–19.

58 Jarboe, C.H. Zirvi, K.A. Nicholson, J.A. et al., 1967. 'Scopoletin, an antispasmodic component of *Viburnum opulus* and *prunifolium*', *J Med Chem* **10**, pp. 488–9.

59 Peyer, W. and Gstirner, F. 1931. 'Cortex *Viburni prunif*. and its fluid extract', *Pharm Zentralhalle* **72**, pp. 626–8.

60 Nicholson, J.A. Darby, T.D. and Jarboe, C.H. 1972. 'Viopudial, a hypotensive and smooth muscle anti-spasmodic from *Viburnum opulus*', *Proc Soc Exp Biol Med*, **140**(2), pp. 457–61.

61 Iwamoto, H.K. Evans, W.E. and Krantz, J.C. 1945. 'Characterization of the glycosidal principle of *Viburnum prunifolium*', *J Am Pharm Assoc Sci Ed* **34**, pp. 205–7; Evans, W.E. Iwamoto, H.K. and Krantz, J.C. 1945. 'A note on the pharmacology of *Viburnum prunifolium* and its glycoside', *J Am Pharm Assoc Sci Ed* **34**, pp. 207–8.

62 Raszeja, W. 1962. '*Viburnum opulus* bark. IV. Evaluation of *Viburnum opulus* bark and its official preparations', *Biul Inst Roslin Leczniczych* **8**, pp. 122–33.

63 Nicholson, J.A. Darby, T.D. and Jarboe, C.H. 1972. 'Viopudial, a hypotensive and smooth muscle anti-spasmodic from *Viburnum opulus*', *Proc Soc Exp Biol Med* **140**(2), pp. 457–61; Evans, W.E. Harne, W.G. and Krantz, J.C. 1942. 'A uterine principle from *Viburnum prunifolium*', *J Pharmacol Exptl Therapy* **75**, pp. 174–7.

64 Miura, H. Inoue, E. Kitamura, Y. et al., 1985. 'Examination and determination of arbutin in the leaves of *Viburnum* and *Ilex spp, Shoyakugaku Zasshi* **39**(3), pp. 181–4.

65 Tuttle, R.S. Marmelstein, L. Trad, T. et al., 1989. 'In vitro uterine response to tetramethylpyrazine, the active constituent of Chung Chong (a traditional Chinese medicine)', *Am J Obstet Gynecol* **161**(5), pp. 1319–23.

66 Ozaki, Y. and Ma, J.P. 1990. 'Inhibitory effects of tetramethylpyrazine and ferulic acid on spontaneous movement of rat uterus in situ', *Chem Pharm Bull* Tokyo **38**(6), pp. 1620–3.

67 Chen, H.C. Hsieh, M.T. and Shibuya, T.K. 1986. 'Suanzaorentang versus diazepam: a controlled double-blind study in anxiety', *Int J Clin Pharm, Ther and Tox* **24**(12), pp. 646–50.

68 Hoffmann, D. 1991. *Thorson's Guide to Medical Herbalism*, Thorson's, UK, p. 146.

69 Bremness, L. 1988. *The Complete Book of Herbs*, R.D. Press, Surry Hills, NSW, p. 122.

70 Mills, S.Y. 1985. *The Dictionary of Modern Herbalism*, Lothian Publishing Company Pty Ltd, Melbourne, p. 185.

71 Mabey, R. 1988. *The Complete New Herbal*, Penguin, London, p. 111.

72 Elisabetsky, E. Coelho de Souza, G.P. Dos Santos, M.A.C. et al., 1995. 'Sedative properties of linalool', *Fitoterapia* **66**(5), pp. 407–14.

73 ibid. pp. 407–14.

74 Nieschulz, O. and Schneider, G. 1965. '[Pharmalogical findings of the alkaloids of *Ruta graveolens*]', *Naturwissenschaften* **52**(13), pp. 394–5 (Germ.); Sovak, I. Buzas, G. Minker, M. et al., 1967. '[Active components of *Ruta graveolens*. IV]', *Planta Med* **15**(2), pp. 132–9 (Germ.); Minker, E. Bartha, C. Koltai, M. et al., 1980. 'Effect of secondary substances isolated from *Ruta graveolens* L. on the coronary smooth muscle', *Acta Pharmaceutica Hungarica* **50**, pp. 7–11.

75 ibid. pp. 7–11.

76 Bohuslavizki, K.H. Hinck-Kneip, C. Kneip, A. et al., 1993. 'Reduction of MS-related scotomata by a new class of potassium channel blockers from *Ruta graveolens*', *Neuro-ophthalmology* **13**(4), pp. 191–8.

77 Bohuslavizki, K.H. Hansel, W. Kneip, A. et al., 1992. 'Potassium blockers from *Ruta*—a new approach for the treatment of multiple sclerosis', *Gen Physiol Biophys* **11**, pp. 507–12.

78 Riddle, J.M. 1992. *Contraception and Abortion from the Ancient World to the Renaissance*, Harvard University Press, Massachusetts, p. 89.

79 Conway, G.A., and Slocumb, J.C. 1979. 'Plants used as abortifacients and emmenagogues by Spanish New Mexicans', *J. Ethnopharm* **1**, pp. 241–61.

80 Gandhi, M. Lal, R. Sankaranarayanan, A. et al., 1991. 'Post-coital activity of *Ruta graveolens* in female rats and hamsters', *J Ethnopharm* **34**, pp. 49–59.

81 Kong, Y.C. Lau, C.P. Wat, K.H. et al., 1989. 'Antifertility principle of *Ruta graveolens*', *Planta Medica* **55**, pp. 176–8.

82 Nieschulz, O. and Schneider, G. 1965. '[Pharmacological findings of the alkaloids of *Ruta graveolens*]', *Naturwissenschaften* **52**(13), pp. 394–5 (Germ.).

83 Kong, Y.C. Lau, C.P. Wat, K.H. et al., 1989. 'Antifertility principle of *Ruta graveolens*', *Planta Medica* **55**, pp. 176–8.

84 McIntyre, A. 1994. *The Complete Woman's Herbal*, Hodder & Stoughton, Rydalmere, NSW, p. 9.

85 Mills, S.Y. 1988. *The Dictionary of Modern Herbalism*, Lothian Publishing Company Pty Ltd, Melbourne, p. 154.

86 Evans, S. 1996. *Notes on Materia Medica*, Southern Cross University, East Lismore, p. 20.

87   Riddle, J.M. 1992. *Contraception and Abortion from the Ancient World to the Renaissance*, Harvard University Press, Massachusetts, p. 122.

88   Mills, S.Y. 1988. *The Dictionary of Modern Herbalism*, Lothian Publishing Company Pty Ltd, Melbourne, p. 11.

89   Evans, S. 1996. *Notes on Materia Medica*, Southern Cross University, East Lismore, pp. 133–4.

90   Riddle, J.M. 1992. *Contraception and Abortion from the Ancient World to the Renaissance*, Harvard University Press, Massachusetts, p. 83.

91   Mills, S.Y. 1991. *Out of the Earth,* Penguin UK, p. 399.

92   Chandler, R.F., Hooper, S.N., Harvey, M.J. 1982. 'Ethnobotany and Phytochemistry of Yarrow', *Achillea millefolium*, Compostitae, *Econ Bot* **36**(2), pp. 203–23.

93   Bisset, N.G. (ed.) 1994. *Herbal Drugs and Phytopharmaceuticals*, Medpharm Scientific Publishers, Stuttgart, (orig. pub: Wichtl, M. (ed.), CRC Press, pp. 342–4.

94   Scientific Committee, British Herbal Medicine Association, ed. P.R. Bradley, 1992. *British Herbal Compendium*, British Herbal Medicine Association, Dorset UK, pp. 227–9.

95   Weiss, R. 1988. *Herbal Medicine*, A.B Arcanum, Sweden, p. 315.

96   Heron, Silena 1989. 'Botanical Treatment of Chronic Gynecological Conditions: Infertility, Endometriosis, and Symptoms of Menopause', pp. 122–43. In *American Herbalism*. ed. Michael Tierra, The Crossing Press, USA, 1992.

97   Mills, S.Y. 1991. *Out of the Earth,* Penguin UK, p. 292.

98   Miclea, A. and Boldisteanu, A. 1993. 'Antihaemorrhoidal suppositories comprising *Alchemilla extract*', *Chem Abst* **119**, p. 529.

99   Jonadet, M. Meunier, M.T. Villie, F. et al., 1986. 'Flavonoids extracted from *Ribies nigrum L* and *Alchemilla vulgaris L*, I. In vitro inhibitory activities on the enzyme elastase, trypsin and α-chymotrypsin. II. Angioprotective activities compared in vivo', *J Pharmacol* **17**(1), pp. 21–7.

100   Petcu, P. Andronesca, E. and Gheorgheci, V. 1979. 'Treatment of juvenile menomenorrhagia with *Alchemilla vulgaris L* fluid extract', *Clujul Med.* **52**(3), pp. 266–70.

101   McIntyre, A. 1995. *The Complete Woman's Herbal*, Hodder Headline Australia Pty Ltd, Rydalmere, NSW, p. 110.

102   Kielczynski, W. 1997, personal communication.

103   Kuroda, K. and Kaku, T. 1969. 'Pharmacological and chemical studies on the alcohol extracts of *Capsella bursa pastoris*', *Life Sci* **8**, pp. 151–5; Kuroda, K. and and Takagi, K. 1968. 'Physiologically active substances in *Capsella bursa pastoris*', *Nature* **220**, pp. 707–8.

104   Kuroda, K. Akao, M. Kanisawa, M. et al., 1976. 'Inhibitory effect of *Capsella bursa pastoris* extract on growth of Ehrlich solid tumor in mice', *Cancer Res* **36**, pp. 1900–2; Kurado, K. Akao, M. Kanisawa, M. et al., 1974. 'Inhibitory effect of *Capsella bursa-pastoris* on hepatocarcinogenesis induced by 3'-methyl–4-(dimethylamino)azobenzene in rats', *Gann* **65**, pp. 317–21.

105   El-Abyad, M.S. Morsi, N.M. Zaki, D.A. et al., 1990. 'Preliminary screening of some Egyptian weeds for antimicrobial activity'. *Microbios* **62**, pp. 47–57.

106   Schumann, E. 1939. 'Newer concepts of blood coagulation and control of haemorrhage', *Am J Ob Gyn* **38**, pp. 1002–7.

107   Weiss, R. 1988. *Herbal Medicine*, A.B Arcanum, Sweden, p. 311.

108   Mills, S. 1991. *Out of the Earth*, Penguin, England, p. 316.

109   Weiss, R. 1988. *Herbal Medicine*, A.B Arcanum, Sweden, p. 314.

110   Holmes, P. 1989. *The energetics of western herbs*, Artemis Press, Boulder, Colorado, pp. 313–15.

111   Bisset, N.G. (ed.), 1994. *Herbal drugs and phytopharmaceuticals*, Medpharm Scientific Publishers, Stuttgart, (Original publication: Witchtl, M. (ed.), CRC Press) pp. 288–91.

112 Edwards, G.H. 1984. 'Neglected herbs: *Lamium*', *New Herbal Practitioner*, Vol. 11, No. 2, Oct. pp. 18–32.

113 Leung, A.Y. and Foster, S. 1996. *Encyclopedia of Common Natural Ingredients*, John Wiley and Sons, Inc., New York. pp. 495–8.

114 Zhao, G. and Wang, X. 1986. '[Hemostatic constituent of *Sanchi (panax notoginseng)*-Dencichin.]' *Zhongcaoyao* 17(6), pp. 74–5, 260.

115 Li, L. Wang, Z. Li, S. et al., 1988. '[Effects of *Panax notoginseng* saponins on hemorrhagic shock in rabbits.]' *Zhongguo Yaoli Xuebao* 9(1), pp. 52–5.

116 Pan, X. Yan, Q. and Lui, T. 1993. '[Inhibitory effects of total saponins extracted for *Panax ginseng*, *Panax quinquefolium* and *Panax notoginseng* on platelet function and thrombosis in rats.]' *Zhongguo Yaoluixue Yu Dulixue Zashi* 7(2), pp. 141–4.

117 Lei, X.L. and Chiou, G.C. 1986. 'Cardiovascular pharmacology of *Panax notoginseng* (burk) F.H. Chen and *Salvia miltiorrhiza*', *Am J Chin Med* 14(3–4), pp. 145–52.

118 Wang, J. and Chen, J. 1984. '[Cardiac and hemodynamic effects of the total saponins of *Panax notoginseng*]' *Zhongguo Yaoli Xuebao* 5(3), pp. 181–5.

119 Xu, Q. Zhao, and Y. Cheng, G.R. 1993. '[Blood-lipid decreasing action of total saponins of *Panax notoginseng* (Burk.) F.H. Chen.]' *Chung Kuo Chung Yao Tsa Chih*, 18(6), pp. 367–8, 383.

120 Leung, A. Mo, Z. and Zheng, Y. 1991. 'Reduction of cellular damage induced by cerebral ishaemia in rats', *Neurochem Res* 16(6), pp. 687–92.

121 Wu, J.X. and Sun, J.J. 1992. '[Comparative effects of *Panax notoginseng* saponins, verapamil, and norepinephrine on cerebral circulation in anesthetized rats and rabbits.]' *Chung Kuo Yao Li Hsueh Pao* 13(6), pp. 520–3.

122 Zhang, L. and Zhang, J.T. 1987. '[Memory facilitation induced by *Panax ginseng* and pseudoginseng in mice.]' *Chung Hsi I Chieh Ho Tsa Chih* 7(10), pp. 582, 610–12.

123 Grove, D.C. Jenkins, G.L. and Thompson, M.R. 1938. 'A phytochemical and pharmacological investigation of *Trillium erectum*', *J Am Pharm Assoc* 27(6), pp. 457–66.

124 Lieberman, S. Chang, F.C. Barusch, M.R. et al., 1942. 'Saponins and sapogenins. XX. Bethogenin and trillogenin, new sapogenins from *Trillium erectum*', *J Am Chem Soc* 64, pp. 2581–3.

125 Marker, R.E. Wagner, R.B. Goldsmith, D.P.J. et al., 1943. 'Sapogenins. 67. Pennogenin, nologenin and fesogenin, three new sapogenins from Beth root', *J Am Chem Soc* 65, p. 128.

126 Cassidy, A. Bingham, S. and Setchell, K.D.R. 1994. 'Biological effects of a diet of soy protein rich in isoflavones on the menstrual cycle of premenopausal women' *Am J Clin Nutr* 60, pp. 333–40.

127 Amann, W. 1967. '[Improvement of acne vulgaris following therapy with *Agnus castus* (Agnolyt, Reg. trademark).]' *Therapie d Gegenw* 106(1), pp. 124–6; Amann, W. 1975. '[Acne vulgaris and *Agnus castus* (Agnolyt, Reg. trademark).]' *Z Allg Med* 51(35), pp. 1645–8.

128 Ecker, G. 1964. 'Pramenstruelles syndrom als schrittmacher einer post-traumatischen epilepsie', *Landarzt* 40, pp. 872–4.

129 Hillebrand, H. 1964. 'Die behandlung der pramenstruelles stomatitis aphthosa ulcerosa mit Agnolyt (Reg. trademark)', *Landarzt* 40, p. 1577.

130 Albus, G.A. 1964. 'Herpes simplex recidivans als fragmentares zeichan eines pramenstruellen syndroms', *Z Haut-und Gesch* 36, pp. 220–3.

131 Amman, W. 1979. '[Premenstrual water retention. Favourable effect of *Agnus castus* (Agnolyt, Reg. trademark).]' *Z Allg Med* 55(1), pp. 48–51.

132 Opitz, G. and Liebl, A. 1980. '[The conservative treatment of mastopathy with Mastodynon (Reg. trademark).]' *Therapie der Gegenw* 119(7), pp. 804–9; Wuttke,

W. Jarry, H. and Leonhardt, S. 1994. '[*Agnus castus* as dopaminergic activity principle in premenstrual mastodynia.]' *Ars Medici* **84**(13), pp. 850, 853–4, 856.

133   Amann, W. 1982. [Amenorrhea. 'Favourable effect of *Agnus castus* (Agnolyt, Reg trademark) on amenorrhea.]' *Z Allg Med* **58**(4), pp. 228–31.

134   Peters-Welte, C. and Albrecht, M. 1994. ['Menstrual cycle disorders and PMS. Study on the use of *Vitex agnus castus*.'] *TW Gynakologie* **7**(1), pp. 49–52 (Germ.).

135   Roeder, D. 1994. ['Therapy of cyclical disorders with *Vitex agnus-castus*'] *Z Phytother* **15**(3), pp. 157–63.

136   Roeder, D. 1994. ['Therapy of cyclical disorders with *Vitex agnus castus*.'] *Zeiterschrift fur Phytotherapie* **15**(3), pp. 157–63 (Germ.).

137   Milewicz, A. Gejdel, E. Sworen, H. et al., 1993. ['*Vitex agnus castus* extract in the treatment of luteal phase defects due to latent hyperprolactinaemia. Results of a randomised placebo-controlled double-blind study.'] *Arzneim-Forsch/Drug Res* **43**(II)(7), pp. 752–6.

138   Jarry, H. Leonhardt, S. Gorkow, C. et al., 1994. 'In vitro prolactin but not LH and FSH release is inhibited by compounds in extracts of *agnus castus*: direct evidence for a dopaminergic principle by the dopamine receptor assay', *Exp Clin Endocrinol* **102**(6), pp. 448–54; Sliutz, G. Speiser, P. Schultz, A.M. et al., 1993. '*Agnus castus* extracts inhibit prolactin secretion of rat pituitary cells', *Horm Metab Res* **25**, pp. 253–5.

139   Cahill, D.J. Fox, R. Wardle, P.G. et al., 1994. 'Multiple follicular development associated with herbal medicine', *Human Reproduction* **9**(8), pp. 1469–70.

140   Mohr, W. 1957. 'Gedanken zur Forderung des Stillens durch Medikamente', *Hippokrates* **28**, pp. 586–91.

141   Merz, P.G. Schrodter A., Rietblrock, S., et al., 1995. 'Prolaktinsekretion and vertraglichkeit under der behandlung mit einem *Agnus-castus*-Spezialextrakt (BP1095E1). Erste ergebnisse zum einflub auf die prolakinsekretion, *Phytopharmaka in Forschung und Klinischer Anwendung*, ed. D. Loew and N. Rietbrock, Darmstadt, Skein Kopff.

142   Dittmar, F.W. et al., in Snow, J.M. 1996. '*Vitex agnus-castus* L. (Verbenaceae)', *Protocol J Bot Med* Spring: pp. 20–3.

143   Ota, H. and Fukishima, M. 1988. 'Stimulation by Kanpo prescriptions of aromatase activity in rat follicle cell cultures', *Recent Advances in the Pharmacology of Kanpo (Japanese Herbal) Medicines*, eds E. Hosoya and Y. Yamamura, Excerpta Medica, Amsterdam. pp. 177–83.

144   Ota, H. and Fukishima, M. 1988. 'Stimulation by Kanpo prescriptions of aromatase activity in rat follicle cell cultures', *Recent Advances in the Pharmacology of Kanpo (Japanese Herbal) Medicines*, eds E. Hosoya and Y. Yamamura. Excerpta Medica, Amsterdam. pp. 177–83.

145   Takeuchi, T. 1988. ['Effect of shakuyaku-kanzo-to, shakuyaku, kanzo, paeoniflorin, glycyrrhetinic acid and glycyrrhizin on ovarian function in rats']. *Nippon Naibunpi Gakkai Zasshi* **64**(11), pp. 1124–39; Takeuchi, T. Nishii, O. Okamura, T. et al., 1989. 'Effect of traditional herbal medicine, shakuyaku-kanzo-to on total and free serum testosterone levels'. *Am J Chin Med (USA)* **17**(1–2), pp. 35–44.

146   Takahashi, K. and Kitao, M. 1994. Effect of TJ-68 (shakuyaku-kanzo-to) on polycystic ovarian disease. *Int J Fertil Menopausal Stud* **39**(2), pp. 69–76; Takahashi, K. Yoshino, K. Shirai, T. et al., 1988. 'Effect of a traditional herbal medicine (shakuyaku-kanzo-to) on testosterone secretion in patients with polycystic ovarian syndrome detected by ultrasound'. *Nippon Sanka Fujinka Gakkai Zasshi* **40**(60), pp. 789–92.

147   Fukushima, M. and Ota, H. 1988. 'Endocrinological effects of Shakuyaku-kanzo-to (TJ-68) and Toki-shakuyaku-san (TJ-23) in sulpiride-induced hyperprolactinemic rats', *Recent Advances in the Pharmacology of Kanpo (Japanese Herbal) Medicines*, eds E. Hosoya and Y. Yamamura, Excerpta Medica, Amsterdam. pp. 155–62.

148 Mori, T. Sakamoto, S. Singtripop, T. et al., 1993. 'Suppression of spontaneous development of uterine adenomyosis by a Chinese herbal medicine, Keishi-bukuryo-gan, in mice'. *Planta Med* **59**, pp. 308–11.

149 Sakamoto, S. Yoshino, H. Shirahata, Y. et al. 1992. 'Pharmacotherapeutic effects of Kue-chih-fu-ling-wan (Keishi-bukuryo-gan) on human uterine myomas'. *Am J Chin Med* **20**(3–4), pp. 313–17.

150 Inoue, M. 1988. 'The treatment of benign mastopathies with traditional Sino-Japanese medicine (Kanpo)', *Kanpo Igaku* **12**(5), p. 127.

151 Sakamoto, S. 1988. 'Actions of Keishi-bukuryo-gan (TJ–25) on the rat gonadal system', *Recent Advances in the Pharmacology of Kanpo (Japanese Herbal) Medicines*, eds E. Hosoya and Y. Yamamura. Excerpta Medica, Amsterdam. pp. 170–4.

152 Bensky, D. and Gamble, A. 1986. *Chinese Herbal Medicine Materia Medica*, Eastland Press, Seattle. p. 399.

153 Harada, M. 1969. 'Pharmacological studies on peony root. IV. Analysis of therapeutic effects of peony- and liquorice-containing common prescriptions in Chinese medicine and comparison with effects of experimental pharmacological tests'. *Yakugaku Zasshi* **89**(7), pp. 899–908.

154 Genazanni, E. and Sorrentino, L. 1962. 'Vascular action of actein: active constituent of *Actaea racemosa L. Nature* **194**, pp. 544–5.

155 Duker, E.M., et al., 1991. 'Effects of extracts from *Cimicifuga racemosa* on gonadotrophin release in menopausal women and ovariectomised rats'. *Planta Medica* **57** pp. 420–4.

156 Harnischfeger, G. Stolze, H. 1980. 'Proven active substances from natural materials. Black snake root'. *Notabene Medici* **10**(5), pp. 76–83.

157 Jarry, H. Harnischfeger, G. and Duker, E. 1985. 'Studies on the endocrine efficacy of the constituents of *Cimicifuga racemosa*: 2. In vitro binding of constituents to oestrogen receptors'. *Planta Med* **4**(9), pp. 94–8.

158 Duker, E. Lothar, K. Hubertus, J. et al., 1991. 'Effects of extracts from *Cimicifuga racemosa* on gonadotrophin release in menopausal women and ovariectomized rats'. *Planta Med* **57**(5) pp. 420–4.

159 Daiber, W. 1985. 'Climacteric complaints: success without using hormones!' *Arztl Prax* **35**(65), pp. 1946–7.

160 Vorberg, G. 1984. 'Treatment of menopausal complaints'. *Z Allgeinmed* **60**(13), pp. 626–9.

161 Stoll, W. 1987. 'Phytopharmacon influences atrophic vaginal epithelium. Double blind study—*Cimicifuga* vs estrogenic substances'. *Therapeutikon* **1**, p. 23.

162 Lehmann-Willenbrock, E. and Riedel, H. 1988. 'Clinical and endocrinologic examinations concerning therapy of climacteric symptoms following hysterectomy with remaining ovaries'. *Zent B.l Gynakol* **110**, pp. 611–18.

163 Stolze, H. 1982. 'An alternative to treat menopausal complaints'. *Gyne* **3**(1), pp. 14–16.

164 Petho, A. 1987. 'Menopausal complaints. Change-over of a hormone treatment to a herbal gynecological remedy practicable?' *Arztl Praxis* **38**(47), pp. 1551–3.

165 Warnecke, G. 1985. 'Influencing menopausal symptoms with a phytotherapeutic agent. Successful therapy with *Cimicifuga* mono-extract'. *Medwelt* **36**(22), pp. 186–95.

166 Mascolo, N. Jain, R. Jain, S.C. and Capasso, F. 1989. 'Ethnopharmacologic investigations of ginger (*Zingiber officinale*). *Journal of Ethnopharmacology* **27** (1–2), pp. 129–40.

167 Denyer, C.L et al., 1994. 'Isolation of antirhinoviral sesquiterpenes from ginger (*Zingiber officinale*)'. *Journal of Naural Products* **57**(5), pp. 658–62.

168 Fischer-Rasmussen, W. Kjaer, S.K. Dahl, C. et al., 1990. 'Ginger treatment of hyperemesis gravidarum'. *Eur J Obst Gynec Reprod Biol* **38**, pp. 19–24.

169　Stewart, J.J. Wood, M.J. Wood C.D. et al., 1991. 'Effects of ginger on motion sickness susceptibility and gastric function'. *Pharmacology* **42**, pp. 111–20.

170　Phillips, S. Ruggier, R. and Hutchison, S.E. 1993. '*Zingiber officinale* (ginger)—an antiemetic for day case surgery'. *Anaesthesia* **48**(8), pp. 715–17; Bone, M.E. Wilkinson, D.J. Young, J.R. et al., 1990. 'Ginger root—a new antiemetic. The effect of ginger root on postoperative nausea and vomiting after major gynaecological surgery'. *Anaesthesia* **45**(8), pp. 669–71.

171　Yamahara, J. Huang, Q. Li, Y. et al., 1990. 'Gastrointestinal motility effect of ginger and its active constituent'. *Chem Pharm Bull* **38**(2), pp. 430–1.

172　Sertie, J.A.A. Basile, A.C. Oshiro, T.T. et al., 1992. 'Preventive anti-ulcer activity of the rhizome extract of *Zingiber officinale*'. *Fitoterapia* **113**(1), pp. 55–9.

173　Giri, J. Devi, T.K.S. and Meerani, S. 1984. 'Effect of ginger on serum cholesterol levels'. *Indian J Nutr Diet* **21**(12), pp. 433–6.

174　Guh, J.H. Jo, F.N. Jong T.T., et al., 1995. 'Antiplatelet effect of gingerol isolated from *zingiber officinale*', *J Pharm Pharmacol* **47**(4), pp. 329–32.

175　Srivastava, K.C. 1989. 'Effect of onion and ginger consumption on thromboxane production in humans'. *Prostaglandins, Leukotrienes and Essential Fatty Acids* **35**(3), pp. 183–5.

176　Kiuchi, F. Iwakami, S. Shibuya, M. et al., 1992. 'Inhibition of prostaglandin and leukotriene biosynthesis by gingerols and diarylheptanoids'. *Chem Pharm Bull Tokyo* **40**(2), pp. 387–91; Kiuchi, F. Shibuya, M. Sankawa, U. et al., 1982. 'Inhibitors of prostaglandin biosynthesis from ginger'. *Chem Pharm Bull* **30**(2), pp. 754–7.

177　Srivastava, K.C. and Mustafa, T., 1992. 'Ginger (*Zingiber officinale*) in rheumatism and musculoskelatal disorders'. *Med Hypothesis* **39**, pp. 342–8.

178　Mustafa, T. and Srivastava, K.C. 1990. Ginger (*Zingiber officinale*) in migraine headache'. *J Ethnopharmacol* **29**(3), pp. 267–73.

179　Hashim, S. Aboobaker, V.S. Madhubala, R. et al., 1994. 'Modulatory effects of essential oils from spices on the formation of DNA adduct by aflatoxin B1 in vitro'. *Nutrition and Cancer* **21**(2), pp. 169–75.

180　Suekawa, M. Ishige, A. Yuasa, K. et al., 1984. 'Pharmacological studies on ginger. I. Pharmacological actions of pungent constituents, (6)-gingerol and (6)-shogaol'. *J Pharmacobiodyn* **7**(11), pp. 836–48.

181　*The British Herbal Pharmacopoeia*, pt II, 1979. British Herbal Medicine Association, Cowling, West Yorkshire, pp. 55–7.

182　Willard, T. 1991. *The Wild Rose Scientific Herbal*, Wild Rose College of Natural Healing, Calgary, Canada, pp. 85–7.

183　Leung, Ay, and Foster, S. 1996. *Encyclopedia of Common Natural Ingredients Used in Foods, Drugs, and Cosmetics, 2nd edn.* John Wiley and Sons, Inc., New York, p. 215.

184　Auxence, E.G. 1953. 'A pharmacognostic study of *Piscidia erythrina*'. *Econ Botany* **7**, pp. 270–84.

185　The BHMA Scientific Committee, P.R. Bradley, ed., 1992. *British Herbal Compendium.* British Herbal Medicine Association, Dorset. pp. 139–40.

186　Pilcher, J.D. Burman, G.E. and Delzell, W.R. 1916. 'The action of the so-called female remedies on the excised uterus of the guinea pig'. *Arch Int Med* **18**(5), pp. 557–83.

187　Costello, C.H. and Butler, C.L. 1948. 'An investigation of *Piscidia erythrina* (Jamacia dogwood)'. *J Am Pharm Assoc* **37**(3), pp. 89–97.

188　The BHMA Scientific Committee, P.R. Bradley, ed., 1992. *British Herbal Compendium.* British Herbal Medicine Association, Dorset. pp. 139–40.

189　Hoffman, D. 1996. *Therapeutic Herbalism.* Correspondence course, self-published, California.

190 Heptinstall, S. 1988. 'Feverfew—an ancient remedy for modern times?' *J Royal Soc Med* **8**, pp. 373–4.

191 Pugh, W.J. and Sambo, K. 1988. 'Prostaglandin synthetase inhibitors in feverfew'. *J Pharm Pharmacol* **40**(10), pp. 743–5.

192 Heptinstall, S. White, A. Williamson, L. et al., 1985. 'Extracts from feverfew inhibit granule secretion in blood platelets and polymorphonuclear leucocytes'. *Lancet* **1**(8437), pp. 1071–4.

193 Bohlmann, F. and Zdero, C. 1982. 'Sesquiterpene lactones and other constituents from *Tanacetum parthenium*'. *Phytochem* **21**, pp. 2543–9.

194 Barsby, R.W.J. Salan, U. Knight, D.W. et al., 1993. 'Feverfew and vascular smooth muscle: Extracts from fresh and dried plants show opposing pharmacological profiles, dependent upon sesquiterpene lactone content'. *Planta Med* **59**, pp. 20–5.

195 Murphy, J.J. Heptinstall, S. and Mitchell, J.R.A. 1988. 'Randomised double-blind placebo-controlled trial of feverfew in migraine prevention'. *Lancet* **2**(8604), pp. 189–92; Johnson, E.S. Kadam, N.P. Hylands, D.M. et al., 1985. 'Efficacy of feverfew as prophylactic treatment of migraine'. *BMJ* **291**, pp. 569–73.

196 Heptinstall, S. White, A. Williamson, L. et al., 1985. 'Extracts of feverfew inhibit granule secretion in blood platelets and polymorphonuclear leucocytes'. *Lancet* **1**(8437), pp. 1071–4.

197 McIntyre, A. 1994. *The Complete Woman's Herbal*. Hodder & Stoughton, Rydalmere, NSW. p. 131.

198 Bergner, P. 1988. 'Botanical Medicine: Two herbs for migraine'. *Townsend Letter for Doctors* January: pp. 22–3.

199 Barsby, R.W.J. Salan, U. Knight, D.W. et al., 1993. 'Feverfew and vascular smooth muscle: Extracts from fresh and dried plants show opposing pharmacological profiles, dependent upon sesuiterpene lactone content'. *Planta Med* **59**, pp. 20–5.

200 Mitchell, J.C. Geissman, T.A. Dupuis, G. et al., 1971. 'Allergic contact dermatitis caused by *Artemesia* and *Chrysanthemum* species. Role of sesquiterpene lactones'. *J Invest Dermatol* **56**(2), pp. 98–101.

201 Linde, K. Ramirez, G. Mulrow, C. et al., 1996. 'St John's wort for depression—an overview and meta-analysis of randomised clinical trials'. *British Medical Journal* **313**, pp. 253–8.

202 Mills, S.Y., 1991. *Out of the Earth*. Penguin, UK. p. 513.

203 Linde, K. Ramirez, G. Mulrow, C. et al., 1996. 'St John's wort for depression—an overview and meta-analysis of randomised clinical trials'. *British Medical Journal* **313**, pp. 253–8.

204 ibid. pp. 253–8.

205 De Smet, P. and Nolen, W. 1996. 'St John's wort as an anti-depressant'. *British Medical Journal* **313**, pp. 241–2.

206 Hiller, K.O. and Rahlfs, V. 1995. *Forschende Komplementarmedizin* **2**, pp. 123–32.

207 Panijel, M. 1995. *Therapiewoche* **35**, pp. 4659–68.

208 Lavie, G. Valentine, F., Levin, B., et al., 1989. 'Studies of the mechanisms of action of the antiretro-viral agents hypericin and pseudohypericin,' *Proc Natl Acad Sci USA* **86**(15), pp. 5963–7; Weiner, D.B. Lavie, G. Williams W.V et al., 1989. 'Hypericin mediates anti-HIV effects *in vitro*', *Int Conf AIDS*, **5** p. 659 (abstract no. C.608); Tang J. Calacino, J.M. Larsen, S.H. et al., 1990. 'Virucidal activity of hypericin against enveloped and non-enveloped DNA and RNA viruses', *Antiviral Res* **13**(6), pp. 313–25.

209 Mills, Simon, 1991. *Out of the Earth*. Penguin UK. pp. 512–14.

210 Gerhard, I. et al., 1995. 6th Phytotherapy Conference, Berlin, October, pp. 5–7.

211 Weiss, R.F. 1988. *Herbal medicine*. A.B Arcanum, Gothenburg, Sweden and Beaconsfield, London. p. 279.

212 Culpeper, N. (Reprint) *Culpeper's Complete Herbal*. W. Foulsham & Co. Ltd, New York. p. 239.

213 Yeung, H.W. Kong, Y.C. Lay, W.P. et al., 1977. 'The structure and biological effect of leonurine'. *Planta Med* **31**, pp. 51–6.

214 Wohlfart, R. Haensel, R. and Schmidt, H. 1982. 'An investigation of sedative-hypnotic principles in hops. Part 3'. *Planta Med* **45**, p. 224; Wichtl, M. 1993. 'Lupuli strobulus/glandula'. In *Herbal Drugs and Phytopharmaceuticals*. ed. N.G. Bisset. CRC Press, Boca Raton. pp. 305–8.

215 Caujolle, F. Pham Huu Chanh, Duch-Kan, P. et al., 1969. 'Etude de l'action spasmolytique du houblon (*Humulus lupulus, Cannabinacees*)'. *Agressologie* **10**(5), pp. 405–10.

216 Zenisek, A. and Bednar, J. 1960. 'Contribution to the identification of the estrogen activity of hops'. *Am Perfumer Aromat* **75**(5), pp. 61–2; Chury, J. 1960. '[*Phytoestrogen content of plants*]'. *Experientia* **16**, pp. 194–5; Bednar, J. Zenisek, A. 1961. 'Identification of the estrogenic activity of hops'. *Brauwissenschaft* **14**, pp. 4–7.

217 Bravo, L. Cabo, J. Fraile, A. et al., 1971. ['Pharmacodynamic study of hops (*Humulus lupulus*). II. Estrogenic action'.] *Ars Pharm* **12**(11–12), pp. 421–5; Fenselau, C. and Talalay, P. 1973. 'Is oestrogenic activity present in hops?' *Food and Cosmetic Toxicology* **11**, pp. 597–603.

218 Weiss, R.F. 1988. *Herbal medicine*. A.B Arcanum, Gothenburg, Sweden and Beaconsfield, London. p. 285.

219 Sopporo Breweries Ltd, 1985. 'Extraction of antigonadotrophic glycoproteins'. *Chem Abst* **103**, p. 330; Okamoto, R. and Kumai, A. 1992. Antigonadotrophic activity of hop. extract. *Acta Endocrinol* **127**(4), pp. 371–7.

220 Cabo Torres, J. and Bravo Diaz, L. 1971. ['Pharmacodynamic study of hops (*Humulus lupulus*). IV. Antioxytocic activity'.] *Ars Pharm* **12**(3-4-5-6), pp. 191–201.

221 Zufall, C.J. and Richtmann, W.O. 1943. 'A pharmacognostical study of certain American species of Verbena'. *Pharm Arch* **14**(5), pp. 65–80.

222 *British Herbal Pharmacopoeia*. pt 1, 1976. British Herbal Medicine Association, Cowling, West Yorks. pp. 74–5.

223 Mills, S. 1988. *The Dictionary of Modern Herbalism*. Healing Arts Press, Vermont. pp. 212–13.

224 Wichtl, M. 1993. 'Verbenae Herba'. In *Herbal Drugs and Phytopharmaceuticals*. ed. N.G. Bisset. CRC Press, Boca Raton. pp. 520–2.

225 Valnet, J. 1983. 'Phytotherapie'. In Hunter, A. 1995. *Verbena officinalis, Australian Journal of Medical Herbalism* **7**(4), pp. 105–7.

226 Auf'mkolk, M. Ingbar, J. Kubota, K. et al., 1985. 'Extracts and auto-oxidised constituents of certain plants, inhibit the receptor-binding and the biological activity of Graves' immunoglobulins. *Endocrinology* **116**(5) pp. 1687–93.

227 Research Group on Reproductive Physiology, 1974. 'Effect of Verbena herb on the uterus: II. Interaction between Verbena herb and prostaglandins'. *Tung Wu Hsueh Pao* **20**(4), pp. 340–5.

228 Hunter, A. 1995. '*Verbena officinalis*'. *Australian Journal of Medical Herbalism* **7**(4), pp. 105–7.

229 Houghton, P.J. 1988. 'The biological activity of valerian and related plants'. *Journal of Ethnopharmacology* **22**, pp. 121–42.

230 Leathwood, P.D. et al., 1982. 'Effect of *Valeriana officinalis* L on subjective and objective sleep parameters'. *Pharmacology, Biochemistry and Behaviour* **17**, pp. 65–71

231 Klich, R. and Gludbach, B. 1975. 'Verhaltenstorungen im kindesarter und deren therapie'. *Med. Welt* **26**, pp. 1251–4.

232 Leung, A. and Foster, S. 1996. *Encyclopedia of common natural ingredients used in food, drugs and cosmetics*. John Wiley, New York. pp. 475–6.

233 Chen, H.C. Hsieh, M.T. and Shibuya, T.K. 1986. 'Suanzaorentang versus diazepam:

a controlled double-blind study in anxiety'. *International Journal of Clinical Pharmacology, Therapy and Toxicology* **24**(12), pp. 646–50.

234　Chen, H.C. and Hsieh, M.T. 1985. 'Clinical trial of suanzaorentang in the treatment of insomnia'. *Clinical Therapeutics* **7**(3), pp. 334–7.

235　Chen, H.C. Hsieh, M.T., and Shibuya, T.K. 1986. 'Suanzaorentang versus diazepam: a controlled double-blind study in anxiety'. *International Journal of Clinical Pharmacology, Therapy and Toxicology* **24**(12), pp. 646–50.

236　Chen, H.C., and Hsieh, M.T. 1985. 'Studies on Suanzaorentang in the treatment of anxiety'. *Psychopharmacology* **85**, p. 486.

237　Leung, A. and Foster, S. 1996. *Encyclopedia of common natural ingredients used in food, drugs and cosmetics.* John Wiley, New York. pp. 330–1.

238　Mathews, J.D. Riley, M.D. Fejo, L. et al., 1988. 'Effects of the heavy use of kava on physical health: summary of a pilot study in an aboriginal community', *Med J Aust* **148**(11), pp. 548–55.

239　Monograph Piperis methystici rhizoma, Bundesanzeiger, no. 101, June 1, 1990. In Leung, A. and Foster, S. 1996. *Encyclopedia of common natural ingredients used in food, drugs and cosmetics.* John Wiley, New York. pp. 330–1.

240　Volz, H.P. 1995. 6th Phytotherapy Conference, Berlin, October 5–7.

241　Weiss, R.F. 1988. *Herbal medicine* A.B. Arcanum, Gothenburg, Sweden and Beaconsfield, London. p. 298.

242　Warneke, G. 1991. '[Psychosomatic dysfunctions in the female climacteric. Clinical effectiveness and tolerance of kava Extract WS 1490' *Fortschr Med* **109**(4), pp. 119–22.

243　Fulder, S. 1980. *The Root of Being.* Hutchinson, London, pp. 243–5.

244　Baranov, A.L. 1982. 'Medical uses of ginseng and related plants in the Soviet Union: recent trends in the Soviet literature', *J Ethnopharmacology* **6**(3), pp. 339–53.

245　Jie, Y.H. Cammisuli, S. and Baggiolini, M. 1984. 'Immunomodulatory effects of *Panax Ginseng* C.A. Meyer in the mouse', *Agents Actions* **15**(3–4), pp. 386–91.

246　Popov, I.M. and Goldwag, W.J. 1973. 'A review of the properties and clinical effects of ginseng', *Am J Chin Med* **1**(2), pp. 263–70; D'Angelo, L. Grimaldi, R. Caravaggi, M. et al., 1986. 'A double blind, placebo-controlled clinical study on the effect of standardised ginseng extract on psychomotor performance in healthy volunteers', *J Ethnopharmacol* **16**(1), pp. 15–22.

247　Lui, C.X. and Xiao, P.G. 1992. 'Recent advances on ginseng research in China', *J Ethnopharmacol* **36**(1), pp. 27–38.

248　Punnonen, R. and Lukola, A. 1980. 'Oestrogen-like effect of ginseng'. *BMJ* **281**(6248), p. 1110.

249　Greenspan, E.M. 1984. 'Ginseng and vaginal bleeding' [letter] *JAMA.* Apr. **249**(15), p. 2018.

250　Palmer, B.V. Montgomery, A.C.V. and Monterio, J.C.M.P. 1978. 'Ginseng and mastalgia'. *BMJ* i, p. 1284.

251　Bensky, D. and Gamble, A. 1986. *Chinese Herbal Medicine Materia Medica.* Eastland Press, Seattle. p. 455.

252　Shideman, F.E. 1950. 'A review of the pharmacology and therapeutics of *Hydrastis* and its alkaloids hydrastine, berberine, and canadine'. *Bulletin of the National Formulary Commission* **18**, pp. 3–19.

253　Khursheed, H. and Hafiz, A. 1986. 'In vivo antibacterial activity of *Berberis asiatica*'. *Journal of the Pakistan Medical Association* Jan. pp. 5–7.

254　Kumazawa, Y. Itagaki, A. Fukumoto, M. et al., 1984. 'Activation by peritoneal macrophages by berberine-type alkaloids in terms of induction of cytostatic activity'. *International Journal of Immunopharmacology* **6**(6), pp. 587–92; Sabir, M. and Bhide, N.K. 1971 'Study of some pharmacological actions of berberine'. *Indian Journal of Physiology and Pharmacology* **15**(3), pp. 111–32.

255 Pedersen, M. 1987. *Nutritional herbology*. Pedersen Publishing, Bountiful, Utah. p. 273.

256 Kumazawa, Y. Itagaki, A. Fukumoto, M. et al., 1984. 'Activation by peritoneal macrophages by berberine-type alkaloids in terms of induction of cytostatic activity'. *International Journal of Immunopharmacology* 6(6), pp. 587–92.

257 Willuhn, G. 1993. '*Taraxaci radix* cum herba'. in *Herbal Drugs and Phytopharmaceuticals*. ed. N.G. Bisset. CRC Press, Boca Raton.

258 Baba, K. Abe, S. and Mizuno, D. 1981. '[Antitumor activity of hot water extract of dandelion, *Taraxacum officinale*—correlation between antitumor activity and timing of administration]', *Yakugaku Zasshi* 101(6), pp. 538–43.

259 Madaus, G. 1976. *Lehrbuch der Biologischen Heilmittel* Georg Olms Verlag, Hildesheim, p. 2675.

260 Culpeper, N. '*Culpeper's Complete Herbal*, W. Fousham & Co. Ltd, New York, p. 368.

261 Wagner, H. and Seligman, O. 1985. 'Liver therapeutic drugs from *Silybum marianum*', in *Advances in Chinese Medicinal Materials Research*. eds. H.M. Chang, H.W. Cheung, W.-W. and Tso, A. Koo World Scientific Publishing Co., Singapore.

262 Vogel, G. 1977. 'Natural substances with effects on the liver'. *New Natural Products and Plant Drugs with Pharmacological, Biological or Therapeutical Activity*. eds H. Wagner and P. Wolff. Springer-Verlag, Berlin. pp. 249–65.

263 Magliulo, E. Carosi, P.G. Minoli, L. et al., 1973. 'Studies on the regenerative capacity of the liver in rats subjected to partial hepatectomy and treated with silymarin'. *Arzneimittel Forschung* 23, pp. 161–7.

264 Rui, Y.C. 1991. 'Advances in pharmacological studies of silymarin'. *Mem Inst Oswaldo Cruz* 86(Suppl. 2), pp. 79–85.

265 Bosisio, E. Benelli, C. and Pirola, O. 1992. 'Effect of the flavonolignans of *Silybum marianum L.* on lipid peroxidation in rat liver microsomes and freshly isolated hepatocytes'. *Pharmacology Research* 25(2), pp. 147–54.

266 Chang, H.M. and But, P.P. 1987. *Pharmacology and Applications of Chinese Materia Medica* Vol. 2. World Scientific, Singapore.

267 Wu, C. and Yu, Q. 1985. 'Pharmacological studies on *Bupleurum chinensis* and its active ingredient, crude saikosaponin'. *Chem Abst* 103, p. 25.

268 Shibata, S. 1977. 'Saponins with biological and pharmacological activity', in *New Natural Products and Plant Drugs with Pharmacological, Biological or Therapeutic Activity*. eds H. Wagner and P. Wolff Springer-Verlag, Berlin. pp. 177–96.

269 Nose, M. Amagaya, S. and Ogihara, Y. 1989. 'Corticosterone secretion-inducing activity of saikosaponin metabolites formed in the alimentary tract'. *Chemistry and Pharmacology Bulletin* 37(10), pp. 2736–40; Yuchi, S. Uchida, Y. and Fujikawa, A. 1986. 'Enhancement of the effectiveness of cortsicosteroid by *Bupleurum falcatum* root extracts'. *Chem Abst* 104, p. 141.

270 Yu, Q. and Wan, L. 1986. 'Mechanism of the antiinflammatory effect of *Bupleurum chinense* crude saikosaponin'. *Chem Abst* 104, p. 43.

271 Tang, W. and Eisenbrand, G. 1992. *Chinese Drugs of Plant Origin*. Springer-Verlag, Berlin.

272 Chang, H.M. and But, P.P. 1987. *Pharmacology and Applications of Chinese Materia Medica* Vol. 2, World Scientific, Singapore.

273 Yen, M.H. Lin, C.C. Chuang, C.H. et al., 1994. 'Anti-inflammatory and hepatoprotective activity of saikosaponin-f and the root extract of *Bupleurum kaoi*, *Fitoterapia* LXV(5), pp. 409–17.

274 Ye, R.G. Ren, G.H. and Li, H.Q. 1995. '[Observation of therapy of integrated TCM-WM on repeatedly relapsed primary nephrotic syndrome in adults.]' *Chung Kuo Chung Hsi I Chieh Ho Tsa Chih* 15(1), pp. 15–17.

275 Wei, J. 1992. ['Treatment of 100 children with infantile nephrotic syndrome by

integrated traditional Chinese medicine and Western medicine.]' *Chung Kuo Chung Hsi I Chieh Ho Tsa Chih* **12**(8), pp. 452, 465–8.

276 Bensky, D. and Gamble, A. 1986. *Chinese Herbal Medicine Materia Medica.* Eastland Press, Seattle.

277 Vollmer, H. and Giebel, A. 1938. 'The diuretic action of several combinations of juniper berry and ononis root'. *Archiv Experimentell Pathologie und Pharmakologie* **190**, pp. 522–34.

278 Leung, A.Y. and Foster, S. 1996. *Encyclopedia of Common Natural Ingredients Used in Foods, Drugs, and Cosmetics.* 2nd edn John Wiley and Sons, Inc., New York. p. 205.

279 Hook, I. McGee, A. and Henman, M. 1993. 'Evaluation of dandelion leaf for diuretic activity and variation in potassium content'. *Int J Pharmacog* **31**(1), pp. 29–34.

280 Racz-Kotilla, E. Racz, G. and Solomon, A. 1974. 'The action of *Taraxacum officinale* extracts on the bodyweight and diuresis of laboratory animals'. *Planta Med* **26**, pp. 212–17.

281 Sanchez de Medina, F. Gamez, M.J. Jimenez, I. et al., 1994. 'Hypoglycaemic activity of juniper 'berries'.' *Planta Med* **60**, pp. 197–200; Swanston-Flatt, S.K. Day, C. Bailey, C.J. et al., 1990. 'Traditional plant treatments for diabetes. Studies in normal and streptozotocin diabetic mice'. *Diabetologia* **33**(8), pp. 462–4.

282 Heil, B.M. and Schilcher, H. 1993. Poster presentation, 24th International Symposium on Essential Oils, Berlin.

283 Riddle, J.M. 1992. *Contraception and Abortion from the Ancient World to the Renaissance.* Harvard University Press, Cambridge.

284 Prakash, A.O. Saxena, V. Shukla, S. et al., 1985. 'Anti-implantation activity of some indigenous plants in rats'. *Acta Eur Fertil* **16**(6), pp. 441–8.

285 Agrawal, O.P. Bharadwaj, S. and Mathur, R. 1980. Antifertility effects of the fruits of *Juniperus communis. Planta Med* (Suppl), pp. 98–101.

286 British Herbal Medicine Association, 1976. *British Herbal Pharmacopoeia, pt. 1* British Herbal Medicine Association, Cowling, West Yorks. pp. 74–5.

287 Grases, F. Melero, G. Costa-Bauza, A. et al., 1994. 'Urolithiasis and phytotherapy' *Int Urol Nephrol* **26**(5), pp. 507–11.

288 Gibelli, C. 1931. 'The hemostatic action of *Equisetum*'. *Arch Int Pharmacodyn* **41**, pp. 419–29.

289 Capasso, F. Mascolo, N. Morrica, P. et al., 1983. 'Phytotherapeutic profile of some plants used in folk medicine'. *Boll Soc Ital Biol Sper* **59**; pp. 1398–404.

290 Weiss, R.F. 1988. *Herbal Medicine.* Arcanum, Gothenburg, Sweden. pp. 238–9.

291 D'Agostino, M. Dini, A. Pizza, C. et al., 1984. 'Sterols from *Equisetum arvense*'. *Boll Soc It Biol Sper* **LX**(12), pp. 2241–5.

292 Nakabayashi, T., 1957 'Thermostable antithiamine factor. II. Thiamine-decomposing substances of horsetail'. *Vitamins* **12**, pp. 20–4.

293 Weiss, R.F. 1988. *Herbal Medicine.* Arcanum, Gothenburg, Sweden, pp. 238–9.

294 D'Agostino, M. Dini, A. Pizza, C. et al., 1984. 'Sterols from *Equisetum arvense*'. *Boll Soc It Biol Sper* **LX**(12), pp. 2241–5.

295 Smith, S.K. Abel, M.H. Kelly, R.W. et al., 1981. 'A role for prostacyclin (PGI2) in excessive menstrual bleeding'. *Lancet* **1**, pp. 522–5; Kelly, R.W. Lumsden, M.A. et al., 1984. 'The relationship between menstrual blood loss and prostaglandin production in the human: evidence for increased availability of arachidonic acid in women suffering from menorrhagia'. *Prost Leuk Med* **16**, pp. 69–77.

296 Bruneton, J. 1995. *Pharmacognosy, Phytochemistry, Medicinal Plants.* Lavoisier Publishing Inc, c/o Springer-Verlag, Secausus, NY. p. 292.

297 Markaverich, B.M. and Gregory, R.R. 1993. 'Preliminary assessment of luteolin as an affinity ligand for type II estrogen-binding sites in rat uterine nuclear extracts'. *Steroids* Jun. **58**(6), pp. 268–74.

298 Tong, S. 1995. *A preliminary report: A randomized pre-clinical double-blind trial*

to assess effectiveness of Echinacea 2000+ in the prevention and treatment of colds and influenza. Dept of Health Service Management, School of Health, University of New England.

299 Muller-Jakic, B. Breu, W. Probstle, A. et al. 1993. 'In vitro inhibition of cyclooxygenase and 5-lipoxygenase by alkamides from *Echinacea* and *Achillea* species'. *Planta Medica* **60**, pp. 37–40.

300 Bauer, R. Juric, K. Puhlmann, J. et al., 1988. '[Immunologic *in vivo* and *in vitro* studies on *Echinacea* extracts]', *Arzneimittel Forschung V* **38**, pp. 276–81.

301 Mose, J.R. 1983. 'The effect of echinacin on phagocytosis and natural killer cells'. *Die Mediz. Welt* **34**, pp. 1463–7.

302 Busing, K.H. 1952. 'Hyaluronidase-hemmung durch echinacin'. *Arzneimittel Forschung* **1**, p. 194. In Willard, T. 1991. *The Wild Rose Scientific Herbal.* Wild Rose College of Natural Healing, Alberta. pp. 113–15.

303 Amin, A.H. Subbaiah, T.V. and Abbasi, K.M. 1969. 'Berberine sulfate: Antimicrobial activity, bioassay and mode of action'. *Canadian Journal of Microbiology* **15**, pp. 1067–76; Johnson C.C. Johnson, G. et al., 1952. 'Toxicity of alkaloids to certain bacteria'. *Acta Pharm. Tox* **8**, pp. 71–8; Ghosh, A.K. 1983. 'Effect of Berberine chloride on *Leishmania donovani*'. *Indian Journal of Medical Research* **78**, pp. 407–16.

304 Kumazawa, Y. Itagaki, A. Fukumoto, M. et al., 1984. 'Activation of peritoneal macrophages by berberine-type alkaloids in terms of induction of cytostatic activity'. *International Journal of Immunopharmacology* **6**(6), pp. 587–92.

305 Boucaud-Maitre, Y. Algernon, O. and Raynaud, J. 1988. 'Cytotoxic and antitumoural activity of *Calendula officinalis* extracts'. *Pharmazie* **43**, pp. 220–1; Klouchek-Popova, E. Popov, A. Pavlova, N. et al., 1982. 'Influence of the physiological regeneration and epithelialization using fractions isolated from *Calendula officinalis*'. *Acta Physiol Pharmacol Bulg* **8**(4), pp. 63–7.

306 Boucaud-Maitre, Y. Algernon, O. and Raynaud, J. 1988. 'Cytotoxic and antitumoural activity of *Calendula officinalis* extracts'. *Pharmazie* **43**, pp. 220–1.

307 Wagner, H.. Proksch, A. Riess-Maurer, I. et al., 1985. 'Immunostimulating action of polysaccharides (heteroglycans) from Higher plants'. *Arzneimittelforschung* **35**(7), pp. 1069–75.

308 *British Herbal Pharmacopoeia*, part 1, 1976. British Herbal Medicine Association, West Yorks. pp. 38–9.

309 Kielczynski, W. 1995. Personal communication.

310 Cartier, A. Chan, H. Malo, J.L. et al., 1986. 'Occupational asthma caused by eastern white cedar (*Thuja occidentalis*) with demonstration that plicatic acid is present in this wood dust and is the causal agent', *J Allergy Clin Immunol* **77**(4), pp. 639–45.

311 Gohla, S.H. Haubeck, H.D. and Neth R.D. 1988. 'Mitogenic activity of high molecular polysaccharide fractions isolated from *Cupressaceae Thuja occidentale* L.I. Macrophage—dependent induction of CD-4-positive T-helper (Th+) lymphocytes', *Leukemia* **2**(8), pp. 528–33; Gohla, S.H. Haubeck, H.D Schrum S. et al., 1989. 'Activation of CD-4 positive T cells by poly-saccharide fractions isolated from *Cupressaceae Thuja occidentalis* L. (Arborvitae)', *Haematol Bluttransfus* **32**, pp. 268–72.

312 Gerhausser, C. Leonhardt, K. Tan, G.T. et al., 1992. 'What is the active antiviral principle of *Thuja occidentalis* L?', *Pharm Pharmacol Lett* **2**, pp. 127–30.

Chapter 20

1 Drife, J. 1990. 'Benefits and risks of oral contraceptives', *Adv Contracept* Dec; **6** Suppl, pp. 15–25.

2 Kaunitz, A.M. 1993. 'Combined oral contraception with desogestrel/ethinyl estradiol: tolerability profile', *Am J Obstet Gynecol* **168**(3 Pt 2), pp. 1028–33.

3   Long, C.A. 1994. 'Amenorrhoea', *'Manual of Clinical Problems in Obstetrics and Gynecology'*, eds M.E. Rivlin and R.W. Martin, Little, Brown and Company, Boston, p. 385–8.

4   Steinberg, S. 1991. 'The treatment of late luteal phase dysphoric disorder', *Life Sci* **49**, pp. 767–802.

5   Rose, D.P. and Braidman, I.P. 1971. 'Oral contraceptives and tryptophan metabolism: effects of oestrogen in low dose combined with progestagen and of a progestagen (megestrol acetate) given alone', *J Clin Path* **25**, pp. 252–8.

6   Andersch, B. and Hahn, L. 1981. 'Premenstrual complaints: II. Influence of oral contraceptives', *Acta Obstet Gynecol Scand* **60**, pp. 579–83.

7   Vorherr, H. 1986. 'Fibrocystic breast disease: pathophysiology, pathomorphology, clinical picture, and management', *Am J Obstet Gynecol* **154**(1), pp. 161–79.

8   ibid, pp. 161–79.

9   Vessey, M.P. Villard-Mackintosh, L. and Painter, R. 1993. 'Epidemiology of endometriosis in women attending family planning clinics', *BMJ* **306**(6871), pp. 182–4.

10   Barbieri, R.L. 1990. 'Endometriosis', *Drugs* **39**(4), pp. 502–10.

11   Vercellini, P. Trespidi, L. and Colombo, A. 1993. 'A gonadotrophin-releasing hormone agonist versus a low-dose oral contraceptive for pelvic pain associated with endometriosis', *Fertil Steril* **60**(1), pp. 75–9.

12   ibid. pp. 75–9.

13   Israel, R. 1994. 'Endometriosis: treatment', *'Management of common problems in obstetrics and gynecology'*, eds D.R. Mishell and P.F. Brenner, Blackwell Scientific Publications, Boston, USA, p. 750.

14   Friedman, A.J. and Thomas, P.P. 1995. 'Does low-dose combination oral contraceptive use affect uterine size or menstrual flow in premenopausal woman with leiomyomas?' *Obstet Gynecol* **85**(4), pp. 631–5.

15   Thomas, J. ed, 1995. *Australian Prescription Products Guide*, Australian Pharmaceutical Publishing Company, Melbourne.

16   Smith, S.K. Abel, M.H. Kelly, R.W. et al., 1981. 'A role for prostacyclin (PGI2) in excessive menstrual bleeding', *Lancet* **1**, pp. 522–5.

17   Thomas, J. ed, 1995. *Australian Prescription Products Guide*, Australian Pharmaceutical Publishing Company, Melbourne.

18   Ota, H. Maki, M. Shidara, Y, et al., 1992. 'Effects of danazol at the immunologic level in patients with adenomyosis, with special reference to autoantibodies: a multi-center cooperative study', *Am J Obstet Gynecol* **167**(2), pp. 481–6.

19   Watts, J.F. Butt, W.R. and Logan Edwards, R. 1987. 'A clinical trial using danazol for the treatment of premenstrual tension', *Br J Obs Gynaecol* **94**, pp. 30–4.

20   Kenton, L. 1995. *Passage to Power*, Ebury Press, London; Lee, J.R. 1993. *Natural Progesterone: The Multiple Roles of a Remarkable Hormone*, BLL Publishing, Sebastapol, USA; Dalton, K. *PMS: The Essential Guide to Treatment Options*, Thorsons, London.

21   Freeman, E. Rickels, K. Sondheimer, S.J. et al., 1990. 'Ineffectiveness of progesterone suppository treatment for premenstrual syndrome', *JAMA* **264**, pp. 349–53; Van der Meer, Y.G. Benedek, Jaszmann, L.J. and Van Loenen, A.C. 1983. 'Effect of high dose progesterone on the premenstrual syndrome: a doubleblind cross-over trial', *J Psychomat Obstet Gynaec* **2–4**, pp. 220–1.

22   Brenner, P.F. 1988. 'The menopausal syndrome', *Obstet Gynecol* **72**(5 Suppl), pp. 6–11.

23   Hillard, T.C. Whitcroft, S. Ellerington, M.C. et al., 1991. 'The long term risks and benefits of hormone replacement therapy', *J Clin Pharm Ther* **16**(4), pp. 231–45.

24   Breckwoldt, M. Keck, C. and Karck, U. 1995. 'Benefits and risks of hormone replacement therapy (HRT)', *J Steroid Molec Biol* **53**(1–6), pp. 205–8; Adami, H.O. 1992. 'Long-term consequences of estrogen and estrogen-progestin replacement', *Cancer Causes Control* **3**(1), pp. 83–90; Hillard, T.C. Whitcroft,

S. Ellerington, M.C. et al., 1991. 'The long term risks and benefits of hormone replacement therapy', *J Clin Pharm Ther* **16**(4), pp. 231–45; Hulka, B. 1994. 'Links between hormone replacement therapy and neoplasia', *Fertil Steril* **62**(6 Suppl 2), pp. 168–175

25   Hulka, B. 1994. 'Links between hormone replacement therapy and neoplasia', *Fertil Steril* **62**(6 Suppl 2), pp. 168–75.

26   Hunt, K. Vessey, M. McPherson, K. et al., 1987. 'Long-term surveillance of mortality and cancer incidence in women receiving hormone replacement therapy', *Br J Obstet Gynaecol* **94**(7), pp. 620–35.

27   Gambrell, R.D. 1987. 'Hormone replacement therapy and breast cancer', *Maturitas* **9**(2), pp. 123–33.

28   van-Leeuwen, F.E. 1991. 'Epidemiological aspects of exogenous progestagens in relation to their role in pathogenesis of human breast cancer', *Acta Endocrinol Copenh* **125** (Suppl 1), pp. 13–26.

29   Hulka, B. 1994. 'Links between hormone replacement therapy and neoplasia', *Fertil Steril* **62**(6 Suppl 2), pp. 168–175.

30   Colditz, G.A. Stampfer, M.J. Willett, W.C. et al., 1992. 'Type of postmenopausal hormone use and risk of breast cancer: 12-year follow-up from the Nurses' Health Study', *Cancer Causes Control* **3**(5), pp. 433–9.

31   Hulka, B. 1994. 'Links between hormone replacement therapy and neoplasia', *Fertil Steril* **62**(6 Suppl 2), pp. 168–175.

32   Shelley, J.M. Smith, A.M.A. and Dudley, E. 1995. 'Use of hormone replacement therapy by Melbourne women', *Aust J Public Health* **19**, pp. 387–92.

33   Recker, R.R. Davies, K.M. Hinders, S.M. et al., 1992. 'Bone gain in young adult women', *JAMA* **268**(17), pp. 2403–8.

34   Law, M.R. Wald, N.J. et al., 1991. 'Strategies for prevention of osteoporosis and hip fracture', *BMJ* **303**, pp. 453–59.

35   Rebar, R.W. 1994. 'Unanswered questions in hormonal replacement therapy', *Exp-Gerontol* **29**(3–4), pp. 447–61.

36   Ravn, S.H. Rosenberg, J. and Bostofte, E. 1994. 'Postmenopausal hormone replacement therapy—clinical implications', *Eur J Obstet Gynecol Reprod Biol* **53**(2), pp. 81–93.

37   Posthuma, W.F. Westendorp, R.G. and Vandenbroucke, J.P. 1994. 'Cardioprotective effect of hormone replacement therapy in postmenopausal women: is the evidence biased?' *BMJ* **308**(6939), pp. 1268–9; Kafonek, S.D. 1994. 'Postmenopausal hormone replacement therapy and cardiovascular risk reduction. A review', *Drugs* **47** (Suppl 2), pp. 16–24.

38   Everson, G.T. McKinley, C. and Kern, F. 1991. 'Mechanisms of gallstones formation in women. Effects of exogenous estrogen (Premarin) and dietary cholesterol on hepatic lipid metabolism', *J Clin Invest* **87**(1), pp. 237–46.

39   Rock, J.A. Truglia, J.A. Caplan, R.J. et al., 1993. 'Zoladex (goserelin acetate implant) in the treatment of endometriosis: a randomised comparison with danazol', *Obstet Gynecol* **82**(2), pp. 198–205; Trabant, H. Widdra, W. and de Looze, S. 1990. 'Efficacy and safety of intranasal buserelin acetate in the treatment of endometriosis, a review of six clinical trials and comparison with danazol', *Prog Clin Biol Res* **323**, pp. 357–82.

40   Donnez, J. Nisolle, M. Grandjean, P. et al., 1993. '[The role of GnRH agonists in the endoscopic treatment of endometriosis and fibromyomas.]' *Contracept Fertil Sex* **21**(1), pp. 59–62.

41   Kauppila, A. 1993. 'Changing concepts of medical treatment of endometriosis', *Acta Obstet Gynecol Scand* **72**(5), pp. 324–36.

42   Mortolla, J.F. Girton, L. and Fischer, U. 1991. 'Successful treatment of severe premenstrual syndrome by combined use of gonadotrophin releasing hormone agonist and estrogen/progestin', *J Clin Endocrinol Metab* **72**(2), pp. 252A–252F.

43 Van-Leusden, H.A. 1994. 'Impact of different GnRH analogs in benign gyneco-logical disorders related to their chemical structure, delivery systems and dose', *Gynecol Endocrinol* **8**(3), pp. 215–22.

44 Dawood, M.Y. 1994. 'Hormonal therapies for endometriosis: implications for bone metabolism', *Acta Obstet Gynecol Scand Suppl* **159**, pp. 22–34.

45 Waibel-Treber, S. Minne, H.W. Scharla S.H. et al., 1989. 'Reversible bone loss in women treated with GnRH-agonists for endometriosis and uterine leiomyoma', *Hum Reprod* **4**(4), pp. 384–8.

46 Andersch, B. Hahn, L. Wenderstam, C. et al., 1978. 'Treatment of premenstrual syndrome with bromocriptine', *Acta Endocrinol* **88**(S 216), pp. 165–74.

47 Steinberg, S. 1991. 'The treatment of late luteal phase dysphoric disorder', *Life Sci* **49**, pp. 767–802.

48 Kauppila, A. and Ronnberg, L. 1985. 'Naproxen sodium in dysmenorrhea second-ary to endometriosis', *Obstet Gynecol* **65**(3), pp. 379–83.

49 Rees, M.C.P. 1990. 'Human menstruation and eicosanoids', *Reprod Fertil Dev* **2**, pp. 467–76.

50 Fraser, I.S. Shearman, R.P. McIlveen, J. et al., 1981. 'Efficacy of mefenamic acid in patients with a complaint of menorrhagia', *Obstet Gynecol* **58**(5), pp. 543–51.

51 Mezrow, G. 1994. 'Treatment of dysfunctional uterine bleeding', *'Management of Common Problems in Obstetrics and Gynecology'*, eds D.R. Mishell and P.F. Brenner, Blackwell Scientific Publications, Boston, USA. p. 444.

52 Mira, M. McNeil, D. Fraser, I.S. et al., 1986. 'Mefanamic acid in the treatment of premenstrual syndrome', *Obstet Gynecol* **68**(3), pp. 395–8.

53 Thomas, J. ed, 1995. *Australian Prescription Products Guide*, Australian Pharma-ceutical Publishing Company, Melbourne.

54 ibid.

55 Steinberg, S. 1991. 'The treatment of late luteal phase dysphoric disorder', *Life Sci* **49**, pp. 767–802.

56 Pariser, S.F. Stern, S.L. Shank, M.L. et al., 1985. 'Premenstrual syndrome: concerns, controversies, and treatment', *Am J Obstet Gynecol* **153**(6), pp. 599–604.

57 Friedman, A.J. and Haas, S.T. 1993. 'Should uterine size be an indication for surgical intervention in women with myomas'? *Am J Obstet Gynecol* **168**(3 Pt 1), pp. 751–5.

58 Vergani, P. Ghidini, A. Strobelt, N. et al., 1994. 'Do uterine leiomyomas influence pregnancy outcome'? *Am J Perinatal* **11**(5), pp. 356–8.

59 Starks, G.C. 1988. 'CO2 laser myomectomy in an infertile population', *J Reprod Med* **33**(2), pp. 184–6.

60 Werbach, M. 1987. *Nutritional Influences on Illness*, Thorsons, London, p. 447.

61 Rayner, H. Lovelle Allen, S. and Braverman, E.R. 1991. 'Nutrition and wound healing', *J Nutr Environ Med*, Aug, pp. 8–13.

62 Hamilton, K., 1995. 'Wound healing and nutrition', *J Nutr Environ Med*, Nov, p. 15.

63 Phillips, S. Ruggier, R. and Hutchison, S.E. 1993. *'Zingiber officinale* (ginger)—an antiemetic for day case surgery', *Anaesthesia* **48**(8), pp. 715–7.

64 Bone M.E. Wilkinson, D.J. Young, J.R. et al., 1990. 'Ginger root—a new anti-emetic. The effect of ginger root on postoperative nausea and vomiting after major gynaecological surgery', *Anaesthesia* **45**(8), pp. 669–71.

Index

allergic rhinitis, 417
allergies, 417; *see also* sneezing (allergic)
  acute, 288
  to dairy products, 287–9
almond smoothie, recipe for, 407–8
Aloe barbadensis, 230
5 alpha reductase, 215
alpha-linolenic acid (ALA), 82, 83, 282, 283
Amanita phalloides, 372
amenorrhoea, 37, 43, 73, 110, 157, 158, 170–3, 203, 208–22, 255, 265, 270
  primary, 209, 212–13
  secondary, 209–12
  treatment, 324, 325, 333, 338, 339, 347, 356, 374
  see also post-Pill amenorrhoea
amiloride, 369
amino acids, 280, 289
amitryptoline *see* Tryptanol
amphoteric, 325
anabolic herbs, 367
anabolic steroids, 218
anaemia, 44, 95, 103, 176, 180, 188, 221, 222, 278, 290
  effect of the Pill, 385
  symptoms of, 190
  treatment, 189–91, 326, 368, 370, 396
anaesthetics, 365
analgesics, 254, 355, 373
anatomy, female, 23–34
ANDI *see* aberrations of normal development and involution
Androcur, 219
androgen-insensitivity syndrome, 212
androgenic alopecia, 64, 65, 136, 218, 219, 261, 265, 268, 349, 389
  treatment of, 220–1, 350
androgenic effects *see* masculinisation
androgens, 55, 57, 60, 64–5, 66, 69, 70, 101, 102, 136, 141, 187, 213, 215, 261, 265–6, 309, 311, 315, 349
  excess, 196, 211, 217–21, 264, 265, 267, 268, 270–1, 309, 349, 350
androgens, adrenal *see* adrenal androgens
androgens, ovarian *see* ovarian androgens
androstenediol, 65
androstenedione, 65, 136, 268, 312
Anemone pulsatilla, 119, 228, 254, 356
Angelica sinensis, 119, 133, 144, 163, 180, 182, 183, 198, 202, 222, 227, 235, 250, 253, 254, 270, 320, 322–5, 331, 348, 349–50, 354, 355, 366, 368, 374
angina pectoris, treatment for, 331, 343, 355
anima, 422
animal spirit *see* anima
anodynes, 228, 354–9

anorexia nervosa, 110, 165, 166, 167, 194
  treatment, 334
anovulation *see* ovulation, failure of
ANTA *see* Australian Natural Therapists Association
anti-bacterial herbs, 335, 368
antibiotics, 73, 101, 102, 181, 206, 310, 332, 378
  and the Pill, 386
anti-coagulant drugs, 172
anti-convulsants, 373
anti-depressants, 148, 400
  and the Pill, 387
anti-diuretic hormone and alcohol, 375
anti-epileptic drugs and the Pill, 386
antigonadotrophic herbs, 362
anti-haemorrhagic herbs *see* astringents
anti-hypertensive drugs, 210, 215
anti-infective herbs, 370, 378–83
anti-inflammatory herbs, 339, 341, 345, 350, 355, 357, 370, 371, 373, 377, 381
antimicrobial herbs, 341, 354, 365, 370, 377, 380, 381, 382
anti-oxidants, 202, 204, 235, 256, 286
  and prevention of cancer, 295, 297
  sources, 279, 285, 286, 369
antiseptic creams, 206
antiseptic herbs, 335, 376, 377, 378–83
antispasmodic herbs *see* spasmolytics
antithiamine, 377
antithyrotopic activity, 363
anti-tumour herbs, 381
anti-ulcer drugs, 215
anti-ulcer herbs, 341
anti-viral herbs, 368, 382
anxiety, 76, 97, 108, 111, 112, 128, 141, 148, 160, 162, 234, 247, 293
  treatment, 98–100, 112, 118–19, 122, 143, 163–4, 331, 359–65, 390, 400
anxiolytics, 400
apigenin, 338
appendicitis, treatment for, 315
appetite stimulants, 333, 354, 370, 371
appetite suppressants, 390
apricots, 297
arachidonic acid, 79, 82, 83, 84, 126, 284, 357
arbor vitae *see* Thuja occidentalis
arbutin, 330
Arctium lappa, 102–3
Arctostaphylos uva-ursi, 330
aromatase enzyme, 60, 217, 264, 309, 349
aromatherapy, 19–20
  to treat dysmenorrhoea, 233
aromatic herbs, 354
aromatisation, 60, 265; *see also* peripheral oestrogen conversion

arrhythmia, treatment for, 323, 355
Artemesia vulgaris, 203, 227, 251, 334–5
arthritis, treatment for, 315, 333, 353, 357;
    see also rheumatoid arthritis
artichoke *see Cynara scolymus*
asafoetida *see Ferula asafoetida*
Asherman's syndrome, 209
asparagus, 313
aspirin, 398
asthma, 367, 399
    treatment, 283, 324, 335, 355, 363, 379
Astragalus membranaceus, 143–4, 235, 368
astringents, 47, 48, 163, 181, 182, 188, 204, 206, 207, 337–45, 354, 377, 381
atherosclerosis, 285
atherosclerotic plaque, 284, 285
ATMS *see* Australian Traditional Medicine Society
Atractylodes macrocephala, 144, 366
Australian Natural Therapists Association (ANTA), 20
Australian Traditional Medicine Society (ATMS), 20
auto-immune disease, 133, 212, 241
auto-transfusion, 403–4
Avena sativa, 143, 147, 252
avocadoes, 282, 287
azulene, 338

Ba Wei Di Huang Tang *see* Rehmannia Eight Combination
Ba Zen Tang, 366
Bach flower essences, 163
bacteriostatic herbs, 332
bad breath, 410, 414
bai shao *see Paeonia lactiflora*
baldness *see* androgenic alopecia
bananas, 122, 291
Baptista tinctoria, 382
barberry *see Berberis vulgaris*
barley, 280
Bartholin's glands, 25–6
basal body temperature, 75–6, 179, 269
    graph, 117
bean sprouts, 306–7
beans, 71, 257, 279, 280, 290, 291, 306–7, 308
    recommended daily intake, 300
bearberry *see Arctostaphylos uva-ursi*
beer: and colon cancer, 299
    and prolactin levels, 215, 217, 345
beetroot, 297, 405
benign breast disease *see* breast disease, benign
benzo[a]pyrene, 308
benzodiazapines *see* Valium
benzoyl peroxide, 101

berberine, 370, 380
Berberis vulgaris, 229, 230, 254, 257, 370–1
berry drink, recipe for, 408
beta-carotene, 167, 204, 256, 286
    and cancer prevention, 295, 297
    and the Pill, 387
    sources, 297
3 beta-dehydrogenase, 180
beta-glucuronidase, 60, 68, 69
beta-lactoglobulin, 287, 288
betamethasone, 172
beta-sitosterol, 316, 323
beth root *see Trillium erectum*
bethogenin, 344
Betula pendula, 375
bilateral salphingo-oopherectomy, 133, 179, 404
bile, 60, 64, 71, 255, 369, 421
    acids, 280
    effect of oestrogen, 393
    to improve bile flow, 256, 291, 370, 371, 373
biochanin A, 306–8
bioflavonoids, 144, 146, 147, 181, 188, 235, 236
    deficiency, 183–4
Bioglan MaxEPA, 84
birch *see Betula pendula*
birth control *see* contraceptives
bitter foods, 291
bitter greens, 254, 257, 291
bitters, 71, 119, 120, 126, 147, 167, 182, 183, 190, 229, 230, 231, 235, 250, 256, 257, 271, 279, 324, 325, 327, 355, 358, 363, 367, 369–74, 380, 381
Black Bile (humour), 6, 255, 420, 421, 422
black cohosh *see Cimicifuga racemosa*
black haw *see Viburnum prunifolium*
blackcurrant seed oil, 82, 127, 284
bladder, 175
    and endometriosis, 238, 246
bladder cancer, link with coffee, 299
bleeding, abnormal, 140, 155–8, 173, 312
    causes, 192–5, 200, 367, 409, 410
    definition, 155, 192–207
    treatment, 320, 338, 388, 390, 397
    see also bleeding, erratic;
        break-through bleeding
bleeding, erratic, 197–207
bloating, 279, 292, 399, 412, 415
    and lactose intolerance, 288, 289
    PMS bloating *see* fluid retention
        treatment, 371
blocked nose/ears, 289, 398
Blood (humour), 6, 419, 420
blood deficiency, 221–2, 324, 335

blood disorders, 176; *see also* anaemia;
leukaemia
blood, excess of *see* plethora
blood fat levels *see* blood lipid levels
blood flow *see* circulation
blood in urine *see* haematuria
blood lipid levels, 269, 292
effect of coffee, 293
effect of noresthisterone, 392
effect of the Pill, 388
regulation of, 271, 279
blood pressure, 149
regulation of, 368, 374
blood pressure, high *see* hypertension
blood quality, 221–2
blood stagnation, 344
blood sugar level, 100, 113, 114, 120,
122, 128–9, 160, 265, 269, 280
regulation of, 271, 279, 370, 376
blood tonics, 323, 324, 331, 366
blood tonification, 323
blood vessels, 282
blue cohosh *see* *Caulophyllum
thalictroides*
blueberries, 236
BMI *see* body mass index
body mass index, 165, 167, 171, 204,
266, 268
body weight: excess, 268, 269; *see also*
obesity
influence of, 89–90, 266–7, 392
and menopause, 136, 141, 145, 149
see also body mass index; weight
gain; weight reduction
body weight, low, 72–3, 138, 164–7,
170, 209, 266–7
treatment of, 167–8
boils, treatment for, 379
bone density, 72, 73, 74, 133, 149, 168,
172, 215, 266–7, 272
effect of exercise, 169, 171, 392
effect of the Pill, 386, 387, 390, 392
and GnRH agonists, 397
and oestrogens, 392, 398
and phyto-oestrogens, 309–10
bowel, 68, 73, 112, 308, 312, 313, 319
and dysmenorrhoea, 225, 254
and endometriosis, 175, 238, 245–6,
247
function, 421
pain, 247, 338
and recovery from surgery, 405–6
regulation of, 230–1, 279, 310, 370
see also bowel cancer; constipation;
peristalsis
bowel cancer, 296, 298, 299
brain, 282
bran, 281
and magnesium absorption, 273
see also rice bran oil; wheat bran

bread, 279, 280, 302, 406
breakfast cereals *see* cereals
breakfast menus, 301; *see also* seed
breakfast
break-through bleeding, 385, 389, 396;
see also spotting
breast cancer, 62, 63, 68, 69, 70, 71,
86, 124–5, 133, 134, 278, 293, 299
effect of HRT, 391–2, 393, 396
prevention of, 280, 289, 295–9, 300,
310
treatment for, 173, 308
breast disease, benign 75, 123–5, 293
fibrocystic, 68, 123, 256
and the Pill, 385
treatment, 126–30, 172, 173
breast examination, 17, 18, 50–1;
see also breast self-examination (BSE)
breast-feeding, 74, 323, 356
effect of, 125, 211, 214, 221, 240,
243
herbs to assist, 365–6
herbs to avoid, 382
see also galactogogues; lactation
breast milk, 82, 282, 288, 322
production in non-pregnant women
see galactorrhoea
breast pain *see* mastalgia
breast self-examination (BSE), 50–1, 149
breasts, 308
development of, 64, 70, 212, 213
reduction in size, 219, 261, 389
breathing difficulties, 97, 260, 288, 324,
368, 416;
see also asthma
Brenner cysts *see* Brenner tumours
Brenner tumours, 212, 259
Brevinor, 387
brewers's yeast, 102, 204
Broadbent, John, 12–13
broccoli, 296
bromocriptine, 115, 126, 215, 216,
397–8
side-effects, 398
bronchitis, treatment for, 307, 333, 335,
350
brussels sprouts, 257, 296
BSE *see* breast self-examination
buckwheat leaf tea, 184, 235
bulimia nervosa, 165, 166, 167, 194
Bupleurum falcatum, 119, 144, 199,
235, 348, 368, 370, 373–4
butter, lactose levels in, 288

cabbages, 250, 254, 257, 279, 291, 296,
407
Caesarean section, 243
and fibroids, 402
caffeine: effect of, 99, 122, 128, 231,
243, 255, 293–4, 367, 407

coriander, 292
corn oil, 284, 316
corpus albicans, 31
corpus luteum, 31, 39–41, 56, 58, 64,
    136, 263, 349
    insufficiency, 74, 75
corticosteroid drugs, 369
corticosteroids, 64, 172, 211, 218, 219,
    311, 315, 373
    effect of stress, 160
    see also aldosterone; corticosterone;
        cortisol; cortisone; glucocorticoids
corticosterone, 373–4
corticotrophins, 218
cortisol-binding globulin (CBG), 66
cortisol, 66, 110, 369
cortisone, 311
    effect of, 211
Corydalis ambigua, 228, 251, 254, 354–5
Cos lettuce, 257
coughing, 410
    treatment, 307, 355
coumarins, 330, 333
coumestans, 305, 306–7, 313
    sources of, 317
coumestrol, 74, 306–7, 310
counselling, 252
cramp bark see Viburnum opulus
cravings (food), 108, 114, 119–20, 128,
    247, 279, 415
croup, treatment for, 333
cryosurgery, 209
CT scan, 215
cultured milk products see yoghurt and
    cultured milk products
cumin, 292
Curcuma longa, 228–9
curds see casein
curette, 174, 178, 193, 195, 197, 200,
    209, 322, 400
Cushing's syndrome, 66, 134, 172, 211,
    218, 264
cyclophosphamide, 133, 172
Cynara scolymus, 257
cyproterone acetate see Androcur
cystadenocarcinomas, 212, 260
cystadenomas, 259–60
cystic hyperplasia, 123, 200
cystitis, 145
    treatment, 356, 377
cysts, follicular, 262–3
cysts, functional see cysts, physiological
cysts, hormone-producing, 212, 262, 264
cysts, luteal see luteal cysts, 262, 263
cysts, physiological, 259, 261, 262–5
    treatment, 263–4
cytotoxic drugs, 172–3

D&C see curette
daidzein, 306, 307, 308

dairy products, 113, 119, 122, 127,
    272, 281, 287–9, 290
    intolerance to, 287–9
    low-fat, 290
Damp (TCM quality), 4, 335, 414
danazol, 115, 126, 187, 218, 219, 220,
    249, 348, 389–90
    side effects, 389, 390, 397
dandelion see Taraxacum officinale
dandelion 'coffee', 371
Dang gui see Angelica sinensis
Danocrine see danazol
Daucus carota, 10
DDT and fibroids, 186
De Materia Medica (Dioscorides), 9, 362
deadly nightshade family, 313
death cap toadstool see Amanita
    phalloides
Deca-Durabolin, 218
Decadron see dexamethasone
Deer Massage, 214
dehydroepiandrosterone (DHEA), 65, 219
delayed period see period, late
Democritus, 35
demulcents, 368
dental caries, 293
Depo-Provera, 194
depression, 96–100, 108, 110, 113, 114,
    146, 148, 162, 251–2, 255, 413
    and dairy intolerance, 289
    and the Pill, 385
    treatment, 98–100, 112, 120–1, 122,
        163, 333, 351, 356, 359–65, 390
dermatitis, 101
dermoid cysts, 258, 259, 260
DES see diethylstilboestrol
desogesterol, 219
detoxification diets, 168
dexamethasone, 172, 219
DGLA see dihomogamma-linolenic acid
DHA see docosahexaenoic acid
DHEA see dehydroepiandrosterone
DHT see dihydrotestosterone
diabetes mellitus, 134, 200, 211
    and HRT, 396
    treatment, 280, 368, 376
Diane, 219, 387
diaphoretics, 363
diaphragm, 176
diarrhoea, 225, 226, 237, 247, 279,
    292, 370, 374, 399, 405, 414, 415
    and lactose intolerance, 288–9
    treatment, 227, 322, 338, 339, 346,
        354
diathermy, 205, 249, 401
diazepam see Valium
diet, 277–303, 409
    during adolescence, 95–6, 99, 102
    and bone density, 392
    detoxification, 168

endometrial ablation, 179, 402
endometrial cancer, 62, 68, 200, 201,
    270
  and HRT, 392, 395, 396
  and the Pill, 385
endometrial cysts see endometriomas
endometrial hyperplasia, 77, 186, 193,
    197, 199, 200–4, 270, 398
  prevention, 309
endometriomas, 244, 246, 248, 254, 262
  treatment, 397
endometriosis, 27, 28, 29, 49, 62, 67,
    68, 69, 75, 78, 85–6, 132, 134, 142,
    157, 169, 170, 172, 173, 175, 186,
    197, 224, 238–55, 258, 262, 314, 344
  and alcohol, 294
  and bleeding, 177, 195, 197
  causes, 239–44, 293, 313
  and cervical eversion, 205
  and Chinese herbs, 217
  and emmenagogues, 203, 250
  and fibroids, 186
  and HRT, 396
  incidence, 239
  and the Pill, 386
  and prolactin, 216
  and progestogens, 201
  symptoms, 247–8
  treatment, 249–53, 255, 349, 350,
    371, 372, 388, 389, 396–7, 399,
    401, 402, 404
endometrium, 27, 29, 32–4, 38, 39, 59,
    64, 75, 140, 157, 175, 178, 179, 180,
    181, 185, 193, 195, 196, 200, 201,
    202, 238, 240, 247, 250, 400
  and oestrogen, 394, 395
  and the Pill, 388
  protection of, 203–4, 269–70
endorphins, 111
enemas, 225
energy drinks see high-protein drinks
enterodiol, 281, 308
entero-hepatic circulation of oestrogens
    see liver and oestrogens
enterolactone, 281, 308
enuresis, treatment for, 37; see also
    incontinence
enveloped viruses, treatment for, 360
environmental oestrogens see
    xeno-oestrogens
EPA see eicosapentaenoic acid
ephedra, 9
epilepsy: and hyperprolactinaemia, 214
  treatment, 333, 334, 335, 346
epinephrine, 109, 159, 160
Equisetum arvense, 181, 182, 188, 198,
    377–8
equol, 307
ergot alkaloids, 357
erratic bleeding see bleeding, erratic

erythromycin, 101
Esberitox, 382
Eschscholtzia californica, 99
essential fatty acids, 80–6, 112, 122,
    232, 251, 253, 254, 255, 279, 282,
    287
  deficiency, 282
  sources, 290
essential oils, 163, 233, 376
Estigyn, 391, 394
Estraderm, 394
ethinyl oestradiol, 386
evening meal menus see dinner menus
evening primrose oil, 77, 82, 83, 84–5,
    86, 114, 120, 121, 127, 144, 145,
    146, 147, 232, 252–3, 284
  and the Pill, 388, 389
exercise: negative effect of, 73, 92, 138,
    165, 170–1, 194, 204, 209, 210, 214,
    242
  positive effect of, 71, 125, 128, 135,
    148, 149, 168–70, 220, 227, 235,
    236, 242, 250, 254, 255, 392, 407
  see also aerobic exercise; long, slow,
    distance exercise
exhaustion see fatigue
expectorants, 368
extraglandular oestrogen conversion see
    peripheral oestrogen conversion
extra-uterine fibroids see fibroids,
    extra-uterine
eye disorders, treatment of, 329, 333

facial hair, 64
  cause of, 136
  see also hirsutism
faintness, 114, 120, 226, 247
  treatment, 364
Fallopian tubes, 27, 85, 170, 175, 213
  abnormalities, 243
  and endometriosis, 238, 239, 240, 245
  and fibroids, 185
  patent, 239
false unicorn root see *Chamaelirium
    luteum*
fatigue, 96, 120, 128, 140, 141, 142,
    143, 148, 162, 190, 222, 234,
    251, 272, 280, 290, 400, 410, 411,
    412, 414, 416
  treatment for, 163, 336, 351, 390, 399
  see also chronic fatigue syndrome;
    post-viral fatigue syndrome
fats: and cancer, 299
  intake, 68, 122, 125, 126, 227, 250,
    281–7, 290
  recommended daily intake, 301
  see also essential fatty acids; saturated
    fats; unsaturated fats
febrile conditions see fever
Femoden, 219

158, 176–7, 193, 195, 197, 198, 211, 213, 265, 267, 270, 308, 313, 316, 325, 344
herbs which influence, 345–52, 367
see also hypothalamus; pituitary gland
hypothalamus, 39, 40, 56, 57, 58, 59, 70, 75, 110, 141, 157, 159, 160, 165, 170, 171, 314, 398
dysfunction, 210, 211, 212, 214; *see also* hyperthyroidism; hypothyroidism
hypothyroidism, 126, 127, 134, 157, 214, 215
treatment, 307, 341
Hysone *see* hydrocortisone
hysterectomy, 133, 134, 179, 187, 226, 235, 249, 403–4
recovery from, 142, 327, 352
hysteria, 106
treatment, 119, 333
hysteroscope, 185, 193, 400
hysteroscopy, 174, 178, 197, 200, 396, 400–1

idiopathic thrombocytopaenia (ITP), 343
illness (definition), 15
immune system, 141, 415
effect of stress, 162
and endometriosis, 240–1, 249, 252–3
to improve function, 367, 370, 378, 379, 380, 382, 389
imperforate hymen *see* hymen, imperforate
implantation bleeds, 195
incontinence, 145
treatment, 340
see also enuresis
indigestion, 399, 415
treatment, 292, 361, 370, 371
indoles, 70, 255, 256, 279, 341
and cancer prevention, 296
infertility, 27, 74, 75, 76, 85, 86
and Asherman's syndrome, 209
causes, 133, 171, 173, 175, 184, 239, 243, 253, 255, 282, 293, 308, 311, 422
and endometriosis, 239, 241, 243, 248, 252
and polycystic ovarian disease, 261, 265, 269, 270
treatment, 263, 270, 312, 314, 327, 347, 349
inflammatory mediators, 357
influenza, treatment for, 360, 373, 378, 379
inositol, 375
insanity, 255
historical treatment, 346
insect repellents, 333

insomnia, 121, 128, 137, 143, 148, 160, 234, 272, 293, 417
treatment, 164, 217, 253, 331, 339, 351, 361, 362, 363, 364, 390
insulin, 113, 119
insulin resistance, 267, 271
intercourse *see* sexual activity
inter-menstrual bleeding *see* metrorrhagia
internal examinations *see* pelvic examinations
intestinal lactase, 288
intramural fibroids *see* fibroids, myometrial
intra-uterine device (IUD), 157, 176, 205
and endometriosis, 243
in-vitro fertilisation (IVF), 252, 347
iodothyromines, 307
iron, 95–6, 170, 188, 222, 257
absorption of, 190–1
and auto-transfusions, 404
deficiency, 148, 157, 180, 183, 189–90, 290
effect of the Pill, 386, 387
sources of, 191, 290, 322, 370, 376
irritability, 76, 106, 107, 111, 114, 119, 128, 146, 160, 179, 221, 229, 251, 255, 280
treatment, 71, 112, 113, 122, 183, 351, 358, 364
irritable bowel syndrome, 225, 253–4
treatment, 229–31, 361
ischaemia, 224, 328, 343; *see also* uterine ischaemia
isoflavones, 305, 306–8, 309, 310, 313
sources of, 317
isoflavonoids, 304, 306–11
isotretinoin, 101–2
to treat pigmentation disorders, 387
ITP *see* idiopathic thrombocytopaenia
IUD *see* intra-uterine device
IVF *see* in-vitro fertilisation

Jamaican dogwood *see* Piscidia erythrina
jaundice, causes, 389
juniper *see* Juniperus communis
Juniperus communis, 10, 375, 376–7

Kalms (Nutricare), 164
kava-kava *see* Piper methysticum
kava-kava abuse syndrome, 365
keloid scar tissue, 405
kidneys, 61, 110, 113, 136, 282, 369, 375
effect of fibroids, 185
effect of juniper berries, 376
effect of stress, 160
failure of, 210, 285
and HRT, 396
treatment of diseases/disorders, 374, 377

201, 215, 216, 217, 246, 253, 314, 346
luteinised unruptured follicle syndrome, 75, 252, 253
luteinising hormone (LH), 39, 56, 57, 58, 75, 76, 111, 136, 141, 143, 160, 171, 209, 210, 211, 212, 213, 215, 265, 267, 270, 312, 345, 350, 351, 362, 396
luteolin, 378
lycopene, 297
Lycopus virginiana, 271
lymphatic congestion, 252
lymphocytes, 382; *see also* T-lymphocytes; T-helper lymphocytes
lymphokines, 241

macrophages, 240–1, 246, 371, 380
magnesium, 77, 95, 114, 119, 120, 121, 147, 149, 163, 170, 232, 257, 271, 272–3, 397, 406
    deficiency, 110, 111, 112, 113, 119, 122, 272, 294
    sources, 273, 289, 376
malabsorption, 371
male-pattern baldness *see* androgenic alopecia
malnutrition
    effect of, 194
    treatment, 370
mammary dysplasia, 123
mammary hyperplasia, benign, 123
mammogram, 124, 149
manganese, 271, 322
mannitol, 375
MAO *see* monoamine oxidase
margarine, 282, 286
marigold *see Calendula officinalis*
marshmallow, 9
Marvelon, 219
masculinisation, 65, 219, 261, 269
    effect of the Pill, 385, 388, 389
    treatment, 269–70, 309
    see also androgenic alopecia; hirsutism
massage oil (recipe), 233
massage therapy, 19–20
    to treat dysmenorrhoea, 233
mastalgia, 75, 86, 107, 110, 112, 113, 123, 125, 146, 247, 312, 349, 350, 367, 388, 395
    treatment, 120, 122, 126–30, 169, 315, 346, 386, 390, 397, 398, 399, 400
Mastodynon N, 347
Materia Medica (Chinese), 228
Matricaria chamomilla, 199
Matricaria recutita, 99, 119, 143, 228, 230, 405
measles, treatment for, 360
meat, 82, 84, 127, 204, 232, 281, 290

mechlorethamine, 133, 172
Medicago sativa, 167, 306–7, 311
medroxyprogesterone acetate, 388
mefenamic acid *see* Ponstan
Melaleuca alternifolia, 103, 206, 382–3
Melancholic temperament, 4, 6, 255, 413, 417, 422
melasma, 387
Melipramine and the Pill, 387
Melissa officinalis, 230, 405
Melleril, 214
melons, 291
menarche, 74, 89, 134, 158, 170, 186, 197, 209, 268
    early, 200
    delayed, 218
menopausal symptom index, 138–9
menopause, 32, 37, 46, 60, 62, 72, 73, 74, 107, 131–58, 169, 196, 197, 209, 218–19; *see also* peri-menopause
    age at, 132
    bleeding after, 193, 200, 201
    definition of, 132
    effect on fibroids, 186
    late, 200
    medically induced, 133, 173, 178
    premature, 132–3, 173
    and progestogens, 389
    pseudo, 397
    surgically induced, 133–4
    temporary *see* pseudo
    treatment for symptoms, 138–49, 312, 324, 340, 349, 351, 360, 363, 365–6, 367, 369, 388; *see also* Hormone Replacement Therapy
menorrhagia, 68, 83–4, 103, 140, 157, 158, 163, 172, 173, 174, 175, 176, 177, 221, 222
    functional, 177–8, 195, 196, 199
    treatment, 178–84, 197, 322, 325, 339, 340, 341, 343–4, 345, 355, 380, 385
menses *see* period
menstrual cycle, 29, 32–4, 38–50, 67, 71, 79–80, 91
    effect of stress on, 160
    and endometriosis, 246–7
    irregularities, 65, 69, 74, 75, 95, 159, 160, 170, 171, 172, 173, 179, 196, 210, 215, 217, 218, 219, 222, 255, 261, 263, 264–5, 268, 269, 417
    length of, 43–4, 156, 158, 242, 309, 345, 346
    at menopause, 137, 140
    regulation of, 197, 202, 203, 215, 216, 305, 312, 314, 324, 325, 326, 338, 340, 342, 345, 347, 348, 357, 362, 397, 398
menstrual flow: colour & consistency, 47–8, 251

natural killer cells , 241
natural medicine,
    history, 1–21
    training, 19
    see also herbal medicine; Traditional
        Chinese Medicine
'natural' progesterone, 313, 314–16
natural spirit, 422
naturopathy, 19–20
nausea, 140, 272, 330, 374, 388, 398,
    399, 415
    treatment, 292, 405
neck of the womb see cervix
needle aspiration, 124
neoplasia, 50
nephrotic syndrome, 374
nervine sedatives, 359
nervine stimulants, 359
nervine tonics, 359
nervines, 4, 99, 119, 142, 147, 163,
    167, 199, 228, 231, 334, 339, 354,
    359–65, 400
neuralgia, treatment for, 333, 355, 363,
    374
neurasthenia, treatment for, 364
neutral herbs, 364, 368
NHAA see National Herbalists
    Association of Australia
night sweats, 137, 160
    treatment, 143, 336, 361, 364
nitriles, 341
nitrosamine, 295
nologenin, 344
non-steroidal anti-inflammatory drugs
    (NSAIDs), 358
noradrenaline, 109, 111
norepinephrine, 109
norethindrone acetate, 386
norethisterone, 388, 392
norgestimate, 219
nose bleeds, treatment for, 343
nose, blocked see blocked nose/ears
NSAIDs see non-steroidal
    anti-inflammatory drugs
Nurofen, 398
Nurses' Health Study (1976), 391–2
nutritionally depleted blood see blood
    deficiency
nutritive tonics, 366
nuts, 82, 279, 280, 282
    fibre content, 303
    recommended daily intake, 300, 302

oatmeal, 406, 407
oats, 163, 280
obesity, 66, 68, 200, 201, 202, 218,
    219, 268, 269, 281, 292, 293, 309,
    349
    and Cushing's syndrome, 211
    definition, 165

and fibroids, 186
and polycystic ovarian disease, 264,
    265, 267, 270, 271
and SHBG level, 268
treatment, 168
oedema, 415
    treatment, 127, 376
oestradiol, 56, 59–60, 61, 71, 73, 136,
    180, 215, 246, 265, 305, 306, 307,
    312, 314, 316, 349, 393, 394, 395,
    398; see also ethinyl oestradiol
oestradiol valerate see Progynova
oestriol, 59, 61, 71, 394
oestrogen-binding affinity, 306
oestrogen receptors, 305–6, 313, 316,
    398
oestrogenic herbs, 143
oestrogenicity, 306
oestrogens, 27, 31, 32, 33, 34, 39, 40,
    42, 47, 55–7, 58, 59–63, 66, 67–74,
    90, 110, 111, 113, 123, 141, 148,
    193, 194, 196, 201, 213, 219, 281,
    284, 397
    and cancer, 69, 142, 200, 261, 305,
        391–2, 398
    deficiency, 72–4, 134, 135–7, 138,
        140, 145, 149, 171, 210, 211, 219,
        349, 366, 395
    and endometriosis, 239–40, 241, 246
    excess, 67–9, 70, 71, 84, 85, 86, 109,
        112, 118–19, 122, 125, 126, 157,
        168, 177, 182, 183, 186, 188–9,
        200, 215, 239–40, 241, 249, 250,
        251, 266, 267–8, 309, 313, 314,
        350, 372, 373
    excretion of, 47, 296, 305, 386
    and fibroids, 186, 187–8
    and HRT, 391–6
    levels in the Pill, 385–7
    see also conjugated oestrogens;
        endogenous oestrogens;
        phyto-oestrogens; synthetic
        oestrogens; xeno-oestrogens
oestrone, 59–60, 61, 136, 141, 265–6,
    267, 268, 393
Ogen, 393
oily fish see fish, oily
oligohypermenorrhoea, 158
oligohypomenorrhoea, 158
oligomenorrhoea, 158, 203, 208–22
oligomeric procyanidins, 236, 253
olive oil, 146, 282, 287
omega-3 pathway, 80–2, 84, 85, 251,
    282
omega-3 polyunsaturated fatty acids,
    282–3, 285, 287, 299
omega-6 pathway, 80–2, 83, 282
omega-6 polyunsaturated fatty acids,
    125, 282, 284–5, 287
onions, 71, 257, 279

polyps, 16, 157, 178, 193, 237, 398
  treatment, 382, 401
polysaccharides, 323, 371, 381
polyunsaturated fats, 282–5, 299
  effect of heat on, 286
  see also essential fatty acids
pomegranate see Punica granatum
Ponstan, 84, 172, 178, 398–9
Poria cocos, 188, 350, 366
post-menopausal women, 218, 307, 308, 309
  physical complaints, 310, 349
post-operative fatigue see surgery, recovery from
post-Pill amenorrhoea, 210, 385, 387
post-viral fatigue syndrome, 128, 368
pot marigold see Calendula officinalis
potassium, 160, 170
  depletion, 162, 294, 369, 400, 406
  sources of, 122, 375, 376
potatoes, 74, 279, 287, 313, 406
pouch of Douglas, 29, 245
prana, 4
prawns, 232
prednisolone, 172, 374
pregnancy, 26, 38, 42, 49, 61, 73, 110, 114, 156, 171, 208, 234, 321–2, 324, 327–31, 335, 336, 340, 343, 349, 350, 353, 376
  change in skin pigmentation, 387
  and fibroids, 403
  herbs, contraindicated, 356, 358, 376, 377, 382
  and HRT, 396
  see also ectopic pregnancy; partus praeparators; termination of pregnancy (TOP)
pregnancy, phantom see pseudocyesis
pregnenolone, 56, 64
Premarin, 310, 391, 393
premenstrual syndrome (PMS), 16, 67, 68, 74, 75, 77, 78, 85, 99, 106–22, 128, 137, 147, 155, 162, 168, 169, 172, 179, 215, 234, 247, 250, 251, 252, 254, 255–6, 414, 416
  causes, 109–12
  incidence, 108
  and the Pill, 385, 389
  treatment, 272, 286, 293, 345, 346, 349, 358, 359, 366, 370, 374, 376, 390, 398, 399
  see also acne; anxiety; cravings (food); depression; dizziness; faintness; fatigue; fluid retention; forgetfulness; headache; hot flushes; irritability; mastalgia; mood changes; palpitations
premenstrual tension (PMT) see premenstrual syndrome
prepuce, 25, 58

primary amenorrhoea see amenorrhoea, primary
primary dysmenorrhoea see dysmenorrhoea, primary
Primolut N, 178, 197, 220, 235, 314, 348
proanthocyanidins, 235
  see also grape seed extract; oligomeric procyanidins
progesterone, 10, 27, 31, 32, 33, 39, 40, 42, 55–7, 63–4, 66, 67, 70, 84, 85, 113, 119, 123, 138, 140, 178, 193, 194, 197, 201, 235, 243, 246, 263, 269, 284, 311, 312, 313, 316, 362, 386, 395, 395, 397, 399
  effect on premenstrual stress, 390
  imbalances, 74–7, 86, 109, 119, 122, 125, 126, 147, 157, 196, 217, 250, 251, 253, 314, 349, 350
  during menopause, 136
  see also 'natural' progesterone
progestogen-only pill see Mini Pill
progestogens, 66, 126, 172, 178, 194, 201, 215, 218, 219, 220, 249, 314, 385, 387, 388–90, 392
  side effects, 388, 389, 396
Progynova, 393
prolactin inhibiting hormone (PIH) see dopamine
prolactin, 58, 59, 86, 110–11, 125, 209, 213, 349
  effect of stress on, 217
  excess of, 75, 208, 210, 211, 213, 346, 349
  normal level, 216
  regulation of, 57, 85, 111, 112, 126, 173, 216, 271, 312, 345, 347, 350, 397, 398
  see also hyperprolactinaemia
prolactinoma, 209, 210, 213, 214, 215–16, 217
prolapse, uterine/pelvic floor, 332
  treatment, 235, 320, 326, 368, 404
Prostacyclin, series 2 (PGI 2), 80, 84, 177, 178, 399
prostacyclins, 79
prostaglandin inhibiting drugs, 84, 85, 172, 178, 181, 226, 385, 398–9
  side effects, 399
  see also non-steroidal anti-inflammatory drugs
prostaglandin inhibiting herbs, 181, 228, 231, 237, 353
prostaglandin synthetase, 377, 378, 398
prostaglandins, 33, 40, 54, 67, 78–86, 111–12, 113, 181–2, 196, 228, 249, 250, 282, 286, 323, 357
  dietary control of, 232, 251
  and endometriosis, 240, 241, 243, 253

sperm and macrophages, 241
spicy food, 143
spinach, 291, 407
spiral arterioles, 180, 196
spironalactone *see* Aldactone
spleen, enlarged, 345
spotting, 40, 44, 95, 140, 157, 179,
    193, 194, 196, 197, 247, 385, 389
sprains, treatment for, 333
squamous epithelium, 205
St John's wort *see Hypericum perforatum*
St Mary's thistle *see Silybum marianum*
Stachys betonica, 119
stagnant blood, 354
Staphylococcus aureus, 93, 335, 380
star flower oil, 82, 85, 86, 114, 120,
    127, 252, 284
Stelazine, 210, 214
Stemetil, 210, 214
steroid hormones, 55–6, 59, 63, 65, 70,
    284, 311, 349; *see also* androgens;
    corticosteroids; oestradiol;
    oestriol; oestrogens; oestrone;
    progesterone; testosterone
steroidal saponins, 70, 74, 121, 198,
    203, 270, 305, 310, 312, 313–14
    sources, 317, 326, 344
sterols, 297
Stillingia sylvatica, 127
stomach ulcers *see* gastro-intestinal ulcers
stomatitis, treatment for, 335
Stoppard, Miriam, 134
strachydrine, 361
Streptococcus thermophilus, 289
stress fractures, 171
stress: effect of, 75, 76, 99, 100, 103,
    110, 128, 141, 145, 159–62, 171,
    196, 197, 199–200, 202, 204, 210,
    214, 235, 342, 351, 356, 406
    treatment, 76, 122, 162–4, 167, 197,
    271, 361, 362, 365, 374
    see also anxiety
strobiles, 362
stroke: and HRT, 396
    and the Pill, 385, 389
    treatment, 331, 343
stroma, 33
Suan Zao Ren Tang, 331, 364
sub-mucus fibroids *see* fibroids,
    sub-mucus
sub-serous fibroids *see* fibroids,
    extra-uterine
sugar, 292–3
sugar, refined, 113, 128–9, 231, 285,
    293, 405, 407
    excess consumption, 293
suicidal symptoms, 98
sulphur compounds, 256
surgery, 384, 400–8
    preparation for, 404–6

recovery from, 366, 368, 372
sweating, 143, 338, 409, 411
    to induce, 346, 353, 357
    to reduce, 351, 364
    see also night sweats
sweet foods, effect of, 292
sweet herbs, 344, 364, 367, 368, 369
sweet potatoes, 297, 387
Synarel, 178, 397
synthetase inhibitors *see* prostaglandin
    inhibiting drugs
synthetic oestrogens, 391, 394, 398
systemic candida *see candida albicans*

T-helper lymphocytes, 241
T-lymphocytes, 240
Tagamet, 215
tahini, 287
tamoxifen, 126, 133, 173, 308, 398
    side effects, 398
tamoxifen citrate, 398
tampons, 92–3
    and endometriosis, 244
Tanacetum parthenium, 121, 228–9,
    251, 355, 357–8
Tanacetum vulgare, 337
tannins, 182, 320, 322, 337, 340, 342,
    345, 380
    effect on iron absorption, 191
Taraxacum officinale, 120, 230, 256,
    257, 291, 369, 370, 371–2, 375–6,
    400
Tazac, 215
TB *see Mycobacterium tuberculosis*
tea, 293–4
    and endometriosis, 243
    and iron absorption, 191
    and irritable bowel syndrome, 231
tea tree oil *see Melaleuca alternifolia*
temperaments (humoral theory), 4, 6,
    421–2
tension *see* stress
teratomas *see* dermoid cysts
terminal phenolic group, 306
termination of pregnancy (TOP), 74,
    183, 332, 333
terpenoids, 127
Tertroxine and the Pill, 386
testosterone, 56, 63, 65, 66, 136, 219,
    268, 284, 312, 349
    in HRT, 393, 395
    reduction of, 220, 350
    see also serum testosterone
tetracycline, 101
tetramethylpyrazine, 331
Tetrex, 101
textured soy protein, 298
theobromine, 128, 293
theophylline, 128, 293
    and the Pill, 386

thiamine *see* Vitamin B1
thinness *see* body weight, low
thirst, 417
three natural faculties, 422
three treasures, 422
threshold bleeding *see* metrorrhagia
throat constriction *see* globus hystericus
thrombophlebitis and HRT, 396
thrombosis, 338; *see also* venous
    thromboembolism
thromboxanes, 78, 79, 80, 82, 282, 353
thrush *see* candida albicans
Thuja occidentalis, 189, 382
thujone, 335, 339, 382
thymoleptics, 363
thyroid gland, 176, 198, 265
    disorders, 44, 143, 196, 200, 202,
        211, 214, 264, 269; *see also*
        hyperthyroidism; hypothyroidism
    effect of stress, 160
thyroid hormone, 66
thyroxine, 114, 160
tienchi ginseng *see* Panax notoginseng
Tilia europa, 163
tiredness *see* fatigue
tobacco *see* smoking
Tofranil and the Pill, 387
tofu, 142, 279, 280, 298, 310, 407
    recipes for drinks, 408
tomatoes, 279, 297
tonsillitis, treatment for, 335
toothache, treatment for, 357
TOP *see* termination of pregnancy
torsion, 185, 259, 261
    treatment, 262
tortilla, 280
toxic shock syndrome, 93–4
toxins, 141, 168; *see also* aflatoxins;
    detoxification diets
Traditional Chinese Medicine (TCM), 5,
    19–20, 217, 235, 255, 331, 343, 354,
    368, 370, 373, 414
tranquillisers (drug), 400
tranquillising herbs, 365, 374
trans-configuration, 286
transcortin *see* cortisol-binding globulin
trans-fatty acids, 285, 286
transitory zone, 205
transverse vaginal septum, 213
Travel Calm TM (Blackmores), 228
tretinoin, 101
Tribestan, 314
Tribulus terrestris, 314
trichomonas, treatment for, 380, 381,
    383
tri-cyclic anti-depressants, 400
Trifolium pratense, 74, 127, 307–8, 311
    and breast cancer, 308, 309
triglycerides, 285–6, 293, 392

Trigonella foenum-graecum, 146, 271,
    313
trillarin, 344
Trillium erectum, 74, 163, 182, 188,
    199, 203, 313, 341, 344–5
trillogenin, 344
Triminulet, 219
Trioden, 219
Triphasil, 22, 387
Triquilar, 220, 387
Trisequens, 394
triterpenoid saponins, 74, 305, 312, 313
true unicorn root *see* Aletris farinosa
Tryptanol, 360
tubal ligation, 134, 176, 239
tuberculosis *see* Mycobacterium
    tuberculosis
tubes *see* Fallopian tubes
tuna, 407
Tunera diffusa, 189
Turkish coffee, effect on cholesterol
    level, 294
Turner's syndrome, 212, 213
Turnera aphrodisiaca, 220
tyramine, 342

ulcers, stomach *see* gastro-intestinal ulcers
ultrasound imaging *see* ultrasound scans
ultrasound scans, 18, 76, 124, 175, 184,
    187, 209, 213, 248, 259, 263, 264,
    265, 330
Unani Tibb system of medicine, 420, 422
underweight *see* body weight, low
unicorn root, false *see* Chamaelirium
    luteum
unicorn root, true *see* Aletris farinosa
unsaturated fats, 281–6
    effect of heat, 286
    see also monounsaturated fats;
        polyunsaturated fats
ureter, 238
    effect of pressure from fibroids, 185
urethra, 25, 29, 145
    and endometriosis, 246
urethritis, treatment for, 377
urinary tract infections, 145
    treatment, 365, 376, 395
urine, 64, 69, 412, 414
    blood in *see* haematuria
uterine cancer, 71, 158, 187, 193
    prevention, 296
    treatment for, 382
uterine fibroids *see* fibroids
uterine ischaemia, 84
uterine leiomyomas *see* fibroids
uterine ligaments, 145, 248
uterine muscle *see* myometrium
uterine myomata *see* fibroids
uterine tissue tone *see* uterine tone
uterine tone, 179–80, 236–7, 250

to improve, 180, 182, 188, 237, 319, 380

uterine tonics, 48, 182, 188, 227, 231, 237, 250, 319–28, 355, 366
  effects of, 324–5

uterosacral nerve, 226

uterus, 26–8, 64, 70, 133, 134, 175, 200, 225, 238, 308, 319, 321, 328, 400
  abnormalities, 179–80, 185, 209, 209, 212–13, 245, 251, 320
  infections, 157, 209
  removal *see* hysterectomy
  retroverted *see* retroverted uterus
  variations in size, 197, 234, 245, 248, 306, 311

Vaccinium myrtillus, 236

vagina, 25–6, 29, 39, 138, 209, 213, 306, 308, 367
  dryness, 72, 74, 133, 135, 137, 142, 143, 145–6, 166, 310, 351, 390, 394–5, 397
  and endometriosis, 246
  irritations/infections, 72, 95, 145, 351, 395, 409; *see also candida albicans*
  treatment of irritations/infections, 378, 379

vaginal candida *see candida albicans*

vaginal discharge, 95, 176, 234, 410, 412, 413, 414, 415
  as indication of cervicitis, 194, 206
  see also candida albicans

valerian *see Valeriana officinalis*

valerian oil, 233

Valeriana edulis, 363

Valeriana officinalis, 99, 119, 143, 164, 228, 360, 363–4

Valium, 360, 364, 400

varicose veins, 235

vasoconstriction, 357

vegans, need for dietary supplements, 290, 388

vegetable oils, 82, 122, 127, 282, 286–7
  effect of heating, 286
  storage of, 287

vegetable shortening, 286

vegetables, 128, 277, 282, 284, 287
  for cancer prevention, 295–8
  fibre content, 303
  proteins, 290
  recommended daily intake, 279, 300, 302
  see also indoles; leafy vegetables; root vegetables

vegetables, root *see* root vegetables

vegetarianism, effect of, 69, 136, 189, 220, 280, 290, 387

venous thromboembolism: as side effect of the Pill, 220, 385, 387, 388, 389

prevention of, 283, 285, 323, 353, 388, 405

Verbena officinalis, 99, 143, 147, 163, 199, 228, 229, 62–3

vertigo, 272

vervain *see Verbena officinalis*

VHA *see* Victorian Herbalists Association

Vibra-Tabs, 101

Viburnum opulus, 227, 254, 328–31, 355, 356

Viburnum prunifolium, 227, 328–31, 355, 356, 361

Viburnum spp., 251

Victorian Herbalists Association (VHA), 20

vincristine, 133, 172–3

Viola odorata, 127

viopudial, 330

virilisation *see* masculinisation

vital energy, 4, 6–7, 412, 422

vital force, 3–4, 422–4

vital spirit, 422

vitalism, 423

vitamin A, 114, 146, 180, 204, 222, 256, 295, 404–5
  and the Pill, 387
  deficiency, 73, 112, 294
  sources of, 307, 320, 322, 375, 405

vitamin B complex, 99, 102, 119, 163, 199, 206, 252, 254, 294, 320, 406
  and the Pill, 387, 388, 389

vitamin B1, 126, 148, 294

vitamin B3, 114

vitamin B5, 406

vitamin B6, 70–1, 77, 102, 112–13, 119, 120, 121, 146, 147, 148, 199, 216–17
  and the Pill, 387, 388

vitamin B12, 146, 290, 323

vitamin C, 114, 144, 147, 190, 204, 222, 235, 256, 286, 294, 295, 297, 307, 320, 322, 404, 406

vitamin E, 77, 112, 113, 120, 122, 126, 144, 147, 189, 204, 253, 254, 256, 285, 286, 295, 307, 320, 324, 386, 405
  and the Pill, 388

vitamin E cream, 146, 206

vitamin K, 146, 180–1, 204, 222, 307

Vitex agnus castus, 76, 103, 119, 126, 147, 163, 167, 198–9, 202, 217, 229, 253, 254, 270–1, 345–8, 366

volatile oils, 337, 338

vomiting, 225, 226, 247, 259, 331, 398
  treatment, 227, 228, 237, 353, 356, 398

von Willebrand's disease, 103, 176

vulva, 25
  and endometriosis, 246

walnut oil, 82, 283
warfarin, 172
Warming foods, 291
Warming herbs, 228, 231, 325, 327,
  331, 334, 337, 342, 344, 352–4, 355,
  357, 364, 367, 369, 372, 377
Warming spices, 292
warts, treatment for, 382
water: importance of, 278
  recommended daily intake, 302
Water (element), 418–20
weight gain, 122, 129, 172, 279, 279
  and the Pill, 385, 388, 389
  and polycystic ovarian disease, 265–6, 268
  see also body weight; obesity
weight reduction, 302
  to control androgen levels, 220–1, 266
  excessive, 165, 194, 210, 268, 278
  to treat insulin resistance, 271
Well Woman's Check List, 49–50
wheat bran, 273, 280, 281
  and irritable bowel syndrome, 231
wheat flour, 310
wheatgerm oil, 316
wheezing see breathing difficulties
whey see beta-lactoglobulin
white deadnettle see Lamium album
whole grains see grains
whooping cough, treatment for, 307, 355
wild yam see Dioscorea villosa
willow, 7
wine, red see red wine
Withania somnifera, 119, 121
women, role of in health care, 10, 12–13
Women's Precious Pills see Ba Zen Tang
women's tonics, 74, 313, 355
worm infestations, treatment for, 334

xanthines, 293, 375
xeno-oestrogens, 60, 62–3, 69

yams, 313
yam, wild see Dioscorea villosa
yarrow see Achillea millefolium
yeast, 102, 112
  and irritable bowel syndrome, 231
  see also brewer's yeast
Yellow Bile (humour), 6, 7, 229, 255,
  418, 420, 421
Yin and Yang, 420
ylang ylang, 163
yoga, 163, 169, 405
  and hyperprolactinaemia, 214
yoghurt and cultured milk products,
  69–70, 73, 181, 204, 250, 287, 288,
  289, 310, 405, 407
  and prevention of cancer, 298–9
  recommended daily intake, 300
Yunnan Bai Yao, 342

Zantac, 215
zearalenone, 305, 316
zinc, 95, 102, 104–5, 114, 120, 121,
  146, 147, 170, 257, 271, 404, 406
  deficiency, 167, 294
  effect of the Pill, 387–8
  recommended daily dosage, 388
  and synthesis of dopamine, 216–17
Zingiber officinale, 103–4, 127, 228,
  251, 254, 292, 325, 331, 352–3, 354,
  355, 405–6
Zizyphus Combination see Suan Zao
  Ren Tang
Zizyphus spinosa, 99, 364
Zoladex, 133, 178, 397